PHARMACEUTICAL ANALYSIS

A TEXTBOOK FOR PHARMACY STUDENTS
AND PHARMACEUTICAL CHEMISTS

Senior Content Strategist: Pauline Graham
Content Development Specialist: Fiona Conn
Project Manager: Srividhya Vidhyashankar
Designer: Miles Hitchen
Illustration Manager: Amy Faith Heyden

Fourth Edition
PHARMACEUTICAL
ANALYSIS

A TEXTBOOK FOR PHARMACY STUDENTS
AND PHARMACEUTICAL CHEMISTS

David G. Watson BSc PhD PGCE

Senior Lecturer in Pharmaceutical Sciences, Strathclyde Institute of Pharmacy
and Biomedical Sciences, University of Strathclyde, Glasgow, UK

With contributions by

RuAngelie Edrada-Ebel BSc MSc DrRerNat AMRSC

Lecturer, Strathclyde Institute of Pharmacy and Biomedical Sciences,
University of Strathclyde, Glasgow, UK

Bhavik A. Patel BSc PhD MRSC

Reader in Clinical and Bioanalytical Chemistry, School of Pharmacy and
Biomolecular Sciences, University of Brighton, Brighton, UK

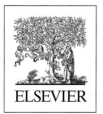

ELSEVIER

Edinburgh London New York Oxford Philadelphia St. Louis Sydney Toronto 2017

ELSEVIER

© 2017, Elsevier Limited. All rights reserved.

First edition 1999
Second edition 2005
Third edition 2012
Fourth edition 2017
ISBN: 978-0-7020-6989-5
ISBN: 978-0-7020-7029-7

Notices

Knowledge and best practice in this field are constantly changing. As new research and experience broaden our understanding, changes in research methods, professional practices, or medical treatment may become necessary.

Practitioners and researchers must always rely on their own experience and knowledge in evaluating and using any information, methods, compounds, or experiments described herein. In using such information or methods they should be mindful of their own safety and the safety of others, including parties for whom they have a professional responsibility.

With respect to any drug or pharmaceutical products identified, readers are advised to check the most current information provided (i) on procedures featured or (ii) by the manufacturer of each product to be administered, to verify the recommended dose or formula, the method and duration of administration, and contraindications. It is the responsibility of practitioners, relying on their own experience and knowledge of their patients, to make diagnoses, to determine dosages and the best treatment for each individual patient, and to take all appropriate safety precautions.

To the fullest extent of the law, neither the Publisher nor the authors, contributors, or editors, assume any liability for any injury and/or damage to persons or property as a matter of products liability, negligence or otherwise, or from any use or operation of any methods, products, instructions, or ideas contained in the material herein.

Printed in China

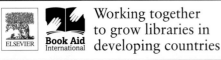

Working together
to grow libraries in
developing countries

www.elsevier.com • www.bookaid.org

Preface

The major revision to this edition is the addition of two new chapters: one on the quality control of biotechnologically produced drugs and the other (thanks to Dr Bhavik Patel) on the use of electrochemical techniques in point of care diagnostics. The applications of both these areas will see rapid expansion in the next few years. Although they are at opposite ends of the spectrum in terms of instrumental complexity they are both important with regard to personalised medicine. They are also connected in the sense that the ability to couple biological sensing to a reading, such as that produced by an electrochemical test, will become increasingly refined as the range of biomolecules produced by biotechnology which can be coupled to such tests expands. The genii of biotechnology is well and truly out of the bottle and will transform our ability to treat currently difficult to manage diseases.

Fortunately for the enthusiastic pharmaceutical analyst this throws up some difficult challenges with regard to the quality control of complex molecules which ensures that both interest and employment in the field will continue and expand. Even large proteins, such as monoclonal antibodies, have fairly well defined structures but perhaps an additional challenge in the future will be with regard to the quality control of stem cell technologies. There may even be a role for the pharmaceutical analyst here, since complex systems always provide a characteristic fingerprint which can be assessed by analytical technologies.

It is approaching 20 years since the first edition of this book and judging by demand, it remains relevant. I continue to learn more about my subject each day and I still like to get out a spanner and tackle the nuts and bolts of making high quality analytical measurements.

Dr Dave Watson, University of Strathclyde

Contents

Learning resources

Animations

Animations are available via the ebook on StudentConsult.com. These animations require Shockwave Player and will work best in Internet Explorer and Mozilla web browsers.

All animations © Dr D. Watson and Dr T.H. Plumridge, 2001-2006 and University of Strathclyde. The authors acknowledge the support of the EPSRC in the creation of these animations.

Chapter 2: Physical and chemical properties of drug molecules
2.1   Ionisation partitioning of drug molecules
2.2   Hydrolysis of ester bond in aspirin
2.3   Measurement of optical rotation

Chapter 3: Titrimetric and chemical analysis methods
3.1   Accuracy and precision in pipetting
3.2   Titration simulation
3.3   Determination of saponification value
3.4   Determination of pKa

Chapter 4: Ultraviolet and visible spectroscopy
4.1   Light wave
4.2   Electromagnetic spectrum
4.3   Ethylene orbitals
4.4   Effect of pH on the spectrum of procaine

Chapter 5: Infrared spectrophotometry
5.1   Fourier transform infrared spectroscopy (FTIR)
5.2   Infrared spectrum of aspirin
5.3   Infrared spectrum of hydrocortisone

Chapter 6: Atomic spectrophotometry
6.1   Spectrum of sodium
6.2   Flame photometer
6.3   Interferences in atomic emission spectrophotometry (AES) and flame emissions spectrophotometry (FES)
6.4   Atomic absorption spectrometry

Chapter 7: Molecular emission spectroscopy
7.1   Fluorescence measurements

1

Control of the quality of analytical methods

Introduction

Pharmaceutical analysis procedures may be used to answer any of the questions outlined in Box 1.1. The quality of a product may deviate from the standard required, but in carrying out an analysis one also has to be certain that the quality of the analysis itself is of the standard required. Quality control is integral to all modern industrial processes, and the pharmaceutical industry is no exception. Testing a pharmaceutical product involves chemical, physical and sometimes microbiological analyses. It has been estimated that £10 billion is spent each year on analyses in the UK alone and such analytical processes can be found in industries as diverse as those producing food, beverages, cosmetics, detergents, metals, paints, water, agrochemicals, biotechnological products and pharmaceuticals. With such large amounts of money being spent on analytical quality control, great importance must be placed on providing accurate and precise analyses (Box 1.2).

Box 1.1 Questions pharmaceutical analysis methods are used to answer

- Is the identity of the drug in the formulated product correct?
- What is the percentage of the stated content of a drug present in a formulation?
- Does this formulation contain solely the active ingredient or are additional impurities present?
- What is the stability of a drug in the formulation and hence the shelf-life of the product?
- At what rate is the drug released from its formulation so that it can be absorbed by the body?
- Do the identity and purity of a pure drug substance to be used in the preparation of a formulation meet specification?
- Do the identity and purity of excipients to be used in the preparation of a formulation meet specification?
- What are the concentrations of specified impurities in the pure drug substance?
- What is the concentration of the drug in a sample of tissue or biological fluid?
- What are the pKa value(s), partition coefficients, solubilities and stability of a drug substance under development?

Box 1.2 International Conference on Harmonisation (ICH) guidelines

The requirements for control of the quality of methods of analysis (validation) have been addressed by the International Conference on Harmonisation of Technical Requirements For Registration of Pharmaceuticals for Human Use, or, more briefly, the ICH (www.ich.org). The ICH was initiated in Brussels in 1990 and brought together representatives of regulatory agencies and industry associations of Europe, Japan and the USA. The purpose of the organisation was to standardise the requirements for medicines regulation throughout the world. The standardisation of the validation of analytical procedures is one area that the ICH has addressed. The ICH indicated that the most important analytical procedures that require validation are:

- Identification tests
- Quantitative tests for impurities
- Limit tests for the control of impurities
- Quantitative tests of the active moiety in samples of drug substance or drug product or other selected component(s) in the drug product.

Thus it is appropriate to begin a book on the topic of pharmaceutical analysis by considering, at a basic level, the criteria which are used to judge the quality of an analysis. The terms used in defining analytical quality form a rather elegant vocabulary that can be used to describe quality in many fields, and in writing this book the author would hope to describe each topic under consideration with accuracy, precision and, most importantly, reproducibility, so that the information included in it can be readily assimilated and reproduced where required by the reader. The following sections provide an introduction to the control of analytical quality. More detailed treatment of the topic is given in the reference cited at the end of the chapter.[1]

Control of errors in analysis

A quantitative analysis is not a great deal of use unless there is some estimation of how prone to error the analytical procedure is. Simply accepting the analytical result could lead to rejection or acceptance of a product on the basis of a faulty analysis. For this reason it is usual to make several repeat measurements of the same sample in order to determine the degree of agreement among them. There are three types of errors which may occur in the course of an analysis: gross, systematic and random. Gross errors are easily recognised since they involve a major breakdown in the analytical process such as samples being spilt, wrong dilutions being prepared or instruments breaking down or being used in the wrong way. If a gross error occurs the results are rejected and the analysis is repeated from the beginning. Random and systematic errors can be distinguished in the following example:

A batch of paracetamol tablets are stated to contain 500 mg of paracetamol per tablet; for the purpose of this example it is presumed that 100% of the stated content is the correct answer. Four students carry out a spectrophotometric analysis of an extract from the tablets and obtain the following percentages of stated content for the repeat analysis of paracetamol in the tablets:

Student 1: 99.5%, 99.9%, 100.2%, 99.4%, 100.5%
Student 2: 95.6%, 96.1%, 95.2%, 95.1%, 96.1%
Student 3: 93.5%, 98.3%, 92.5%, 102.5%, 97.6%
Student 4: 94.4%, 100.2%, 104.5%, 97.4%, 102.1%

The means of these results can be simply calculated according to the formula:

$$\bar{x} = \sum_i \frac{x_i}{n}$$

[Equation 1]

where $\bar{x}$ is the arithmetic mean, x_i is the individual value and n is the number of measurements.

These results can be seen diagrammatically in Figure 1.1.

Student 1 has obtained a set of results which are all clustered close to 100% of the stated content and with a mean for the five measurements very close to the correct answer. In this case the measurements made were both precise and accurate, and obviously the steps in the assay have been controlled very carefully.

Fig. 1.1
Diagrammatic representation of accuracy and precision for analysis of paracetamol in tablet form.

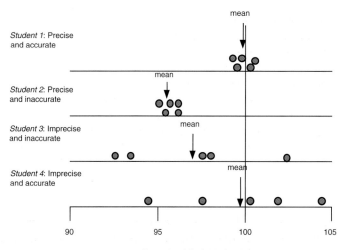

Student 1: Precise and accurate

Student 2: Precise and inaccurate

Student 3: Imprecise and inaccurate

Student 4: Imprecise and accurate

Paracetamol % of stated content

Student 2 has obtained a set of results which are closely clustered but which give a mean that is lower than the correct answer. Thus, although this assay is precise, it is not completely accurate. Such a set of results indicates that the analyst has not produced random errors, which would produce a large scatter in the results, but has produced an analysis containing a systematic error. Such errors might include repeated inaccuracy in the measurement of a volume or failure to zero the spectrophotometer correctly prior to taking the set of readings. The analysis has been mainly well controlled except for probably one step, which has caused the inaccuracy and thus the assay is precisely inaccurate.

Student 3 has obtained a set of results which are widely scattered and hence imprecise and which give a mean which is lower than the correct answer. Thus the analysis contains random errors or, possibly, looking at the spread of the results, three defined errors which have been produced randomly. The analysis was thus poorly controlled, and it would require more work than that required in the case of student 2 to eliminate the errors. In such a simple analysis the random results might simply be produced by, for instance, a poor pipetting technique, where volumes both higher and lower than that required were measured.

Student 4 has obtained a set of results which are widely scattered yet a mean which is close to the correct answer. It is probably only chance that separates the results of student 4 from those of student 3 and, although the answer obtained is accurate, it would not be wise to trust it to always be so.

The best assay was carried out by student 1, and student 2 produced an assay that might be improved with a little work.

In practice it might be rather difficult to tell whether student 1 or student 2 had carried out the best analysis, since it is rare, unless the sample is a pure analytical standard, that the exact content of a sample is known. In order to determine whether student 1 or 2 had carried out the best assay it might be necessary to get other analysts to obtain similar sets of precise results in order to be absolutely sure of the correct answer. The factors leading to imprecision and inaccuracy in assay results are outlined in Box 1.3.

Self-test 1.1

Suggest how the following might give rise to errors in an analytical procedure:

(i) Analysis of a sucrose-based elixir using a pipette to measure aliquots of the elixir for analysis.
(ii) Weighing out 2 mg of an analytical standard on a four-place analytical balance that weighs a minimum of 0.1 mg.
(iii) Use of an analytical standard that absorbs moisture from the atmosphere.
(iv) Incomplete powdering of coated tablets prior to extraction.
(v) Extraction of an ointment with a solvent in which it is poorly soluble.
(vi) Use of a burette that has not been rinsed free of traces of grease.

Answers: (i) Viscosity leads to incomplete drainage of the pipette; (ii) In any weighing there is an uncertainty of ± 0.05 mg, which in relation to 2 mg is $\pm 2.5\%$; (iii) The degree of moisture absorption is uncertain; (iv) Poor recovery of the analyte; (v) Poor recovery of the analyte; (vi) Distortion of meniscus making reading of the burette inaccurate

---

Accuracy and precision

The most fundamental requirements of an analysis are that it should be accurate and precise. It is presumed, although it cannot be proven, that a series of

> ### Box 1.3 Some factors giving rise to imprecision and inaccuracy in an assay
>
> - Incorrect weighing and transfer of analytes and standards
> - Inefficient extraction of the analyte from a matrix, e.g. tablets
> - Incorrect use of pipettes, burettes or volumetric flasks for volume measurement
> - Measurement carried out using improperly calibrated instrumentation
> - Failure to use an analytical blank
> - Selection of assay conditions that cause degradation of the analyte
> - Failure to allow for or to remove interference by excipients in the measurement of an analyte

Fig. 1.2
The Gaussian distribution.

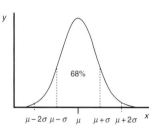

measurements (y) of the same sample will be normally distributed about a mean (μ), i.e. they fall into a Gaussian pattern as shown in Figure 1.2.

The distance σ shown in Figure 1.2 appears to be nearly 0.5 of the width of distribution; however, because the function of the curve is exponential it tends to zero and does not actually meet the x axis until infinity, where there is an infinitesimal probability that there may be a value for x. For practical purposes approximately 68% of a series of measurements should fall within the distance σ either side of the mean and 95% of the measurements should lie with 2σ of the mean. The aim in an analysis is to make σ as small a percentage of the value of μ as possible. The value of σ can be estimated using Equation 2:

$$s = \sqrt{\frac{\sum(x_i - \bar{x})^2}{(n-1)}}$$ **[Equation 2]**

where:

s = standard deviation
n = number of samples
x_i = values obtained for each measurement
$\bar{x}$ = mean of the measurements

Sometimes n rather than $n-1$ is used in the equation but, particularly for small samples, it tends to produce an underestimate of σ. For a small number of values it is simple to work out s using a calculator and the above equation. Most calculators have a function which enables calculation of s directly, and σ estimated using the above equation is usually labelled as σ_{n-1}. For instance, if the example of results obtained by student 1, where the mean is calculated to be 99.9%, are substituted into equation 2, the following calculation results:

$$s = \sqrt{\frac{\begin{array}{c}(99.5-99.9)^2 + (99.9-99.9)^2 + (100.2-99.9)^2 \\ + (99.4-99.9)^2 + (100.5-99.9)^2\end{array}}{(5-1)}}$$

$$= \sqrt{\frac{(-0.4)^2 + (0)^2 + (0.3)^2 + (-0.5)^2 + (0.6)^2}{4}}$$

$$= \sqrt{\frac{0.16+0+0.09+0.25+0.36}{4}} = \sqrt{\frac{0.86}{4}} = \sqrt{0.215} = 0.46$$

$s = 0.46\%$ of stated content

The calculated value for s provides a formal expression of the scatter in the results from the analysis rather than the visual judgement used in Figure 1.1. From the figure obtained for the standard deviation (SD), we can say that 68% of the results of the analysis will lie within the range $99.9 \pm 0.46\%$ ($\pm \sigma$) or within the range 99.44–100.36%. If we re-examine the figures obtained by student 1, it can be seen that 60% of the results fall within this range, with two outside the range, including one only very slightly below the range. The range based on $\pm \sigma$ defines the 68% confidence limits; for 95% confidence $\pm 2\sigma$ must be used, i.e. 95% of the results of student 1 lie within $99.9 \pm 0.92\%$ or 98.98–100.82%. It can be seen that this range includes all the results obtained by student 1.

The precision of an analysis is often expressed as the $\pm$ relative standard deviation ($\pm$ RSD) (Equation 3).

$$RSD = \frac{s}{\bar{x}} \times 100\% \qquad \textbf{[Equation 3]}$$

The confidence limits in this case are often not quoted but, since it is the SD that is an estimate of σ which is being used, they are usually 68%. The advantage of expressing precision in this way is that it eliminates any units and expresses the precision as a percentage of the mean. The results obtained from the assay of paracetamol tablets are shown in Table 1.1.

Self-test 1.2

Four analysts obtain the following data for a spectrophotometric analysis of an injection containing the local anaesthetic bupivacaine. The stated content of the injection is 0.25% weight in volume (w/v).

Analyst 1: 0.245% w/v, 0.234% w/v, 0.263% w/v, 0.261% w/v, 0.233% w/v.
Analyst 2: 0.236% w/v, 0.268% w/v, 0.247% w/v, 0.275% w/v, 0.285% w/v.
Analyst 3: 0.248% w/v, 0.247% w/v, 0.248% w/v, 0.249% w/v, 0.253% w/v.
Analyst 4: 0.230% w/v, 0.233% w/v, 0.227% w/v, 0.230% w/v, 0.229% w/v.

Calculate the mean percentage of stated content and RSD for each set of results at the 68% confidence level. Assuming the content really is as stated on the label, comment on the accuracy and precision of each set of results. Calculate the precision of each assay with regard to 95% confidence limits.

Answers: Analyst 1: 98.9% $\mp$ 5.8%: accurate but imprecise. At 95% confidence RSD = $\mp$ 11.6%; *Analyst 2*: 104.4% $\mp$ 7.7%: inaccurate and imprecise. At 95% confidence RSD = $\mp$ 15.4%; *Analyst 3*: 99.6% $\mp$ 0.9%: accurate and precise. At 95% confidence RSD = $\mp$ 1.8%; *Analyst 4*: 91.9% $\mp$ 0.9%: inaccurate and precise. At 95% confidence RSD = $\mp$ 1.8%.

Table 1.1 Results obtained for the analysis of paracetamol tablets by four analysts

Student	Mean (% of stated content)	S (% of stated content)	± RSD (68% confidence)
1	99.9	0.5	± 0.5%
2	95.6	0.5	± 0.5%
3	96.9	4.0	± 4.4%
4	99.7	4.0	± 4.0%

Validation of analytical procedures

The International Conference on Harmonisation (ICH) has adopted the following terms for defining how the quality of an assay is controlled.

The analytical procedure

The analytical procedure provides an exact description of how the analysis is carried out. It should describe in detail the steps necessary to perform each analytical test. The full method should describe:

(i) the quality and source of the reference standard for the compound being analysed

(ii) the procedures used for preparing solutions of the reference standard

(iii) the quality of any reagents or solvents used in the assay and their method of preparation

(iv) the procedures and settings used for the operation of any equipment required in the assay

(v) the methodology used for calibration of the assay and methodology used for the processing of the sample prior to analysis.

In fact it is difficult to be comprehensive in this short account, since the description of a fully validated method is a lengthy document.

Levels of precision

The ICH guidelines define precision as follows: *"the precision of an analytical procedure expresses the closeness of agreement (degree of scatter) between a series of measurements obtained from multiple sampling of the same homogeneous sample under the prescribed conditions... The precision of an analytical procedure is usually expressed as the variance, standard deviation or coefficient of variation of a series of measurements."*

This is broadly what was described in more detail above for the assay of paracetamol tablets. There is no absolute guideline for how good precision should be for the active ingredient in a formulation, but, in general, a precision of $< \pm 1.0\%$ is desirable. The precision achievable depends on the nature of the sample being analysed. The RSDs achievable in the analysis of trace impurities in a bulk drug or drugs in biological fluids may be considerably greater than $\pm 1.0\%$ because of the increased likelihood of losses when very low concentrations of analyte are being extracted and analysed. The precision of the assay of a particular sample, in the first instance, is generally obtained by repeating the assay procedure a minimum of five times starting from five separate aliquots of sample (e.g. five weights of tablet powder or five volumes of elixir) giving a total of 25 measurements. Repetition of the sample extraction gives a measure of any variation in recovery during extraction from the formulation matrix.

One difficulty in defining the precision of an assay is in indicating which steps in the assay should be examined. Initially an assay will be characterised in detail but thereafter, in re-determining precision (e.g. in order to establish repeatability and intermediate precision), certain elements in the assay may be taken for granted. For example, the same standard calibration solution may be used for several days provided its stability to storage has been established. Similarly there needs to be a limited number of samples extracted for assay, provided it has been established that the recovery of the sample upon extraction does not vary greatly. According to the ICH guidelines, precision may be considered at three levels: repeatability, intermediate precision and reproducibility.

Repeatability

Repeatability expresses the precision obtained under the same operating conditions over a short interval of time. Repeatability can also be termed intra-assay precision. It is likely that the assay would be repeated by the same person using a single instrument. Within repeatability it is convenient to separate the sample preparation method from the instrument performance. Figure 1.3 shows the levels of precision including some of the parameters which govern the system precision of a high-pressure liquid chromatography (HPLC) instrument. It would be expected that the system precision of a well-maintained instrument would be better than the overall repeatability where sample extraction and dilution steps are prone to greater variation than the instrumental analysis step.

An excellent detailed summary of levels of precision is provided by Ermer. For example, Figure 1.4, shows the results obtained from five repeat injections of a mixture of the steroids prednisone (P) and hydrocortisone (H) into a HPLC

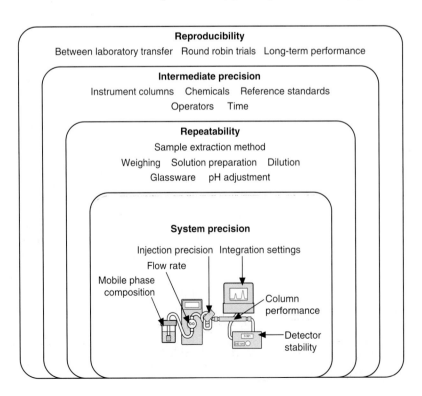

Fig. 1.3
Parameters involved in three levels of precision.

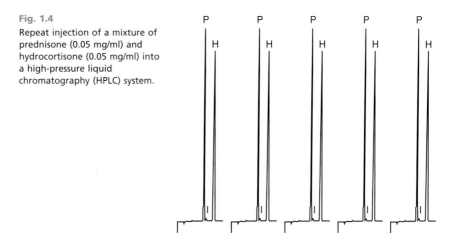

Fig. 1.4

Repeat injection of a mixture of prednisone (0.05 mg/ml) and hydrocortisone (0.05 mg/ml) into a high-pressure liquid chromatography (HPLC) system.

using a manual loop injector. The mixture was prepared by pipetting 5 ml of a 1 mg/ml stock solution of each steroid into a 100 ml volumetric flask and making up the volume with water.

The precision obtained for the areas of the hydrocortisone peak is ± 0.3%; the injection process in HPLC is generally very precise and one might expect even better precision from an automated injection system; thus this aspect of <u>system precision</u> is working well. The precision obtained for the prednisone peak is ± 0.6%; not quite as good, but this is not to do with the injector but is due to a small impurity peak (I) which runs closely after the prednisone, causing some slight variation in the way the prednisone peak is integrated. The integration aspect of the system precision is not working quite as well when challenged with a difficulty in the integration method, but the effect is really only minor. For the repeat, analysis is carried out on a subsequent day on a solution freshly prepared by the same method. The injection precision for hydrocortisone was ± 0.2%. The variation for the means of the areas of hydrocortisone peaks obtained on the two days was ± 0.8%; this indicates that there was small variation in the sample preparation (<u>repeatability</u>) between the two days since the variation in injection precision is ± 0.2% to ± 0.3%. Usually it is expected that instrument precision is better than the precision of sample preparation if a robust type of instrument is used in order to carry out the analysis. Table 1.2 shows the results for the repeat absorbance measurement of the same sample with a UV spectrophotometer in comparison with the results obtained from measurement of five samples by a two-stage dilution from a stock solution. In both cases the precision is good but, as would be expected, the better precision is obtained where it is only instrumental precision that is being assessed. Of course instruments can malfunction and produce poor precision, for example, a spectrophotometer might be nearing the

Table 1.2 Comparison of precision obtained from the repeat measurement of the absorbance of a single sample compared with the measurement of the absorbance of five separately prepared dilutions of the same sample

Sample	Absorbance readings	RSD%
Repeat measurement	0.842, 0.844, 0.842, 0.845, 0.841	± 0.14
Repeat dilution/measurement	0.838, 0.840, 0.842, 0.845, 0.847	± 0.42

end of the useful lifetime of its lamp, and this would result in poor precision due to unstable readings.

A target level for system precision is generally accepted to be $< \pm 1.0\%$.

This should be easily achievable in a correctly functioning HPLC system but might be more difficult in, for instance, a gas chromatography assay where the injection process is less well controlled. The tolerance levels may be set at much higher RSD in trace analyses where instruments are operated at higher levels of sensitivity and achieving 100% recovery of the analyte may be difficult.

Intermediate precision

Intermediate precision expresses within-laboratory variation of precision when the analysis is carried out by different analysts, on different days and with different equipment. Obviously a laboratory will want to cut down the possibility for such variations being large and thus it will standardise on particular items of equipment and particular methods of data handling and make sure that all their analysts are trained to the same standard.

Reproducibility

Reproducibility expresses the precision among laboratories. Such a trial would be carried out when a method was being transferred from one part of a company to another. The data obtained during such method transfer does not usually form part of the marketing dossier submitted in order to obtain a product licence. For new methodologies a popular method for surveying the performance of a method is to carry out a round robin trial, where many laboratories are asked to carry out qualitative and quantitative analysis of a sample where the composition is only known to those organising the trial.

Accuracy

As described above, methods may be precise without being accurate. The determination of accuracy in the assay of an unformulated drug substance is relatively straightforward. The simplest method is to compare the substance being analysed with a reference standard analysed by the same procedure. The reference standard is a highly characterised form of the drug which has been subjected to extensive analysis including a test for elemental composition. The methods for determining the accuracy of an assay of a formulated drug are less straightforward. The analytical procedure may be applied to a drug formulation prepared on a small scale so that the amount of drug in the formulation is more precisely controlled than in a bulk process, a placebo formulation spiked with a known amount of drug or the formulated drug spiked with a known amount of drug. The accuracy of the method may also be assessed by comparison of the method with a previously established reference method such as a pharmacopoeial method.

Accuracy should be reported as percent recovery in relation to the known amount of analyte added to the sample or as the difference between the known amount and the amount determined by analysis. In general, at least five determinations, at 80, 100 and 120% of the label claim for drug in the formulated product, should be carried out in order to determine accuracy.

> **Box 1.4 Extract from a standard operating procedure for the analysis of paracetamol tablets**
>
> 8.   Assay procedure:
> 8.1 Use a calibrated balance
> 8.2 Weigh 20 tablets
> 8.3 Powder the 20 paracetamol tablets and weigh accurately *by difference* a quantity of tablet powder equivalent to 125 ± 10 mg of paracetamol
> 8.4 Shake the tablet powder sample with *ca* 150 ml of acetic acid (0.05 M) for 10 min in a 500 ml volumetric flask and then adjust the volume to 500 ml with more acetic acid (0.05 M).
> 8.5 Filter *ca* 100 ml of the solution into a conical flask and then transfer five separate 5 ml aliquots of the filtrate to 100 ml volumetric flasks and adjust the volumes to 100 ml with acetic acid (0.05 M)
> 8.6 Take two readings of each dilution using a UV spectrophotometer and using the procedure specified in **Section 9**

Standard operating procedure (SOP) for the assay of paracetamol tablets

The terms defined above are perhaps best illustrated by using the example of the simple assay that we mentioned before. The assay in Box 1.4 is laid out in the style of a standard operating procedure (SOP). This particular section of the operating procedure describes the assay itself, but there would also be other sections in the procedure dealing with safety issues, the preparation and storage of the solutions used for extraction and dilution, the glassware required and a specification of the instrumentation to be used.

The assay described in Box 1.4 assesses the precision of some of the operations within the assay. If a single analyst were to assess the *repeatability* of the assay, instructions might be issued to the effect that the assay as described was to be repeated five times in sequence, i.e. completing one assay before commencing another. If *between-day repeatability* were to be assessed, the process used for determining the repeatability would be repeated on two separate days. If the *within-laboratory reproducibility* were to be assessed, two or more analysts would be assigned to carry out the *repeatability* procedure. In arriving at an SOP such as the one described in Box 1.4, there should be some justification in leaving out certain steps in the complete assay. For instance, weighing is often the most precise step in the process, and thus repeat weighings of samples of tablet powder would not be necessary to guarantee precision; the precision of the extraction might be more open to question.

Each of the sections within an assay would have other SOPs associated with them, governing, for instance, the correct use and care of balances, as listed in Box 1.5.

Compound random errors

Systematic errors in analysis can usually be eliminated, but true random errors are due to operations in an assay which are not completely controlled. A common type of random error arises from the acceptance of manufacturers' tolerances for glassware. Table 1.3 gives the RSD values specified for certain items of grades A and B glassware.

Box 1.5 Procedure for the use of a calibrated balance SOP/001A/01

This balance is a high-grade analytical balance. The balance is sited in a vibration-free area, and disturbance by draughts should be avoided. It carries out internal calibration but as a double check it is checked with certified check weights. Any deviation of the check weight values from those expected indicates need for servicing of the balance. Check weight calibration should be carried out once a week according to the instructions in SOP/001C/01.

Caution: The logbook (form SOP/001 AR/01) must be filled in. Any spillages on the balance must be cleaned up immediately and recorded in the log. This balance is to be used only for analytical grade weighings.

Operation

1. When carrying out weighing of amounts < 50 mg use tweezers to handle the weighing vessel.
2. Make sure the door of the balance is shut. Switch on the balance and allow it to undergo its internal calibration procedure. When it is ready the digital read-out will be 0.0000. Wait 30 s to ensure that the reading has stabilised.
3. Introduce the weighing vessel onto the balance pan. Close the door. Wait 30 s to ensure that the reading has stabilised and then send the reading to the printer.
4. If the tare is used in the weighing procedure, press the tare button and wait until the balance reads 0.0000. Wait 30 s to ensure that the reading has stabilised. If it drifts, which under normal circumstances it should not, press the tare button again and wait for a stable reading.
5. Remove the weighing vessel from the balance, introduce the sample into the vessel and put it back onto the balance pan. Close the door and note the reading.
6. Remove the sample and adjust the sample size to bring it closer to the required amount. Re-introduce the sample onto the balance pan. Close the door and note the reading.
7. Repeat step 5 until the target weight is reached. When the required weight is reached wait 30 s to ensure that the reading has stabilised. Send the reading to the printer.

N.B. An unstable reading may indicate that moisture is being lost or gained and that the sample must be weighed in a capped vessel.

Date of issue: 6/10/95   Signature:

Table 1.3 Manufacturers' tolerances on some items of glassware

Item of glassware	Grade A	Grade B
1 ml bulb pipette	± 0.7%	± 1.5%
5 ml bulb pipette	± 0.3%	± 0.6%
100 ml volumetric flask	± 0.08%	± 0.15%
500 ml volumetric flask	± 0.05%	± 0.1%
Full 25 ml burette	± 0.2%	± 0.4%

An estimate of compound random errors is obtained from the square root of the sum of the squares of the RSDs attributed to each component or operation in the analysis. If the analysis of paracetamol described in Box 1.4 is considered, then, assuming the items of glassware are used correctly, the errors involved in the dilution steps can be simply estimated from the tolerances given for the pipette and volumetric flasks. The British Standards Institution (BS) tolerances for the grade A glassware used in the assay are as follows:

500 ml volumetric flask   500 ml ± 0.05%

100 ml volumetric flask   100 ml ± 0.08%

5 ml one mark pipette   5 ml ± 0.3%

$$\text{Standard deviation of error from glassware} =$$

$$\sqrt{0.05^2 + 0.08^2 + 0.3^2} = \sqrt{0.0989} = 0.31\%$$

Thus it can be seen that the compound error from the glassware differs little from the largest error in the process. Of course the glassware errors can be eliminated by calibration of the glassware prior to use, but, in general, analysts will accept manufacturers' tolerances. The tolerated random error from glassware could be readily eliminated; other random errors, such as variation in the extraction efficiency, are more difficult to control.

Self-test 1.3

Estimate the compound random error in the following assay with respect to the dilution steps described, and calculate the error as SD of the w/v percentage of the injection, assuming it is exactly 2% w/v.

A 2% w/v injection was diluted twice using grade A 5 ml bulb pipettes and grade A 100 ml volumetric flasks as follows:

Dilution 1: 5 to 100 ml
Dilution 2: 5 to 100 ml

The uncertainty in the spectrophotometric reading was ± 0.2%.

Answer: ± 0.48% and ± 0.01% w/v

Reporting of results

In calculating an answer from the data obtained in an analysis it is important to not indicate a higher level of precision than was actually possible in the assay. As mentioned in the previous section, when considering the accuracy of glassware used with the assumption that it complied with the BS grade A standard, it was obvious that there was some uncertainty in any figure < 1%. It might be possible to improve on this degree of precision by calibrating glassware; however, any improvement in precision in the real world would take time and hence have cost implications. Thus for the purposes of most analyses, and for the purposes of the calculations in this book, it would seem sensible to report four significant figures, i.e. to 0.1%. In the process of carrying out calculations, five figures can be retained and rounded up to four figures at the end of the calculation. Since in pharmaceutical analyses the percentage of the stated content of a drug in a formulation may be reported as being between 90 and 99.9%, if the first significant figure is 9, then at the end of the calculation a more realistic estimate of precision is given by rounding the answer up to three significant figures. The SD or RSD reported with the answer should reflect the number of significant figures given; since there is usually uncertainty in figures < 1% of the answer, the RSD should not be reported below 0.1%. Taking this into consideration the correct and incorrect ways of reporting some answers are given in Table 1.4.

Table 1.4 Significant figures in the reporting of analytical results

Answer ± S Incorrect	RSD	Answer ± S Correct	RSD
% of stated content = 99.2 ± 0.22	0.22	% of stated content = 99.2 ± 0.2	0.2
% of stated content = 101.15 ± 0.35	0.35	% of stated content = 101.2 ± 0.4	0.4
0.2534 ± 0.00443% w/v	1.75	0.2534 ± 0.0044% w/v	1.7
1.0051 ± 0.0063% w/w	0.63	1.005 ± 0.006% w/w	0.6
1.784 ± 0.1242 μg/ml	6.962	1.784 ± 0.124 μg/ml	7.0

Other terms used in the control of analytical procedures

System suitability

System suitability should not be confused with method validation. System suitability tests are most often applied to analytical instrumentation. They are designed to evaluate the components of the analytical system in order to show that the performance of the system meets the standards required by the method. Method validation is performed once at the end of method development, whereas system suitability tests are performed on a system periodically to determine whether or not it is still working properly and is capable of carrying out the analysis. System suitability relates to the performance of the equipment. In selecting equipment, the four Qs rule can be applied:[2]

(i)   Design qualification (fit for purpose). What is the equipment required to do?
(ii) Installation qualification. Does the equipment work in the way that the manufacturer claims?
(iii) Operational qualification. Does the equipment work for the analyst's particular application?
(iv) Performance qualification. Does the instrument continue to perform to the standard required?

In routine use it is point 4 that is checked, and, for a given procedure, an analyst will use several tests routinely, in order to monitor instrument performance, e.g. the resolution test during chromatography. The system suitability tests that would routinely be carried out on a HPLC are described in Chapter 10.

Analytical blank

This consists of all the reagents or solvents used in an analysis without any of the analyte being present. A true analytical blank should reflect all the operations to which the analyte in a real sample is subjected. It is used, for example, in checking that reagents or indicators do not contribute to the volume of titrant required for a titration, including zeroing spectrophotometers or in checking for chromatographic interference.

Calibration

The calibration of a method involves comparison of the value or values of a particular parameter measured by the system under strictly defined conditions with pre-set standard values. Examples include calibration of the wavelength and absorbance scales of a UV/visible spectrophotometer (Ch. 4), calibration of the wavelength scale of an IR spectrometer (Ch. 5) and construction of chromatographic calibration curves (Ch. 12).

Limit of detection

This is the smallest amount of an analyte which can be detected by a particular method. It is formally defined as follows:

$$x - x_B = 3s_B$$

where x is the signal from the sample, x_B is the signal from the analytical blank and s_B is the SD of the reading for the analytical blank. In other words, the criterion for a reading reflecting the presence of an analyte in a sample is that the difference between the reading taken and the reading for the blank should be three times the SD of the blank reading. The SD of the signal from the sample can be disregarded since the sample and the blank should have been prepared in the same manner so that it and the sample produce a similar SD in their readings. A true limit of detection should reflect all the processes to which the analyte in a real assay is subjected and not be a simple dilution of a pure standard for the analyte until it can no longer be detected. The definition of limit of detection (LOD) above applies mostly to spectrophotometric readings.

In the case of chromatographic separations there is usually a constant background reading called the baseline. According to the EP the limit of detection is where the height of a chromatographic peak is three times the height of the fluctuation of the baseline noise over a distance equal to 20 times width of the peak at half height. Chromatographic software will generally calculate this for the operator; however, manual estimation can be carried out as shown in Figure 1.5 where the LOD is reached where 2H/h is < 3.

Limit of quantification

The limit of quantification is defined as the smallest amount of analyte which can be quantified reliably, i.e. with an RSD for repeat measurement of $< \pm 20\%$. The limit of quantification is defined as: $x - x_B = 10s_B$. In this case the analyte should give a peak at more than ten times the standard deviation of the chromatographic baseline during chromatographic analysis. As shown in Figure 1.5 where the limit of quantification (LOQ) is reached where 2H/h is < 10.

Self-test 1.4

In which of the following cases has the limit of detection been reached?

Signal from sample	Sample SD	Signal from analytical blank	Analytical blank SD
1. Abs 0.0063	0.0003	0.0045	0.0003
2. Abs 0.0075	0.0017	0.0046	0.0018
3. 0.335 ng/ml	0.045 ng/ml	0.045 ng/ml	0.037 ng/ml

Answer: 2

Linearity

Most analytical methods are based on processes where the method produces a response that is linear and that increases or decreases linearly with analyte concentration. The equation of a straight line takes the form:

$$y = a + bx$$

where a is the intercept of the straight line with the y axis and b is the slope of the line. Taking a simple example, a three-point calibration curve is constructed through readings of absorbance against procaine concentration (Table 1.5).

The best fit of a straight line through these values can be determined by determining a and b from the following equations:

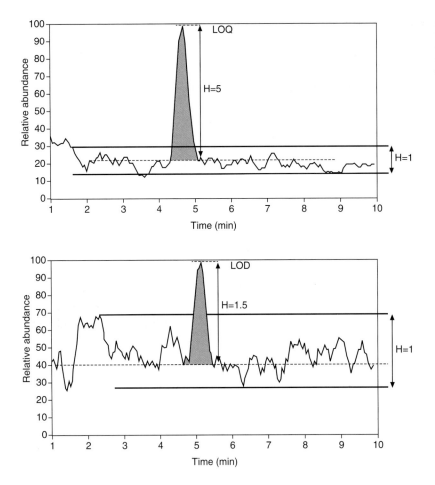

Fig. 1.5
Estimation of limit of detection (LOD) and limit of quantification (LOQ) for a chromatographic system.

Table 1.5 Data used for the construction of a calibration curve for the spectrophotometric determination of procaine

Procaine concentration mg/100 ml	Absorbance reading
0.8	0.604
1.0	0.763
1.2	0.931

$$b = \frac{\sum_i (x_i - \overline{x})(y_i - \overline{y})}{\sum_i (x_i - \overline{x})^2}$$

$$a = \overline{y} - b\overline{x}$$

where x_i is the individual value for x, $\overline{x}$ is the mean value of x_i, y_i is the individual value for y and $\overline{y}$ is the mean of y_i.

From the data in Table 1.4:

$$\bar{x} = \frac{0.8 + 1.0 + 1.2}{3} = 1.0$$

$$\bar{y} = \frac{0.604 + 0.763 + 0.931}{3} = 0.766$$

$$b = \frac{\begin{array}{c}(0.8-1.0)(0.604-0.766) + (1.0-1.0)(0.763-0.766) \\ + (1.2-1.0)(0.931-0.766)\end{array}}{(0.8-1.0)^2 + (1.0-1.0)^2 + (1.2-1.0)^2}$$

$$= \frac{0.0324 + 0 + 0.033}{0.04 + 0.04} = 0.818$$

$$a = 0.766 - 0.818 \times 1.0 = -0.052$$

Thus the equation for the best fit is:

$$y = 0.818x - 0.052$$

The statistical measure of the quality of fit of the line through the data is the correlation coefficient r. A correlation coefficient of > 0.99 is regarded as indicating linearity. The correlation coefficient is determined from the following equation:

$$r = \frac{\sum_i \{(x_i - \bar{x})(y_i - \bar{y})\}}{\sqrt{\sum_i [(x_i - \bar{x})^2] \sum_i [(y_i - \bar{y})^2]}}$$

Substituting the values from Table 1.4:

$$r = \frac{\begin{array}{c}(0.8-1.0)(0.604-0.766) + (1.0-1.0)(0.763-0.766) \\ + (1.2-1.0)(0.931-0.766)\end{array}}{\sqrt{\begin{array}{c}[(0.8-1.0)^2 + (1.0-1.0)^2 + (1.2-1.0)^2] \\ [(0.604-0.766)^2 + (0.763-0.766)^2 + (0.931-0.766)^2]\end{array}}}$$

$$r = \frac{0.0324 + 0 + 0.033}{\sqrt{0.08 \times 0.0534}} = 1.00$$

Thus, to three significant figures, the straight line fit through the values in Table 1.4 is perfect. For a fuller treatment of the mathematical determination and significance of a correlation coefficient see Miller and Miller.[1] The equation for the correlation coefficient is very useful in that it can be applied to correlations between curves of any shape and thus it can be used for spectral comparisons, such as those carried out between diode array spectra obtained during HPLC (Ch. 12).

Range

The term range can be applied to instrument performance (dynamic range), but, when applied to the performance of an assay, it refers to the interval between the upper and lower concentration of an analyte for which an acceptable level of precision and accuracy has been established. Typical ranges are: 80–120% of the stated amount for a finished product; 70–130% of the expected concentration, e.g. for content of single tablets (the range may be even wider for some products, such as doses delivered by a metered dose inhaler) and 0–110% for dissolution tests where the drug is released from the dosage form over a time period.

Robustness

Robustness is evaluated in order to determine how resistant the precision and accuracy of an assay are to small variations in the method. The types of parameters which are assessed in order to determine the robustness of a method include the stability of analytical solutions; the length of the extraction time; the effect of variations in the pH of a HPLC mobile phase; the effect of small variations in mobile phase composition; the effect of changing chromatographic columns; the effect of temperature and flow rate during chromatography.

Selectivity

The selectivity of a method is a measure of how capable it is of measuring the analyte alone in the presence of other compounds contained in the sample. The most selective analytical methods involve a chromatographic separation. Detection methods can be ranked according to their selectivity. A simple comparison is between fluorescence spectrophotometry and UV spectrophotometry. There are many more compounds which exhibit UV absorption than there are those which exhibit strong fluorescence; thus fluorescence spectrophotometry is a more selective method. Because selective methods are based on more complex principles than non-selective methods, they may be less robust, e.g. fluorescence spectrophotometry is more affected by changes in the analytical method than UV spectrophotometry.

Sensitivity

The sensitivity of method indicates how responsive it is to a small change in the concentration of an analyte. It can be viewed as the slope of a response curve and may be a function of the method itself or of the way in which the instrumentation has been calibrated. In Figure 1.6 the method having a *linear* response $y = 2.5x$ is five times more sensitive than the method exhibiting a linear response

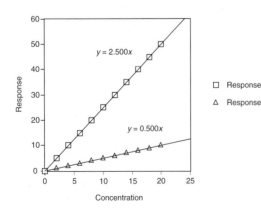

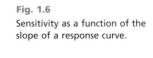

Fig. 1.6
Sensitivity as a function of the slope of a response curve.

$y = 0.5x$. Sensitivity and the *limit of detection* of a method are often confused. The limit of detection is due to a combination of *range* and *sensitivity*.

Weighing by difference

Weighing by difference is used to minimise weighing errors in an analytical procedure. The sample is weighed in a suitable vessel, e.g. a glass weighing boat with a spout, and then transferred immediately to the vessel in which it is going to be analysed or dissolved. The weighing vessel is then reweighed, and the difference between the weights before and after transfer gives the weight of the sample. This method of weighing minimises errors due to, for example, the absorption of moisture onto the surface of the vessel. It also means that there is not a requirement for complete transfer of the sample that is to be analysed.

The points listed in Boxes 1.6 and 1.7 indicate how pharmaceutical preparations may come to be out of specification.

Box 1.6 Sources of impurities in pharmaceutical manufacture

- During the course of the manufacture of a pure drug substance, impurities may arise as follows:
  (i) Present in the synthetic starting materials
  (ii) Result from residual amounts of chemical intermediates used in the synthetic process and from unintended side reactions
  (iii) Result from reagents, solvents and catalysts used in manufacture.
- The process used to produce the formulated drug substance may introduce impurities as follows:
  (i) Particulate matter from the atmosphere, machines and devices used in the manufacturing process and from containers
  (ii) Impurities that are present in the excipients used in the formulation
  (iii) Cross contamination may occur from other processes carried out using the same equipment, e.g. from mixers
  (iv) Microbial contamination may occur
  (v) The drug may react with the excipients used in the formulation
  (vi) Impurities may be introduced from packaging, e.g. polymeric monomers.

Box 1.7 Processes leading to the deviation of the actual content from the stated content of a drug in a formulation

- Incomplete mixing of drug with formulation excipients prior to compression into tablets or filling into capsules
- Physical instability of the dosage form: tablets that disintegrate too readily; creams or suspensions that separate and over- or undercompression of tablets, leading to deviation from the required weight
- Chemical breakdown of the drug resulting from its reaction with air, water, light, excipients in a formulation or packaging materials
- Partitioning of the drug into packaging materials.

Basic calculations in pharmaceutical analysis

The data from an analysis can be obtained using computer-based methods. However, in order to have some idea of the accuracy of an answer, it is necessary to be able to carry out calculations in the traditional manner. There are various units used to express amounts and concentrations in pharmaceutical analysis, and examples of these units will be considered below.

Percentage volume/volume (%v/v)

Percentage volume/volume (%v/v) is most often encountered in relation to the composition of mobile phases used in HPLC. Thus, when 30 ml of methanol is mixed with 70 ml of water, a 30:70 v/v mixture is formed. Since some shrinking in volume occurs when two liquids are mixed, %v/v may only be approximate. Some chromatographers prefer to prepare mixtures of solvents by weighing them rather than by volume measurement, and in this case the solvent mixture can be expressed as % weight in weight (%w/w).

Percentage weight in volume (%w/v)

Percentage weight in volume (%w/v) is normally used to express the content of active ingredient in liquid formulations such as injections, infusions and eye-drops. The density of the solvent in this case is irrelevant; thus, a 1 g/100 ml solution of a drug is 1% w/v whether it is dissolved in ethanol or water.

Self-test 1.5

Convert the following concentrations to % w/v:

(i)   0.1 g/100 ml
(ii) 1 mg/ml
(iii) 0.1 g/ml
(iv) 100 μg/ml

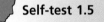

Answers: (i) 0.1% w/v
(ii) 0.1% w/v
(iii) 10% w/v
(iv) 0.01% w/v

Dilutions

In order for an extract from a formulation or a solution of a pure drug substance to be measured it must be diluted so that it falls within the working range of the instrument used to make the measurement. Thus an understanding of dilution factors is fundamental to calculations based on analytical data.

Calculation example 1.1

An infusion stated to contain 0.95% w/v NaCl was diluted so that its Na content could be determined by flame photometry. The following dilutions were carried out:

(i) 10 ml of the sample was diluted to 250 ml with water.
(ii) 10 ml of the diluted sample was diluted to 200 ml with water.

The sample was found to contain 0.74 mg/100 ml of Na.
Atomic weights: Na = 23, Cl = 35.5

(Continued)

Calculation example 1.1 *(Continued)*

Calculate:

The %w/v of NaCl present in the infusion.
The % of stated content of NaCl.

Dilution factor = 10 to 250 ($\times$ 25), 10 to 200 ($\times$ 20). Total dilution = 25 $\times$ 20 = 500.
Therefore, in the original injection, conc. of Na = 0.74 $\times$ 500 mg/100 ml = 370 mg/100 ml.
Conc. of NaCl in the injection = 370 $\times$ (58.5/23) = 941 mg/100 ml = 0.941 g/100 ml = 0.941% w/v.
% of stated content = (0.941/0.95) $\times$ 100 = 99.1%.
In the sample there are 941 mg/100 ml.

Calculation example 1.2

A 2 ml volume of eyedrops contains the local anaesthetic proxymetacaine. HCl is diluted to
100 ml and then 5 ml of the dilution is diluted to 200 ml. The diluted sample was measured by
UV spectrophotometry and was found to contain 0.512 mg/100 ml of the drug. Calculate the
%w/v of the drug in the eyedrops.
Dilution factors 2 to 100 ($\times$ 50), 5 to 200 ($\times$ 40). Total dilution 40 $\times$ 50 = 2000.
Original concentration = 2000 $\times$ 0.512 = 1024 mg/100 ml = 1.024 g/100 ml = 1.024% w/v.

Self-test 1.6

A 5 ml sample of an injection of a steroid phosphate was diluted to 100 ml. Then 10 ml
of the diluted injection was diluted to 100 ml, and this dilution was further diluted
10 to 100 ml. From measurement by UV the diluted sample was found to contain
0.249 mg/100 ml of the steroid. What was the original concentration of the injection
in %w/v and in mg/ml?

Answers: 0.498% w/v, 4.98 mg/ml

Self-test 1.7

A sample of an infusion was diluted 5 ml to 200 ml and then 10 ml to 200 ml. It was
then analysed and was found to contain sodium at 0.789 mg/100 ml. Calculate the
concentration of sodium in the original sample in %w/v. The sample was composed of a
mixture of sodium lactate and sodium bicarbonate in equimolar amounts. Calculate the
amount of sodium lactate and sodium bicarbonate in mg in 10 ml of the sample (Na =
23, lactate = 89, bicarbonate = 61).

Answers: 0.6312% w/v, Na lactate = 153.7 mg/10 ml Na bicarbonate = 115.3 mg/10 ml

---

Preparation of standard stock solutions

In preparing a stock solution of a standard using a standard four-place balance,
assuming there is no lack of availability of standard, it is best to weigh at least
100 mg of material, since an error of 0.1 mg in weight is only 0.1% of the weight
taken.

Calculation example 1.3

Assuming that you wish to avoid pipetting less than a 5 ml volume, starting from a 102.1 mg/100 ml stock solution, how would you prepare the following concentrations for a calibration series?

0.2042 mg/100 ml, 0.4084 mg/100 ml, 0.6126 mg/100 ml,

0.8168 mg/100 ml, 1.021 mg/ml

When a large dilution (> 10) is required it is best to carry it out in two stages.

In this case an initial dilution of 20 ml to 100 ml is carried out, producing a 10.21 mg/100 ml solution. Then 250 ml volumetric flasks can be used to carry out the following dilutions.

5 to 250 ($\times$ 50), 10 to 250 ($\times$ 25), 15 to 250 ($\times$ 16.67), 20 to 250 ($\times$ 12.5),

and 25 to 250 ($\times$ 10), giving the dilution series above.

N.B. Once the volume required for the lowest concentration (5 ml) has been determined, then it can be multiplied $\times$ 2, $\times$ 3, $\times$ 4 and $\times$ 5 to give the series.

Self-test 1.8

A stock solution containing 125.6 mg of standard in 250 ml is prepared. Suggest how the following dilution series could be prepared (pipettes 5 ml or greater must be used).

0.1005 mg/100 ml, 0.2010 mg/100 ml, 0.3015 mg/100 ml, 0.4020 mg/100 ml, 0.5025 mg/100 ml

Answer: Number of possible answers, e.g. dilution 1, 10 ml to 250 ml. Then, from dilution 1, 5, 10, 15, 20 and 25 ml pipettes used to transfer into 100 ml volumetric flasks

Percentage weight/weight (%w/w)

Percentage weight/weight (%w/w) is a common measure used to express the concentration of active ingredient in a formulation such as a cream or to express the content of a minor impurity in a drug substance. Thus, a cream containing 10 mg (0.01 g) of drug per gram is a $(0.01/1) \times 100 = 1\%$ w/w formulation. Equally, if a drug contains 0.5 mg (0.0005 g) per gram of an impurity, the impurity is at a concentration of $(0.0005/1) \times 100 = 0.05\%$ w/w. It is generally accepted that, for a drug, all impurities above 0.05% w/w should be characterised, i.e. their structures should be known and their toxicities should be assessed.

In determining impurities in a drug, 1 g of the drug might be dissolved in 100 ml of solvent. If an analysis was carried out and the drug solution was found to contain 3 mg/100 ml of an impurity, then the %w/w referring back to the original weight of drug substance would be:

$(0.003/1) \times 100 = 0.3\%$ w/w

Parts per million (ppm) calculations

Parts per million (ppm) on a w/w basis is 1 mg/g (1 μg/kg). It is a common measure used for impurities in drug substances, particularly heavy metals and solvents. 1 ppm is also 0.0001% w/w.

Calculation example 1.4

The potassium content of an intravenous infusion containing sodium chloride was determined. The infusion was found to contain 0.9092% w/v NaCl. The undiluted infusion was measured for potassium content in comparison with a potassium chloride standard. The potassium content of the undiluted infusion was found to be 0.141 mg/100 ml. Calculate the potassium content in the sodium chloride in ppm:

$$0.9092\% \text{ w/v} = 0.9092 \text{ g}/100 \text{ ml}$$
$$\text{Potassium content} = 0.141 \text{ mg}/100 \text{ ml} = 141 \text{ } \mu\text{g}/100 \text{ ml}$$

Relative to the sodium chloride, there are 141 μg/0.9092 g = 141/0.9092 ppm = 155 ppm.

Working between weights and molarity

Weights are much easier to appreciate than molar concentrations, but sometimes, particularly in bioanalytical methods, molar concentrations are used.

Definitions

Molar: molecular weight in g/l (mg/ml)
mMolar: molecular weight in mg/l (μg/ml)
μMolar: molecular weight in μg/l (ng/ml)
nMolar: molecular weight in ng/l (pg/ml).

Calculation example 1.5

The metabolism of paracetamol (molecular weight 151.2 amu) by liver microsomes was studied by preparing a 100 μM solution of paracetamol in 1 ml of incubation mixture. A 30.12 mg/100 ml solution of paracetamol in buffer was prepared. What volume of paracetamol solution had to be added to incubation mixture prior to making up the volume to 1 ml:

$$100\ \mu M = 100 \times 151.2 = 15120\ \mu g/l = 15.12\ \mu g/ml.$$

$$30.12\ mg/100\ ml = 30120\ \mu g/100\ ml = 301.2\ \mu g/ml = 0.3012\ \mu g/\mu l.$$

$$\text{Volume of paracetamol solution required} = 15.12/0.3012 = 50.2\ \mu l.$$

Self-test 1.11

(i) Calculate the concentrations in mg/ml and $\mu g/\mu l$ of a 10 μM solution of kanamycin (molecular weight 484.5).
(ii) A solution containing diclofenac sodium (molecular weight 318.1) at a concentration of 79.5 mg/100 ml in buffer was prepared. What volume of this solution was required in order to carry out a microsomal incubation containing a 25 μM concentration of the drug in 1 ml?

Answers: (i) 0.004845 mg/ml, 0.004845 $\mu g/\mu l$
(ii) 10 μl

Additional problems

All answers to be given to four significant figures. e.g. 1% w/v to four significant figures is 1.000% w/v.

1. Convert the following concentrations to %w/v.
   (i)   10 mg/ml
   (ii) 100 mg/l
   (iii) 0.025 g/ml
   (iv) 250 μg/ml
   (v)   20 $\mu g/\mu l$.

Answers: (i) 1.000% w/v
(ii) 0.01000% w/v
(iii) 2.500% w/v
(iv) 0.02500% w/v
(v) 2.000% w/v

2. An infusion which was stated to contain 0.5000% w/v KCl was diluted so that its K content could be determined by flame photometry. The following dilutions were carried out:
   (i)   10 ml of the sample was diluted to 200 ml with water.
   (ii) 10 ml of the diluted sample was diluted to 200 ml with water.
   The sample was found to contain 0.6670 mg/100 ml of K.
   (Atomic weights: K = 39.1 Cl = 35).
   Calculate:
   (i)   The % w/v of KCl present in the infusion
   (ii) The % of stated content of KCl.

Answers: (i) 0.5090% w/v
(ii) 101.8%

(Continued)

Additional problems *(Continued)*

3. Oral rehydration salts are stated to contain the following components:
   Sodium Chloride 3.5 g
   Potassium Chloride 1.5 g
   Sodium Citrate 2.9 g
   Anhydrous Glucose 20.0 g

   8.342 g of oral rehydration salts are dissolved in 500 ml of water. 5 ml of the solution is diluted to 100 ml and then 5 ml is taken from the diluted sample and is diluted to 100 ml.
   The sodium content of the sample is then determined by flame photometry. The sodium salts used to prepare the mixture were:
   Trisodium citrate hydrate ($C_6H_5Na_3O_7,2H_2O$) molecular weight 294.1 and sodium chloride (NaCl) molecular weight 58.5
   Atomic weight of Na = 23
   The content of Na in the diluted sample was determined to be 0.3210 mg/100 ml
   Determine the % of stated content of Na in the sample.

   Answer: 104.5%

4. A 5 ml volume of eyedrops contains the mydriatic drug cyclopentolate. HCl is diluted to 100 ml and then 20 ml of the dilution is diluted to 100 ml. The diluted sample was measured by UV spectrophotometry and was found to contain 20.20 mg/100 ml of the drug. Calculate the %w/v of the drug in the eyedrops.

   Answer: 2.020% w/v

5. 0.5% w/v of an injection is to be used as an anaesthetic for a 2-week-old baby weighing 3.4 kg. The recommended dose for a bolus injection is 0.5 mg/kg. The injection must be given in 1 ml. Calculate the amount of water for injection that must be drawn into the syringe with the appropriate volume of injection.

   Answer: 0.6600 ml

6. 0.0641 g of a semi-synthetic alkaloid was dissolved in 25 ml of 1% w/v acetic acid and was analysed directly by HPLC. The solution was found to contain 0.142 mg/100 ml of an impurity. What is the level of impurity in %w/w and ppm?

   Answers: 0.05538% w/w, 553.8 ppm.

7. The level of ethyl acetate is determined in colchicine by headspace gas chromatography. A solution containing 4.361 g/100 ml of colchicine in water was prepared. An aqueous standard containing 0.5912 mg/100 ml of ethyl acetate was also prepared. Headspace analysis of 2 ml volumes of the two solutions produced GC peaks for ethyl acetate with the following areas:

   Colchicine solution: Peak area 13457
   Ethyl acetate solution: Peak area 14689
   Calculate the ethyl acetate content in the colchicine sample in ppm.

   Answer: 124.2 ppm

References

1. Miller JC, Miller JN. *Statistics and Chemometrics for Analytical Chemistry*. 6th ed. Chichester: Ellis Horwood; 2010.
2. Burgess C. Good spectroscopic practice: science and compliance. *Spectroscopy Europe* 1994;6:10-13.

Further reading

Ermer J, Miller JHM, eds. *Method Validation in Pharmaceutical Analysis*. Weinheim: Wiley-VCH; 2005.
Jones D. *Pharmaceutical Statistics*. London: Pharmaceutical Press; 2002.

Physical and chemical properties of drug molecules

2

Introduction

The physical properties of organic molecules, such as pKa and partition coefficient, are dealt with extensively in pharmacy courses[1,2] but do not feature greatly in analytical chemistry courses. It is often surprising that analytical chemists cannot distinguish between, for instance, basic, weakly basic, acidic, weakly acidic and neutral nitrogen functions. The physical properties of drug molecules, along with simple chemical derivatisation and degradation reactions, play an important part in the design of analytical methods. Drug molecules can be complex, containing multiple functional groups that in combination produce the overall properties of the molecule. This chapter will serve as a starting point for understanding the chemical and physico-chemical behaviour of drug molecules, which influence the development of analytical methods. The latter part of the chapter focuses on some typical drugs that are representative of a class of drug molecules and lists their physical properties and the properties of their functional groups in so far as they are known.

Calcuelation of pH value of aqueous solutions of strong and weak acids and bases

Dissociation of water

The pH of a solution is defined as $-\log [H^+]$, where $[H^+]$ is the concentration of hydrogen ions in solution.

In pure water the concentration of hydrogen ions is governed by the equilibrium:

$$H_2O \underset{Ka}{\rightleftharpoons} H^+ + HO^-$$

Ka is the dissociation constant for the equilibrium, is known as Kw in the case of the dissociation of water and is determined by the following expression:

$$K_w = \frac{[H^+][HO^-]}{[H_2O]} = [H^+][HO^-] = 10^{-14}$$

Since the concentration of water does not change appreciably as a result of ionisation, its concentration can be regarded as not having an effect on the equilibrium and it can be omitted from the equation, and this means that in pure water:

$$[H^+] = [HO^-] = 10^{-7}$$

The pH of water is thus given by $-\log 10^{-7} = 7.00$.

Strong acids and bases

If an acid is introduced into an aqueous solution the $[H^+]$ increases. If the pH of an aqueous solution is known, the $[H^+]$ is given by the expression 10^{-pH}, e.g. $[H^+]$ in pH 4 solution $= 10^{-4}$ M $= 0.0001$ M. Since $[H^+][OH^-] = 10^{-14}$ for water, the concentration of $[OH^-]$ in this solution is 10^{-10} M.

A strong acid is completely ionised in water and $[H^+]$ is equal to its molarity, e.g. 0.1 M HCl contains 0.1 M H^+ (10^{-1} H^+) and has a pH of $-\log 0.1 = 1$. For a solution of a strong base such as 0.1 M NaOH, $[OH^-] = 0.1$ M and $[0.1][H^+] = 10^{-14}$; therefore, $[H^+] = 10^{-13}$ M and the pH of the solution $= 13$. Although the pH range is regarded as being between 0 and 14, it does extend above and below these values, e.g. 10 M HCl, in theory, has a pH of -1.

Self-test 2.1

Calculate the pH of the following solutions:

(i)   0.05 M HCl
(ii) 0.05 M NaOH
(iii) 0.05 M H_2SO_4

Answers: (i) 1.3; (ii) 12.7; (iii) 1.0, since 0.05 M H_2SO_4 contains 0.1 M H^+

Weak acids and bases

Weak acids are not completely ionised in aqueous solution and are in equilibrium with the undissociated acid, as is the case for water, which is a very weak acid. The dissociation constant Ka is given by the expression below:

$$HA \underset{Ka}{\rightleftharpoons} A^- + H^+$$

$$Ka = \frac{[A^-][H^+]}{[HA]}$$

For instance, in a 0.1 M solution of acetic acid ($Ka = 1.75 \times 10^{-5}$), the equilibrium can be written as follows:

$$\underset{(0.1-x)}{COH_3COOH} \underset{Ka}{\rightleftharpoons} \underset{x}{CH_3COO^-} + \underset{x}{H^+}$$

$$Ka = \frac{[CH_3COO^-][H^+]}{[CH_3COOH]}$$

The pH can be calculated as follows:

$$1.75 \times 10^{-5} = \frac{x^2}{(0.1-x)}$$

Since the dissociation of the acetic acid does not greatly change the concentration of the un-ionised acid, the above expression can be approximated to:

$$1.75 \times 10^{-5} = \frac{x^2}{0.1}$$

$$x = [H^+] = \sqrt{1.75 \times 10^{-6}} = 0.00132 \text{ M}$$

$$pH = 29$$

In comparison, the pH of 0.1 M HCl is 1.

The calculation of the pH of a weak base can be considered in the same way. For instance, in a 0.1 M solution of ammonia ($Kb = 1.8 \times 10^{-5}$), the equilibrium can be written as follows:

$$\underset{(0.1-x)}{NH_3 + H_2O} \underset{Kb}{\rightleftharpoons} \underset{x}{NH_4^+} + \underset{x}{HO^-}$$

If the concentration/activity of water is regarded as being 1, then the equilibrium constant is given by the following expression:

$$Kb = \frac{[NH_4^+][HO^-]}{[NH_3]}$$

$$1.8 \times 10^{-5} = \frac{x^2}{(0.1-x)}$$

The concentration of NH_3 can be regarded as being unchanged by a small amount of ionisation, and the expression can be written as:

$$x = [HO^-] = \sqrt{1.8 \times 10^{-6}} = 0.0013 \text{ M}$$

$$[H^+] = \frac{K_w}{0.0013} = \frac{10^{-14}}{0.0013} = 7.7 \times 10^{-12} \text{ M}$$

$$pH = 11.1$$

In comparison, the pH of 0.1 M NaOH is 13.

Acidic and basic strength and pKa

The pKa value of a compound is defined as pKa $= -\log Ka$.

A pKa value can be assigned to both acids and bases.

For an acid, the higher the $[H^+]$ the stronger the acid, e.g.:

$$CH_3COOH \underset{}{\overset{Ka}{\rightleftharpoons}} CH_3COO^- + H^+$$

In the case of a base, it is the protonated form of the base that acts as a proton donor, e.g.:

$$NH_4^+ \underset{}{\overset{Ka}{\rightleftharpoons}} NH_3 + H^-$$

In this case, the lower the $[H^+]$ the stronger the base.

If pKa is used as a measure of acidic or basic strength: *for an acid, the smaller the pKa value the stronger the acid; for a base the larger the pKa value the stronger the base.*

Henderson–Hasselbalch equation

$$Ka = \frac{[A^-][H^+]}{[HA]}$$

Can be rearranged substituting pH for $-\log [H^+]$ and pKa for $-\log Ka$ to give:

$$pH = pKa + \log \frac{[A^-]}{[HA]}$$

For example, when acetic acid (pKa 4.76) is in solution at pH 4.76, the Henderson–Hasselbalch equation can be written as follows:

$$pH = 4.76 + \log \frac{[CH_3COO^-]}{[CH_3COOH]}$$

From this relationship for acetic acid it is possible to determine the degree of ionisation of acetic acid at a given pH.

Thus, when the pH = 4.76, then:

$$4.76 = 4.76 + \log \frac{[CH_3COO^-]}{[CH_3COOH]}$$

$$\log \frac{[CH_3COO^-]}{[CH_3COOH]} = 0$$

$$\frac{[CH_3COO^-]}{[CH_3COOH]} = 10^0 = 1$$

Acetic acid is 50% ionised at pH 4.76. In the case of a weak acid, it is the protonated form of the acid that is un-ionised, and, as the pH falls, the acid becomes less ionised.

For a base, the Henderson–Hasselbalch equation is written as follows:

$$BH^+ \rightleftharpoons B + H^+$$

$$pH = pKa + \log\frac{[B]}{[BH^+]}$$

For example, when ammonia (pKa 9.25) is in a solution at pH 9.25, the Henderson–Hasselbalch equation can be written as follows:

$$9.25 = 9.25 + \log\frac{[NH_3]}{[NH_4^+]}$$

$$\log\frac{[NH_3]}{[NH_4^+]} = 0$$

$$\frac{[NH_3]}{[NH_4^+]} = 10^0 = 1$$

Ammonia is 50% ionised at pH 9.25. In this case, it is the protonated form of the base that is ionised, and, as the pH falls, the base becomes more ionised.

An alternative way of writing the expression giving the percentage of ionisation for an acid or base of a particular pKa value at a particular pH value is:

$$\text{Acid: \% ionisation} = \frac{10^{pH-pKa}}{1 + 10^{pH-pKa}} \times 100$$

$$\text{Base: \% ionisation} = \frac{10^{pKa-pH}}{1 + 10^{pKa-pH}} \times 100$$

Ionisation of drug molecules (see Animation 2.1)

The ionisation of drug molecules is important with regard to their absorption into the circulation and their distribution to different tissues within the body. The pKa value of a drug is also important with regard to its formulation into a medicine and to the design of analytical methods for its determination.

Calculation example 2.1

Calculate the percentage of ionisation of the drugs shown in Figure 2.1 at pH 7.0.

Fig. 2.1
Ionisation of a basic and an
acidic drug.

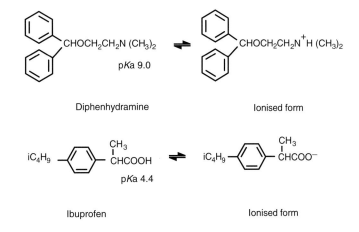

Diphenhydramine   Ionised form

Ibuprofen   Ionised form

Diphenhydramine

This drug contains one basic nitrogen, and, at pH 7.0, its percentage of ionisation can be calculated as follows:

$$\% \text{ Ionisation diphenhydramine} = \frac{10^{9.0-7.0}}{1+10^{9.0-7.0}} \times 100$$

$$= \frac{10^{2.0}}{1+10^{2.0}} \times 100 = \frac{100}{101} \times 100 = 99.0\%$$

Ibuprofen

This drug contains one acidic group, and, at pH 7.0, its percentage of ionisation can be calculated as follows:

$$\% \text{ Ionisation ibuprofen} = \frac{10^{7.0-4.4}}{1+10^{7.0-4.4}} \times 100$$

$$= \frac{10^{2.6}}{1+10^{2.6}} \times 100 = \frac{398}{399} \times 100 = 99.8\%$$

Self-test 2.5

Calculate the percentage of ionisation of the following drugs, which contain 1 group that ionises in the pH range 0–14, at the pH values of (i) 4 and (ii) 9.

(Continued)

Self-test 2.5 *(Continued)*

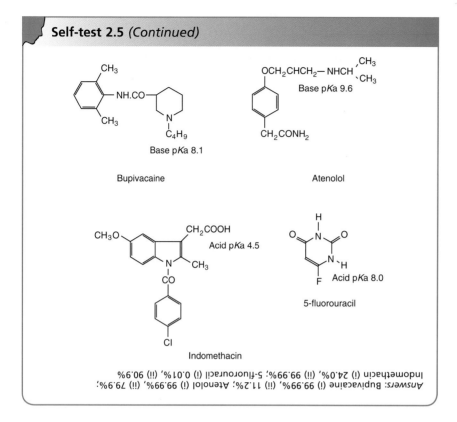

Bupivacaine — Base pKa 8.1

Atenolol — Base pKa 9.6

Indomethacin — Acid pKa 4.5

5-fluorouracil — Acid pKa 8.0

Buffers

Buffers can be prepared from any weak acid or base and are used to maintain the pH of a solution in a narrow range. This is important in living systems; for example, human plasma is buffered at pH 7.4 by a carbonic acid/bicarbonate buffer system.

Buffers are used in a number of areas of analytical chemistry, such as the preparation of mobile phases for chromatography and the extraction of drugs from aqueous solution. The simplest type of buffer is composed of a weak acid or base in combination with a strong base or acid. A common buffer system is the sodium acetate/acetic acid buffer system. The most direct way of preparing this buffer is by the addition of sodium hydroxide to a solution of acetic acid until the required pH is reached. The most effective range for a buffer is 1 pH unit either side of the pKa value of the weak acid or base used in the buffer. The pKa value of acetic acid is 4.76; thus its effective buffer range is 3.76–5.76.

Calculation example 2.2

1 litre of 0.1 M sodium acetate buffer with a pH of 4.0 is required. Molecular weight of acetic acid = 60; therefore, in a litre of 0.1 M buffer there will be 6 g of acetic acid. To prepare the buffer, 6 g of acetic acid are weighed and made up to *ca* 500 ml with water. The pH of the

(Continued)

Calculation example 2.2 *(Continued)*

acetic acid solution is adjusted to 4.0 by addition of 2 M sodium hydroxide solution, using a pH meter to monitor the pH. The solution is then made up to 1 litre with water. Calculate the concentration of acetate and acetic acid in the buffer at pH 4.0.

Using the Henderson–Hasselbalch equation:

$$4.00 = 4.76 + \log \frac{[CH_3COO^-]}{[CH_3COOH]}$$

$$\log \frac{[CH_3COO^-]}{[CH_3COOH]} = -0.76$$

$$\frac{[CH_3COO^-]}{[CH_3COOH]} = \frac{10^{-0.76}}{1} = \frac{0.17}{1}$$

The buffer is composed of 1 part acetic acid and 0.17 part acetate.

The buffer was prepared from 0.1 mole of acetic acid; after adjustment to pH 4.0, the amounts of acetic acid and acetate present are as follows:

$$CH_3COOH = \frac{1}{1.17} \times 0.1 \text{ mole} = 0.085 \text{ mole}$$

$$CH_3COO^- = \frac{0.17}{1.17} \times 0.1 \text{ mole} = 0.015 \text{ mole}$$

Since the acetic acid and acetate are dissolved in 1 litre of water, the buffer is composed of 0.085 M CH_3COOH and 0.015 M CH_3COO^-. Although the concentrations of acetate and acetic acid vary with pH, such a buffer would be known as a 0.1 M sodium acetate buffer.

Note: The 0.1 M buffer should not be prepared by adding acetic acid to a solution of 0.1 M NaOH, since a lot of acetic acid would be required to adjust the pH to 4.0; in fact, 0.1 moles of NaOH would require 0.57 moles of acetic acid to produce a buffer with pH 4.0 and a strength of 0.57 M.

An alternative way of producing 1 litre of 0.1 M acetate buffer would be to mix 850 ml of a 0.1 M solution of acetic acid with 150 ml of a 0.1 M solution of sodium acetate.

Self-test 2.6

1 litre of a 0.1 ammonium chloride buffer with a pH of 9.0 is required. Ammonia has a pKa value of 9.25. If a precise molarity is required this buffer is best prepared from ammonium chloride. The pH of the ammonium chloride may be adjusted to pH 9.0 by addition of a solution of sodium hydroxide (assuming the presence of sodium is not a problem), to avoid adding an excessive amount of the weak base ammonia. A total of 5.35 g (0.1 moles) of ammonium chloride are weighed and dissolved in *ca* 500 ml of water. The pH is then adjusted to pH 9.0 by addition of 5 M NaOH. The solution is then made up to 1 litre with water.

Calculate the concentrations of NH_4^+ and NH_3 in the buffer at pH 9.0, and indicate an alternative method for preparing the buffer.

In this case:

$$pH = pKa + \log \frac{[NH_3]}{[NH_4^+]}$$

Answer: 0.036 M NH_3 and 0.064 M NH_4^+. The buffer could be prepared by mixing 360 ml of a 0.1 M ammonia solution with 640 ml of 0.1 M NH_4Cl.

Some weak acids and bases have more than one buffer range; for example, phosphoric acid has three ionisable protons with three different pKa values and can be used to prepare buffers to cover three different pH ranges. The ionic species involved in the ranges covered by phosphate buffer are:

$$H_2PO_4^-/H_3PO_4 \quad HPO_4^{2-}/H_2PO_4^- \quad PO_4^{3-}/HPO_4^{2-}$$
$$pH\,1.13\text{–}3.13 \quad\quad pH\,6.2\text{–}8.2 \quad\quad pH\,11.3\text{–}13.3$$

The buffering ranges of a weak electrolyte are only discrete if the pKa values of its acidic and/or basic groups are separated by more than 2 pH units. Some acids have ionisable groups with pKa values less than 2 pH units apart, so they produce buffers with wide ranges. For example, succinic acid, which has pKa values of 4.19 and 5.57, can be considered to have a continuous buffering range between pH 3.19 and 6.57.

Self-test 2.7

Determine the buffer range(s) for the following compounds:

(i)   Carbonic acid pKa 6.38, 10.32
(ii) Boric acid pKa 9.14, 12.74
(ii) Glycine 2.34, 9.60
(iv) Citric acid 3.06, 4.74, 5.4

Answers: (i) 5.38–7.38, 9.32–11.32. The lower range is not useful because of the ease with which CO_2 is lost from solution; (ii) 8.14–10.14, 11.74–13.74; (iii) 1.34–3.34, 8.6–10.6; (iv) Continuous buffering range 2.06–6.4

Sometimes a salt of a weak acid with weak base is used in a chromatographic mobile phase to, apparently, set the pH at a defined level, e.g. ammonium acetate or ammonium carbonate. These salts are marginally more effective than a salt of strong acid with a strong base at preventing a change in pH, but they are not truly buffers. Such salts have buffering ranges *ca* 1 pH unit either side of the pKa values of the weak acid and weak base composing them. For example, the pH of a solution of ammonium acetate is *ca* 7.0, but it does not function effectively as a buffer unless the pH either rises to *ca* 8.25 or falls to *ca* 5.76.

A buffer is most effective where its molarity is greater than the molarity of the acid or base it is buffering against.

Calculation example 2.3

If 10 ml of 0.05 M HCl is added to 100 ml of 0.2 M sodium acetate buffer pH 4.5, the resultant pH can be calculated as follows:

Molarity × volume = mmoles

Number of mmoles of acetate + acetic acid in 100 ml of buffer = $0.2 \times 100 = 20$ mmoles.

(Continued)

Calculation example 2.3 *(Continued)*

Using the Henderson–Hasselbalch equation:

$$4.5 = 4.76 + \log\frac{[CH_3COO^-]}{[CH_3COOH]}$$

$$\log\frac{[CH_3COO^-]}{[CH_3COOH]} = -0.26$$

$$\frac{[CH_3COO^-]}{[CH_3COOH]} = \frac{10^{-0.26}}{1} = \frac{0.55}{1}$$

The buffer contains 1 part CH_3COOH and 0.55 parts CH_3COO^-.

$$CH_3COOH = \frac{1}{1.55} \times 20 = 12.9 \text{ mmoles}, \ CH_3COO^- = \frac{0.55}{1.55} \times 20 = 7.1 \text{ mmoles}$$

When HCl is added the following reaction occurs:

$$CH_3COO^- + HCl \rightarrow CH_3COOH + Cl^-$$

The amount of HCl added is $10 \times 0.05 = 0.5$ mmoles

Therefore, after addition of HCl, the amount of acetate remaining is:

7.1 − 0.5 = 6.6 mmoles

The amount of acetic acid now present is:

12.9 + 0.5 = 13.4 mmoles

Therefore, the pH of the buffer after addition of HCl is determined as follows (amounts may be substituted in the equation instead of concentrations since CH_3COO^- and CH_3COOH are present in the same volume):

$$pH = 4.76 + \log\frac{6.6}{13.4} = 4.76 - 0.31 = 4.45$$

The new pH of the buffer is 4.45.

The molarity of the buffer has also changed, since the total amount of CH_3COO^- and CH_3COOH is now contained in 110 ml instead of 100 ml, giving a new molarity of $0.2 \times \dfrac{100}{110} = 0.182$ M.

If 10 ml of 0.05 M HCl were added to 100 ml of water, the pH would be determined as follows:

$$-\log\left(0.05 \times \frac{10}{110}\right) = 2.34$$

Self-test 2.8

10 ml of 0.1 M HCl is added to 20 ml of a 0.5 M sodium acetate buffer with a pH of 4.3. Calculate: the pH of the buffer after addition of the HCl, the molarity of the buffer after addition of the HCl, the resultant pH if the HCl had been added to 20 ml of water.

Answer: pH = 4.04, new molarity = 0.33. Addition of 10 ml of 0.1 M HCl to 20 ml of water would give a pH of 1.48.

Salt hydrolysis

When the salt of a strong acid and a strong base is dissolved in water it produces a pH of *ca* 7.0. When salts of a weak acid and a strong base or of a strong acid and a weak base are dissolved in water, they will produce, respectively, alkaline and acidic solutions.

When sodium acetate is dissolved in water, the acetate ion behaves as a base, removing protons from solution. For a weak electrolyte in water, $Kb \times Ka = Kw$. If a 0.1 M solution of sodium acetate in water is considered:

$$\underset{(0.1-x)}{CH_3COO^-} + H_2O \underset{}{\overset{Kb}{\rightleftharpoons}} \underset{x}{CH_3COOH} + \underset{x}{HO}$$

$$Kb\,(CH_3COO^-) = \frac{Kw}{Ka\,(CH_3COOH)} = \frac{10^{-14}}{1.75 \times 10^{-5}} = 5.7 \times 10^{-10}$$

Regarding the change in the concentration of water as not affecting the equilibrium and regarding the $[CH_3COO^-]$ as being relatively unchanged by hydrolysis.

$$5.7 \times 10^{-10} = \frac{x^2}{0.1}$$

$$[HO^-] = \sqrt{5.7 \times 10^{-11}} = 7.6 \times 10^{-6}$$

$$[H^+] = \frac{10^{-14}}{7.6 \times 10^{-6}} = 1.33 \times 10^{-9}$$

$$pH = 8.9$$

Self-test 2.9

Calculate the pH of a 0.1 M solution of NH_4Cl. Here salt hydrolysis increases $[H^+]$ and the equilibrium in this case is:

$$\underset{(0.1-x)}{NH_4^+} \overset{Ka}{\rightleftharpoons} \underset{x}{NH_3} + \underset{x}{H^+}$$

The Ka for this reaction is 5.6×10^{-10}.

Answer: pH = 5.13

Activity, ionic strength and dielectric constant

The activity of ions in a solution is governed by the dielectric constant of the medium they are dissolved in and by the total concentration of ions in solution. For solutions of electrolytes in water with concentrations < 0.5 M, the activity of the ions present in solution is usually approximated to their individual concentrations. The mean activity coefficient for an ion in solution is defined as:

$$\gamma_\pm = \frac{\text{activity}}{\text{concentration}}$$

Although activity is regarded as 1 in dilute solutions this is still an approximation. The activity of an electrolyte solution in water can be estimated from the following equation:

$$\log \gamma_{\pm} = -0.509(z_+ z_-)\sqrt{I}$$

$$\text{where } I = \frac{1}{2}\sum m_i z_i^2$$

where -0.509 is a constant related to the dielectric constant of the solvent used to prepare the electrolyte solution and to temperature, z is the charge on a particular ion, I is the ionic strength of the solution and m is the molality (moles per kg of solvent) of a particular ion in solution.

Using this equation, the activity of H^+ in 0.1 M HCl can be calculated to be 0.69. Thus, the true pH of 0.1 M HCl is calculated as follows:

$$pH = -\log 0.1 \times 0.69 = 1.2$$

Calculation example 2.4

$$\gamma_{\pm} = \frac{\text{activity}}{\text{concentration}}$$

$$\log \gamma_{\pm} = -0.509|z_+ z_-|\sqrt{I}$$

$$\text{where } I = \frac{1}{2}\sum m_i z_i^2$$

$- 0.509$ is a constant related to the dielectric constant of the solvent used to prepare the electrolyte solution and to temperature.

z is the charge on a particular ion.

I is the ionic strength of the solution.

m is the molality (moles per kg of solvent) of a particular ion in solution.

For dilute solutions the molality can be approximated to the molarity.

Using this equation, the activity of H^+ in 0.1 M HCl can be calculated:

$$\text{where } I = \frac{1}{2}\sum 0.1 \times 1^2 + 0.1 \times 1^2 = 0.1$$

$$\log \gamma_{\pm} = -0.509|1 \times 1|\sqrt{0.1} = -0.509 \times 0.32 = -0.16$$

$$\gamma_{\pm} = 0.69$$

Thus, the true pH of 0.1 M HCl is calculated as follows:

$$pH = -\log 0.1 \times 0.69 = 1.2$$

The ionic strength of buffers varies according to their pH. For instance:

0.1 M sodium phosphate buffer at pH 7.2 is composed of 50 mM $H_2PO_4^-$ + 50 mM HPO_4^{2-} + 150 mM Na^+, having an ionic strength of 0.2.

0.1 M sodium phosphate buffer at pH 8.2 is composed of 9.1 mM $H_2PO_4^-$, 90.9 mM HPO_4^{2-} and 190.9 mM Na^+, having an ionic strength of 0.282.

This slight difference between the pH determined from activity and from concentration is usually ignored. However, from the equation used to calculate the activity coefficient it can be seen that the activity decreases with increasing ionic strength. In addition, the constant (-0.509 for water) increases with decreasing dielectric constant, e.g. water has a dielectric constant of 78.5 and methanol a dielectric constant of 32.6. Addition of methanol to an aqueous solution of an acid or buffer will cause an increase in the pH of the solution through decreasing the activity of all of the ions in solution including H^+. This effect should be noted with regard to the preparation of high-pressure liquid chromatography (HPLC) mobile phases, which are often composed of mixtures of buffers and organic solvents. Ionic strength is important with regard to the preparation of running buffers for capillary electrophoresis, where the greater the ionic strength of the buffer the higher the current through the capillary (Ch. 14).

Partition coefficient

An understanding of partition coefficient and the effect of pH on partition coefficient is useful in relation to the extraction and chromatography of drugs. The partition coefficient for a compound (P) can be simply defined as follows:

$$P = \frac{C_o}{C_w}$$

where C_o is the concentration of the substance in an organic phase and C_w is the concentration of the substance in water.

The greater P the more a substance has an affinity for organic media. The value of P for a given substance of course depends on the particular organic solvent used to make the measurement. Many measurements have been made of partitioning between n-octanol and water, since n-octanol, to some extent, resembles biological membranes and is also quite a good model for reverse-phase chromatographic partitioning. P is often quoted as a log P-value, e.g. a log P of 1 is equivalent to $P = 10$. Where $P = 10$ for a particular compound partitioning into a particular organic solvent, and partitioning is carried out between equal volumes of the organic solvent and water, then ten parts of the compound will be present in the organic layer for each part present in the water layer.

Calculation example 2.5

A neutral compound has a partition coefficient of 5 between ether and water. What percentage of the compound would be extracted from 10 ml of water if (i) 30 ml of ether were used to extract the compound or (ii) three 10 ml volumes of ether were used in succession to extract the compound?

(i) Between water and an equal volume of ether, 5 parts of the drug would be in the ether layer compared with 1 part in the water layer. Where three volumes (30 ml) of ether were used to one volume (10 ml) of water, the distribution would be 15 parts of drug in the ether layer to 1 part in the water layer.

(Continued)

Calculation example 2.5 *(Continued)*

$$\text{Percentage extracted} = \frac{15}{16} \times 100 = 93.75\%$$

(ii) First extraction

5 parts in the ether layer and 1 part in the water layer (total six parts)

At each extraction $\frac{5}{6}$ of the material in the water layer is extracted.

$$\text{Percentage extracted} = \frac{5}{6} \times 100 = 83.3\%$$

Percentage of drug remaining in water layer = 16.7%

Second extraction

$\frac{5}{6}$ of the 16.7% remaining in the water layer is extracted.

$$\text{Percentage extracted} = \frac{5}{6} \times 16.7 = 13.9\%$$

Percentage of drug remaining in water layer = 2.8%

Third extraction

$\frac{5}{6}$ of the 2.8% remaining in the water layer is extracted.

$$\text{Percentage extracted} = \frac{5}{6} \times 2.8 = 2.3\%$$

Percentage of drug remaining in water layer = 0.5%

Total percentage of drug extracted = 83.3 + 13.9 + 2.3 = 99.5%

Self-test 2.10

A drug has a partition coefficient of 12 between chloroform and water. Calculate the percentage of a drug that would be extracted from 10 ml of water with

(i) 30 ml of chloroform; (ii) 3 × 10 ml of chloroform.

Answers: (i) 97.3%; (ii) 99.95%

Effect of pH on partitioning (see Animation 2.1)

Many drugs contain ionisable groups, and their partition coefficient at a given pH may be difficult to predict if more than one ionised group is involved. However, often one group in a molecule may be much more ionised than another at a particular pH, thus governing its partitioning. It is possible to derive from the Henderson–Hasselbalch equation expressions for the variation in the partitioning of organic acids and bases into organic solvent with respect to the pH of the solution that they are dissolved in.

From the Henderson–Hasselbalch equation:

$$\text{For acids: } P\text{app} = \frac{P}{1+10^{\text{pH}-\text{p}K\text{a}}}$$

$$\text{For bases: } P\text{app} = \frac{P}{1+10^{\text{p}K\text{a}-\text{pH}}}$$

*P*app is the apparent partition coefficient, which varies with pH. Thus it can be seen that, when a compound, acid or base, is 50% ionised (i.e. pH = p*K*a), its partition coefficient is half that of the drug in the un-ionised state:

$$P\text{app} = \frac{P}{1+10^0} = \frac{P}{2}$$

As a general rule, for the efficient extraction of a base into an organic medium from an aqueous medium, the p*K*a of the aqueous medium should be at least 1 pH unit higher than the p*K*a value of the base, and, in the same situation for an acid, the pH should be 1 pH unit lower than the p*K*a value of the acid.

Calculation example 2.6

A linctus formulation contains the following components:

Base A p*K*a 6.7, P (chloroform/0.1 M NaOH) = 100	5 mg/ml
Base B p*K*a 9.7, P (chloroform/0.1 M NaOH) = 10	30 mg/ml
Benzoic acid p*K*a 4.2 P (chloroform /0.1 M HCl) = 50	5 mg/ml

In order to selectively extract base A, 5 ml of the linctus is mixed with 15 ml of phosphate buffer pH 6.7 and extracted once with 60 ml of chloroform.

Calculate the percentage and the weight of each component extracted.

Base A

At pH 6.7:

$$P\text{app} = 100/(1+10^{6.7-6.7}) = 100/2 = 50$$

If 20 ml of aqueous buffer phase was extracted with 20 ml of chloroform, there would be 1 part of the base in the aqueous phase to 50 parts in the chloroform layer. Since 60 ml of chloroform is used in the extraction, there will be 1 part of the base remaining in the aqueous phase and 150 parts in the chloroform layer.

Percentage extracted = (150/151) × 100 = 99.3%
Base A is present at 5 mg/ml in the elixir.
Amount of base A in 5 ml of elixir = 5 × 5 mg = 25 mg
Amount of base A extracted = 25 × (150/151) = 24.8 mg

Base B

At pH 6.7:

$$P\text{app} = 10/(1+10^{9.7-6.7}) = 10/1001 = 0.01$$

(Continued)

Calculation example 2.6 *(Continued)*

If 20 ml of aqueous buffer phase was extracted with 20 ml of chloroform, there would be 1 part of the base in the aqueous phase to 0.01 parts in the chloroform layer. Since 60 ml of chloroform is used in the extraction, then 1 part of the base will remain in the aqueous phase while there will be 0.03 parts in the chloroform layer.

Percentage extracted = $(0.03/1.03) \times 100 = 3.0\%$
Base B is present at 30 mg/ml in the elixir.
Amount of base B in 5 ml of elixir = 5×30 mg = 150 mg
Amount of base B extracted = $0.03 \times 150 = 4.5$ mg

Benzoic acid

At pH 6.7 for an acid:

$$P\text{app} = 50/(1+10^{6.7-4.2}) = 50/317 = 0.158$$

If 20 ml of aqueous buffer phase was extracted with 20 ml of chloroform, there would be 1 part of the preservative in the aqueous phase to 0.158 parts in the chloroform layer. Since 60 ml of chloroform is used in the extraction, 1 part of the benzoic acid will remain in the aqueous phase while there will be 0.474 parts in the chloroform layer.

Percentage extracted = $(0.474/1.474) \times 100 = 32.2\%$
Benzoic acid is present at 5 mg/ml in the elixir.
Amount of benzoic acid in 5 ml of elixir = 5×5 mg = 25 mg
Amount of benzoic acid extracted = $(0.474/1.474) \times 25 = 8.0$ mg

The extract is not completely free of the other ingredients in the formulation. If back extraction of the extract with an equal volume of pH 7.7 buffer is carried out, approximately 1% of extracted base A will be removed, but the amount of base B and benzoic acid will be reduced to < 0.5 mg.

Self-test 2.11

A cough mixture contains the following components:

(i) Base 1 $pKa = 9.0$, P (CHCl$_3$/0.1 M NaOH) = 1000		0 mg/5 ml
(ii) Base 2 $pKa = 9.7$, P (CHCl$_3$/0.1 M NaOH) = 10		30 mg/5 ml
(iii) Acidic preservative $pKa = 4.3$, P (CHCl$_3$/0.1 M HCl) = 10		5 mg/5 ml

5 ml of the cough mixture is mixed with 15 ml of phosphate buffer pH 7.0 and extracted with 60 ml of chloroform. Calculate the weight of each component extracted.

Answers: (i) Base 1, 29.0 mg; (ii) Base 2, 1.69 mg; (iii) Preservative, 0.28 mg

---

Drug stability

The purpose of drug stability testing is to provide evidence on how the quality of a drug substance or drug product changes with time under the influence of environmental factors such as temperature, humidity and light. The aim of the testing is to establish a re-test period for the drug substance or a shelf-life for the drug product and recommended storage conditions. ICH guidelines divide the world into four climate zones, I–IV, and stability testing to establish the shelf-life of a product should be carried out in accordance with the climatic conditions in which the drug product is to be sold.

Many drugs are quite stable, but functional groups such as esters and lactam rings, which occur in some drugs, are susceptible to hydrolysis, and functional groups such as catechols and phenols are quite readily oxidised. The most common types of degradation which occur in pure and formulated drugs obey zero- or first-order kinetics.

Zero-order degradation

In zero-order kinetics the rate of degradation is independent of the concentration of the reactants. Thus, if the rate constant for the zero-order degradation of a substance is 0.01 mole h^{-1}, then, after 10 h, 0.1 mole of the substance will have degraded. This type of degradation is typical of hydrolysis of drugs in suspensions or in tablets, where the drug is initially in the solid state and gradually dissolves at more or less the same rate as the drug in solution is degraded, i.e. the equilibrium concentration in free solution remains constant.

First-order degradation

First-order kinetics of drug degradation have been widely studied. This type of degradation would be typical of the hydrolysis of a drug in solution. Such reactions are pseudo first order, since the concentration of water is usually in such large excess that it is regarded as constant even though it does participate in the reaction. In first-order kinetics the rate constant k has the units h^{-1} or s^{-1}, and the rate of the reaction for a drug is governed by the expression:

$$-\frac{d[A]}{dt} = k[A]$$

where A is the concentration of the drug, which will change as degradation proceeds. This expression can be written as:

$$\frac{dx}{dt} = k(a-x)$$

which can also be written as

$$\int_0^s \frac{dx}{(a-x)} = \int_0^t k\,dt$$

where x is the amount of degraded product and a is the starting concentration of the drug. From this expression, by integration and rearrangement, the following expression arises:

$$t = \frac{1}{k}\ln\frac{a}{a-x}$$

The half-life of the drug (the time taken for 50% of a sample drug to degrade, i.e. where x is $a/2$) is thus given by the following expression:

$$t_{0.5} = \frac{1}{k}\ln\frac{a}{a/2} = \frac{1}{k}\ln 2$$

Thus, for aspirin, (see Animation 2.2) which has a rate constant of 0.0133 h^{-1} for the hydrolysis of its ester group at 25°C and pH 7.0, the half-life can be calculated as follows:

$$t_{0.5} = \frac{0.693}{0.0133} = 52.1\,h$$

The shelf-life of a drug, the time required for 10% degradation (where x is 0.1 a), is given by the following expression:

$$t_{0.9} = \frac{1}{k}\ln\frac{a}{0.9a} = \frac{1}{k}\ln 1.11$$

Calculation example 2.7

In a high-pressure liquid chromatography assay of aspirin tablets, ten extracts are made and the extracts are diluted with mobile-phase solution, which consists of acetonitrile/0.1 M sodium acetate buffer pH 4.5 (10:90) and analysed sequentially. If the rate constant for the degradation of aspirin in the mobile phase is 0.0101 h^{-1} at room temperature, how long can the analyst store the solutions at room temperature before the degradation of the analyte is greater than 0.5%?

In this case we are interested in $t_{(0.995)}$: In

$$t_{(0.995)} = \frac{(a/0.995a)}{0.0101} = 0.5\,h$$

Thus, in order for degradation to be < 0.5%, the solutions would have to be analysed within 30 min of their being prepared.

Self-test 2.12

Determine the half-lives of the following drugs, which can undergo hydrolysis of their ester functions in solution, under the conditions specified.

(i)   Atropine at 40°C and pH 7.0 where $k = 2.27 \times 10^{-4}\,h^{-1}$
(ii) Procaine at 37°C and pH 8.0 where $k = 1.04 \times 10^{-2}\,h^{-1}$
(iii) Benzocaine at 30°C and pH 9.0 where $k = 2.27 \times 10^{-3}\,h^{-1}$

Answers: (i) 127.2 d; (ii) 66.6 h; (iii) 12.7 d

Stereochemistry of drugs

The physiological properties of a drug are governed to a great extent by its stereochemistry. In recent years it has emerged that, in some instances, even optical isomers of a drug can have very different physiological effects. Since stereochemistry is concerned with the way in which a drug is orientated in space, this is something that is difficult to visualise on a flat piece of paper and the assignment of absolute configuration to a drug some people find confusing. The three types of isomerisms encountered in drug molecules are geometrical isomerism, optical isomerism and diastereoisomerism.

Geometrical isomerism

Drugs which have a geometrical isomer are relatively uncommon. An example of a drug with a geometrical isomer is the antidepressant zimeldine (Fig. 2.2). The lack of free rotation about the double bond ensures that the stereochemistry of this drug and and its isomer is different. Zimeldine is the only drug used. Other drugs which could also have geometric isomers of this type include amitriptyline and triprolidine.

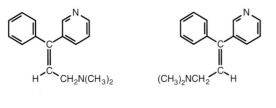

Fig. 2.2
Geometrical isomers.

Zimeldine   Geometrical isomer

Chirality and optical isomerism

Optical isomerism of drug molecules is widespread. Many drug molecules only contain one or two chiral centres. A simple example is the naturally occurring neurotransmitter adrenaline. When a compound has no symmetry about a particular carbon atom, the carbon atom is said to be a chiral centre. When a compound contains one or more chiral centres, it is able to rotate plane-polarised light to the right (+) or the left (−). A chiral centre arises when a carbon atom has four structurally different groups attached to it.

Adrenaline can exist as two enantiomers that are mirror images of each other (Fig. 2.3) and are thus non-superimposable. In Figure 2.3 the wedge-shaped bonds indicate bonds above the plane of the paper, the dotted bonds indicate bonds pointing down into the paper and unbroken lines indicate bonds in the same plane as the paper. In common with all pairs of enantiomers, the adrenaline enantiomers have identical physical and chemical properties; the only difference in their properties is that the enantiomers rotate plane-polarised light in opposite directions. However, the two enantiomers of adrenaline do have different biological properties; the (−) enantiomer exerts a much stronger effect, for instance, in increasing heart rate. It is not possible simply by looking at a structure drawn on paper to say which way it will rotate plane-polarised light – this can only be determined by experiment. In order to describe the configuration about a chiral centre, a set of precedence rules was developed:

(i)   The group of lowest priority attached to the chiral carbon, often hydrogen, is placed behind the plane of the paper with all the other groups pointing forwards.

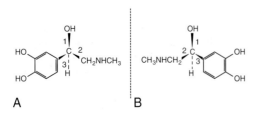

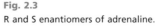

A   B

Fig. 2.3
R and S enantiomers of adrenaline.

(ii) The priorities are assigned to the atoms immediately attached to the chiral centre in order of decreasing atomic mass. For example:

$$Br > Cl > S > F > O > N > C > H$$

(iii) If two atoms attached to the chiral centre are of the same precedence, the priority is assigned on the basis of the atoms attached to these atoms, for example:

$$—C–Cl > —C–S > —C–O > —C–N > —\overset{\overset{\displaystyle C}{|}}{C}–C > —C–C > —C–H$$

(iv) If required, the third atom in a chain may be considered, for example:

$$—CCCl > —CCO > —CCN > —CCC > —CCH$$

Using these rules we can assign the absolute configurations for adrenaline structures A and B. Placing the group of lowest priority behind the paper, in this case H.

For structure A we find moving in a clockwise direction (clockwise = *R*):

$$—O > —CN > —CC$$

Thus the absolute configuration of A is *R* and it follows that its mirror image B must be *S* (the order of precedence moves anti-clockwise).

To relate the (+) (dextrorotatory) and (−) (laevorotatory) forms of a molecule to an absolute (*R* or *S*) configuration is complex and requires preparation of a crystal of the compound suitable for analysis by X-ray crystallography. In contrast, the direction in which a molecule rotates plane-polarised light is easily determined using a polarimeter.

X-ray crystallography of the enantiomers of adrenaline has shown that the (−) form has the *R* configuration and the (+) form has *S* configuration.

It should be noted that in older literature the terms *d* and *l* are used to denote (+) and (−) respectively and *D* and *L* are used to denote *R* and *S* respectively. A mixture containing equal amounts of (+) and (−) adrenaline, or indeed enantiomers of any drug, is known as a racemic mixture and of course will not rotate plane-polarised light. The physical separation of enantiomers in a racemic mixture into their pure (+) and (−) forms is often technically difficult.

Ampicillin (Fig. 2.4) provides a more complex example than adrenaline with regard to assignment of absolute configuration since it contains four chiral centres.

Assignment can be made as follows:

Chiral centre 1:

$$—N > —CO > —CC \quad \text{configuration } R$$

Fig. 2.4

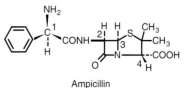

Ampicillin

Chiral centre 2:

$$-N > -CS > -CO \quad \text{configuration } R$$

Chiral centre 3:

$$-S > -N > -CN \quad \text{configuration } R$$

Chiral centre 4: In this case, since the molecule is drawn with the hydrogen pointing forward, it is best to determine the configuration from the molecule as drawn and then assign the opposite configuration.

$$-N > -CS > -CO \quad \text{configuration } R \text{ as drawn, therefore } \textit{configuration}$$
$$\textit{S} \text{ with H behind the plane of the paper}$$

The structures of drugs as drawn on paper do not always lend themselves to ready assignment of absolute configuration, and sometimes a certain amount of thinking in three dimensions is required in order to draw the structures in a form where the absolute configuration can be assigned. In drugs such as steroids, penicillins and morphine alkaloids, which are all based on natural products, chirality is built into the molecules as a result of the action of the stereoselective enzymes present in the plant or micro-organism producing them. However, there are many synthetic drugs where chiral centres are part of the structure. Many of these drugs are used in the form of racemates, since there are technical difficulties in carrying out stereospecific chemical synthesis or in resolving mixtures of enantiomers resulting from non-stereoselective synthesis. In the past, many such racemic mixtures have been used as drugs without regard for the fact that effectively a drug that is only 50% pure is being administered. The so-called 'inactive' enantiomer may in fact be antagonistic to the active form or it may have different physiological effects.[3,4] The most notable example, which gave rise to much of the medicine's legislation in the past 30 years, is the case of thalidomide, which contains one chiral centre and was administered as a racemate in order to alleviate morning sickness during pregnancy. The active enantiomer produced the intended therapeutic effects whilst the 'inactive' enantiomer was responsible for producing birth defects in the children of mothers who took the racemic drug. In fact, administering a pure, therapeutically active enantiomer would not have helped in this case since thalidomide becomes racemised within the body. Current legislation requires a manufacturer seeking to license a new drug in the form of a racemate to justify the use of the racemate as opposed to a pure enantiomer.

Self-test 2.13

Assign absolute configurations to the chiral centres in the following drugs.

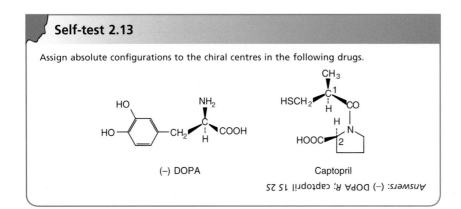

(−) DOPA

Captopril

Answers: (−) DOPA *R*; captopril 1*S* 2*S*

Diastereoisomers

Where more than one chiral centre is present in a molecule, there is the possibility of diastereoisomers, e.g. captopril. Another example of a synthetic drug with two chiral centres is labetalol. The number of diastereoisomers arising from n chiral centres is 2^{n-1}, i.e. 2 in the case of labetalol. In the structure shown in Figure 2.5, chiral centres 1 and 2 in structure A have the configurations R and S respectively; the enantiomer of this structure (B) has the S and R configurations in centres 1 and 2. In addition, there is a pair of enantiomers, C and D, that are diastereoisomers of the structures A and B, and which have the configurations $1R\ 2R$ and $1S\ 2S$.

Fig. 2.5
The stereoisomers of labetalol.

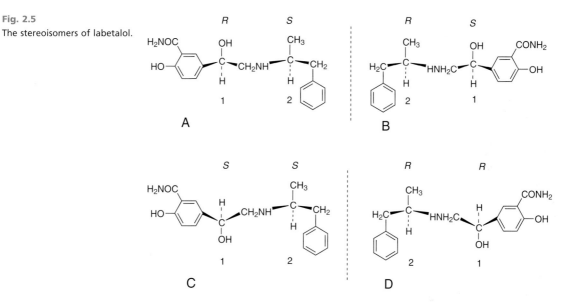

The diastereoisomers in a mixture can usually be separated by ordinary chromatographic methods. In the case of labetalol, two peaks would be seen in a chromatographic trace obtained from a non-chiral phase – one due to the $1R\ 2S$, $1S\ 2R$ pair of enantiomers and the other to the $1R\ 2R$ and $1S\ 2S$ pair of enantiomers. The commercial drug is in fact administered as a mixture of all four isomers, and the BP monograph for labetalol checks the ratio of the two chromatographic peaks produced by the two enantiomeric pairs of diastereoisomers. In order to separate the enantiomeric pairs, a chiral chromatography column would be required, and separation on a chiral column produces four peaks (Ch. 12).

Self-test 2.14

Indicate the configuration of the pairs of enantiomeric diastereoisomers which compose the drug isoxsuprine.

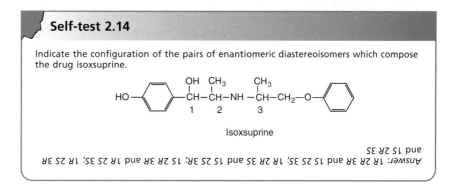

Isoxsuprine

Answer: 1R 2R 3R and 1S 2S 3S; 1R 2R 3S and 1S 2S 3R; 1S 2R 3S and 1R 2S 3R; 1S 2R 3R and 1R 2S 3S

An example of a pair of diastereoisomers used separately as drugs is beta-methasone and dexamethasone, shown in Figure 2.6. With a total of eight chiral centres within the betamethasone and dexamethasone structures, there is the possibility of $2^8 = 256$ isomers of the structure, and these divide into 128 enantiomeric pairs. Both dexamethasone and betamethasone could have corresponding enantiomers, but because they are largely natural products, made by stereospecific enzymes, their optical isomers do not exist. Semi-synthetic steroids are largely derived via microbial fermentation from naturally occurring plant sterols, originally obtained from the Mexican yam. The partially degraded natural products are then subjected to a number of chemical synthetic steps to produce the required steroid.

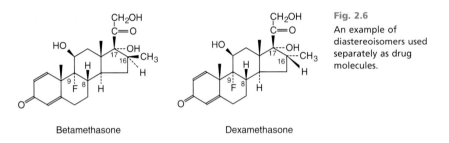

Fig. 2.6

An example of diastereoisomers used separately as drug molecules.

Betamethasone   Dexamethasone

In betamethasone and dexamethasone, the only stereoisomerism is at the synthetically substituted 16 position. In the case of betamethasone, the methyl group is in the β position, i.e. as one looks down on the molecule; it is closer than the hydrogen at position 16 (not necessarily projecting vertically out of the plane of the paper). In dexamethasone, the methyl group is in the α position – farther away than the hydrogen at 16 (not necessarily projecting vertically down into the paper). Of the two steroids, betamethasone has the slightly stronger anti-inflammatory potency. Two other stereochemical terms are *cis* and *trans*, and these refer to the relative orientation of two substituents. In betamethasone, the hydroxyl group at 17 and the methyl group at 16 are *trans* – on opposite sides of the ring; in dexamethasone, the hydroxyl group at 17 and the methyl group at 16 are *cis* – on the same side of the ring. Otherwise the relative orientation of the substituents is the same in both drugs, e.g. fluorine at 9 and hydrogen at 8 are *trans* to each other.

Measurement of optical rotation (see Animation 2.3)

Figure 2.7 shows a schematic diagram of a polarimeter. Light can be viewed as normally oscillating throughout 360° at 90° to its direction of travel. The light source is usually a sodium lamp; the polarising material can be a crystal of Iceland spar, a Nicol prism or a polymeric material such as polaroid. When circularly polarised light is passed through the polariser its oscillations are confined to one plane. In the absence of an optically active material, the instrument is set so that no light is able to pass through the analyser. When the polarised light is passed through an optically active medium, the plane in which the light is oscillating becomes tilted, and light is able to pass through the analyser. The angle of rotation can be measured by correcting for the tilt by rotating the analyser until light again does not pass through it. The angle that the second polariser has to

Fig. 2.7
Schematic diagram
of a polarimeter.

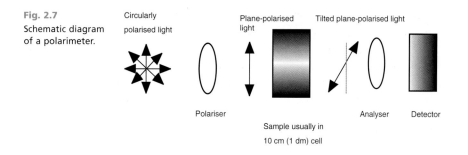

be rotated through to prevent, once again, the passage of light through it gives the measured rotation α. The standard value for the rotation produced by an optically active compound is $[\alpha]$, the specific rotation of a substance where:

$$[\alpha] = \frac{100\alpha}{lc}$$

where α is the measured rotation, l is the pathlength of the cell in which the measurement is made in dm and c is the concentration of the sample solution in g/100 ml.

The observed optical rotation is dependent on both the wavelength of the light and the temperature. The sodium D line (589 nm) is usually used to make measurements. The solvent in which the sample is dissolved may also greatly affect the $[\alpha]$ of a substance. Values for $[\alpha]$ are usually quoted with details of the concentration of the solution used for measurement, the solvent, the temperature and the type of light used. For example, the specific rotation for (−) adrenaline is given as:

$$[\alpha]^{25}\,D = -51°(c = 2, 0.5M\ HCl)$$

The optical rotation was obtained at 25° using the sodium D line with a 2 g 100 ml^{-1} solution in 0.5 M HCl.

If an enantiomer is chemically pure it is possible to determine its degree of enantiomeric purity by measuring its optical rotation relative to a standard value, e.g. if an enantiomeric mixture contains 1% of enantiomer A and 99% of enantiomer B, $[\alpha]$ will be reduced by 2% compared with the value for optically pure B. Examples of the measurement of optical rotation as a quality control check are found in the BP monographs for timolol maleate, tobramycin and phenylephrine hydrochloride.

Self-test 2.15

Optical rotation measurements were made using the sodium D line at 25 °C in a 1 dm cell, and the readings obtained were as follows:

(i) Phenylephrine HCl 2.6% w/v in 0.1 M HCl; $\alpha = -0.98°$
(ii) Timolol maleate 9.8% w/v in 1 M HCl; $\alpha = -0.59°$

Calculate $[\alpha]$ for these drugs and express it in the conventional form.

Answers: (i) $[\alpha]^{25}D = -37.7°$ (2.6, 0.1 M HCl); (ii) $[\alpha]^{25}D = -6.02°$ (9.8, 1 M HCl)

Profiles of physico-chemical properties of some drug molecules
Procaine

C   B   A   **Fig. 2.8**

H_2N—⟨benzene ring⟩—$COOCH_2CH_2N(C_2H_5)_2$

Procaine

Drug type: local anaesthetic.
Functional groups:

- A – Tertiary aliphatic amine, pKa 9.0.
- B – Ester, neutral.
- C – Aromatic amine, very weak base, pKa *ca* 2.

Half-life in water: 26 days at pH 7.0, 37°C.

Additional information: Procaine is formulated in injections and thus susceptible to aqueous-phase hydrolysis; in simple solution its degradation is first order (Fig. 2.9).

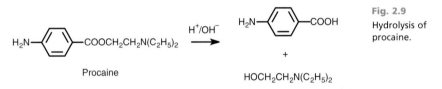

$$H_2N\text{—⟨ring⟩—}COOCH_2CH_2N(C_2H_5)_2 \xrightarrow{H^+/OH^-} H_2N\text{—⟨ring⟩—}COOH$$

Procaine

+

$HOCH_2CH_2N(C_2H_5)_2$

Fig. 2.9
Hydrolysis of procaine.

Closely related drug molecules: Proxymetacaine, benzocaine, tetracaine (amethocaine) butacaine, propoxycaine, procainamide (for stability of an amide group see paracetamol), bupivacaine, lidocaine (lignocaine), prilocaine.

Self-test 2.16

Calculate:

(i) The percentage ionisation of procaine at pH 7.0 (the ionisation of group C at this pH will be negligible)
(ii) The rate constant for its hydrolysis at pH 7.0 and 37 °C

Answers: (i) 99.01 %; (ii) 1.11 × 10³ h⁻¹

Paracetamol

A
$NH.CO.CH_3$

Fig. 2.10

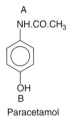

OH
B
Paracetamol

Drug type: analgesic.
Functional groups:

- A – Amide group, neutral.
- B – Phenolic hydroxy group, very weak acid, p*K*a 9.5.

Half-life in water: 21.8 years at pH 6 and 25°C. Most amides are very stable to hydrolysis (Fig. 2.11).

Fig. 2.11
Hydrolysis of paracetamol.

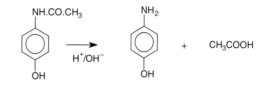

Other drugs containing an amide group: Bupivacaine, procainamide, lidocaine, beclamide, acebutolol.

Aspirin

Fig. 2.12

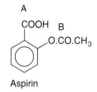

Aspirin

Drug type: analgesic.
Functional groups:

- A – Carboxylic acid, weak acid, p*K*a 3.5.
- B – Phenolic ester, particularly unstable.

Half-life in water: 52 h at pH 7.0 and 25°C; *ca* 40 days at pH 2.5 and 25°C.

Additional information: The rate of HO⁻ catalysed hydrolysis of esters is greater than the rate of H⁺ hydrolysis of esters. Solid aspirin absorbs water from the atmosphere and then hydrolyses (Fig. 2.13).

Fig. 2.13
Hydrolysis of aspirin.

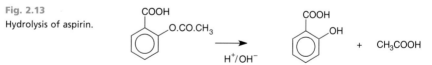

Partition coefficient of un-ionised compound at acidic pH: octanol/water *ca* 631.
Other drugs containing phenolic ester group: metipranolol, vitamin E, benorilate, dipivefrin.

Benzylpenicillin

Fig. 2.14

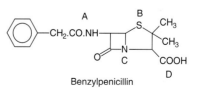

Benzylpenicillin

Drug type: antibiotic.
Functional groups:

- A – Amide, neutral, relatively stable, see paracetamol.
- B – Thioether, neutral, can be oxidised at high levels of oxygen stress.
- C – Lactam ring, neutral, particularly susceptible to hydrolysis (Fig. 2.15).

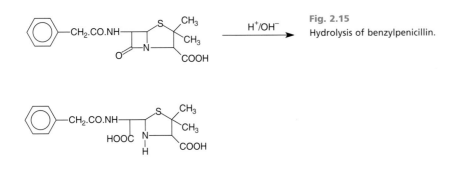

Fig. 2.15
Hydrolysis of benzylpenicillin.

Half-life: 38 days at pH 6.75 and 30°C; ampicillin: 39 days at pH 6.5 and 25°C.

Additional information: Consideration of the stability of these compounds is particularly important since they may be formulated as oral suspensions.

- D – Carboxylic acid, weak acid pKa 2.8 (the strength of the acid is increased by the adjacent lactam ring).

Compounds with similar properties: amoxicillin, cloxacillin, carbenicillin, flucloxacillin, phenoxymethylpenicillin, cefalexin, cefuroxime.

5-Fluorouracil

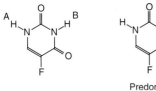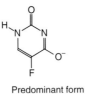

Predominant form
at pH 9.0

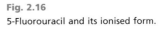

Fig. 2.16
5-Fluorouracil and its ionised form.

Drug type: anticancer.
Functional groups:

- A – Ureide nitrogen, acidic, pKa 7.0.
- B – Ureide nitrogen, very weakly acidic, pKa 13.0.

Additional information: The molecule is quite stable.

Partition coefficient of un-ionised molecule: octanol/water *ca* 0.13.

Compounds containing an acidic nitrogen in a heterocyclic ring: phenobarbital, amobarbital, butobarbital, bemegride, uracil, phenytoin, theophylline, theobromine.

Acebutolol

Fig. 2.17
Acebutolol.

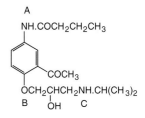

Drug type: β-adrenergic blocker.
Functional groups:

- A – Amide, neutral, susceptible to hydrolysis under strongly acidic conditions (see paracetamol).
- B – Aromatic ether group, potentially oxidisable under stress conditions.
- C – Secondary amine group, pKa 9.4.

Partition coefficient of un-ionised compound: octanol/water *ca* 483.

Fig. 2.18
Sulfadiazine and
its ionised form.

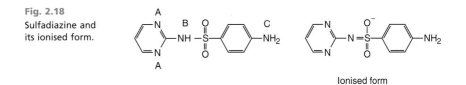

Ionised form

Sulfadiazine

Drug type: antibacterial.
Functional groups:

- A – Diazine ring nitrogens, very weakly basic, pKa < 2.
- B – Sulfonamide nitrogen, weak acid, pKa 6.5.
- C – Weakly basic aromatic amine, pKa < 2.

Partition coefficient of un-ionised compound: octanol/water *ca* 0.55 (log P octanol/water at pH 7.5 = − 1.3).

Closely related compounds: sulfadoxine, sulfamerazine, sulfametopyrazine, sulfquinoxaline, sulfachloropyridazine, sulfamethoxazole, sulfathiazole.

Self-test 2.17

Calculate the % ionisation of sulfadiazine at pH 7.5.

Answer: 90.9%. The weakly basic groups in the molecule are not ionised to any degree at pH 7.5

Isoprenaline

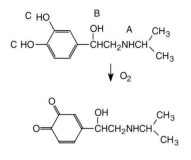

Fig. 2.19
Oxidation of isoprenaline.

Drug type: sympathomimetic.

Functional groups:

- A – Secondary amine, base, pKa 8.6.
- B – Benzyl alcohol group, neutral.
- C – Catechol group, weakly acidic, pKa values *ca* 10 and 12.

Additional information: As indicated in the reaction above, the catechol group is very readily oxidised upon exposure to light or air. Oxidation results in such compounds turning brown, solutions of isoprenaline and related compounds must contain antioxidants as preservatives.

Partition coefficient of the un-ionised drug: The compound is highly water soluble and cannot be extracted to any great extent into an organic solvent since it is ionised to some extent at all pH values.

Closely related compounds: dopamine, adrenaline, noradrenaline, terbutaline, DOPA.

Prednisolone

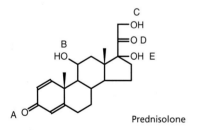

Prednisolone

Fig. 2.20

Drug type: corticosteroid.
Functional groups:

- A and D – Ketone groups, neutral.
- B and C – Secondary and primary alcohol groups, neutral.
- E – Tertiary alcohol group, neutral, prone to elimination by dehydration at high temperatures. Where the hydroxyl group at E is converted to an ester such as valerate, e.g. betamethasone valerate, thermal elimination of the ester can occur quite readily. Another decomposition reaction of the valerate esters is the intramolecular transfer of the ester group from E to C (see the BP tests for betamethasone valerate products).

Partition coefficient: octanol/water *ca* 70. The drug does not ionise so that the partition coefficient is unaffected by pH. Despite being neutral compound the hydroxyl groups in prednisolone give it a water solubility of *ca* 0.5 mg/ml. *Closely related compounds*: dexamethasone, betamethasone, triamcinolone, hydrocortisone, betamethasone valerate, betamethasone dipropionate.

Guanethidine

Fig. 2.21
Guanethidine and
its ionised form.

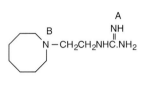
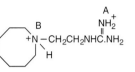

Predominant form of guanethidine
at pH 7.0; charge on A is delocalised
over all three nitrogens

Drug type: anti-hypertensive.
Functional groups:

- A – Guanidine group; one of the strongest nitrogen bases, p*K*a 11.4.
- B – Tertiary amine, p*K*a 8.3.

Compounds containing guanidine group: arginine, creatinine, bethanidine, streptomycin, phenformin, metformin, chlorhexidine.

Pyridostigmine bromide

Fig. 2.22

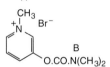

Pyridostigmine bromide

Drug type: anti-cholinergic.
Functional groups:

- A – Salt of strongly basic quaternary ammonium ion. Quaternary ammonium ions are charged at all pH values.
- B – Carbamate group, the nitrogen is neutral as in an amide but the carbamate group is less stable than an amide, having a stability similar to that of a phenolic ester.

Compounds containing a quaternary ammonium group: atracurium besylate, bretylium tosylate, clindium bromide, glycopyrronium bromide.

Additional problems

1. Calculate the pH of the following solutions assuming that the concentration and the activity of the solutions are the same:
   (i)   0.05 M HCl.
   (ii) 0.1 M chloroacetic acid ($Ka = 1.4 \times 10^{-3}$).

(Continued)

Q Additional problems *(Continued)*

(iii) 0.1 M phosphoric acid (first Ka 7.5 × 10^{-3}).
(iv) 0.1 M fumaric acid (Ka 9.3 × 10^{-4}).
(v) 0.1 M di-isopropylamine base (Kb = 9.09 × 10^{-4}).
(vi) 0.1 M imidazole base (Kb = 1.6 × 10^{-7}).

Answers: (i) 1.3; (ii) 1.93; (iii) 1.56; (iv) 2.02; (v) 12.0; (vi) 10.1

2. Calculate the pH of the following salt solutions:
   (i)   0.1 M sodium formate (Ka formic acid = 1.77 × 10^{-4})
   (ii) 0.1 M sodium fusidate (Ka fusidic acid = 4.0 × 10^{-6})
   (iii) 0.1 M ephedrine hydrochloride (Ka of ephedrine = 2.5 × 10^{-10})

Answers: (i) 8.4; (ii) 9.2; (iii) 5.3

3. Calculate what volumes of the salt solutions specified would be required to prepare 1 l of the following buffers:
   (i)   0.1 M phosphoric acid/0.1 M sodium dihydrogen phosphate pH 2.5 (pKa H$_3$PO$_4$ 2.13)
   (ii) 0.1 M sodium dihydrogen phosphate/0.1 M disodium hydrogen phosphate pH 8.0 (pKa H$_2$PO$_4^-$ 7.21)
   (iii) 0.1 M sodium bicarbonate/0.1 M sodium carbonate pH 9.5 (pKa HCO$_3^-$ 10.32)

Answers: (i) 299 ml/701 ml; (ii) 139.5 ml/860.5 ml; (iii) 868.5 ml/131.5 ml

4. Indicate the percentage of ionisation of the functional groups specified in the following drugs at pH 7.0 (Fig. 2.23).

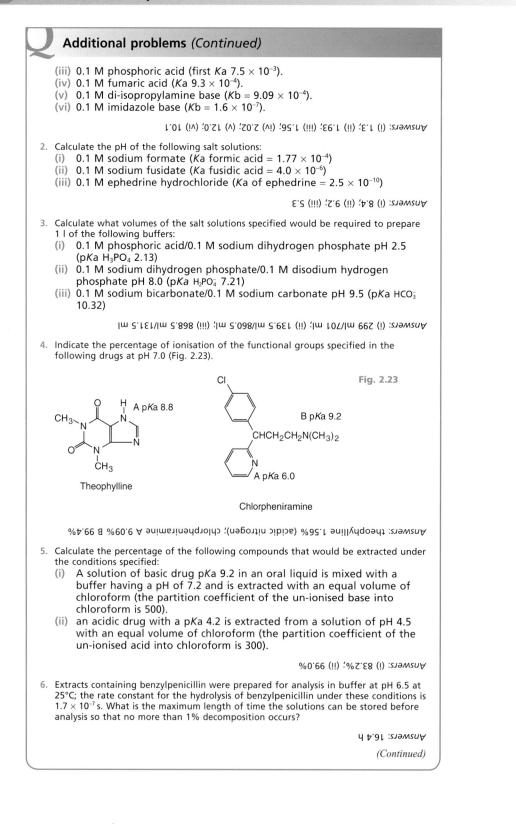

Fig. 2.23

Theophylline

Chlorpheniramine

Answers: theophylline 1.56% (acidic nitrogen); chlorpheniramine A 9.09% B 99.4%

5. Calculate the percentage of the following compounds that would be extracted under the conditions specified:
   (i)   A solution of basic drug pKa 9.2 in an oral liquid is mixed with a buffer having a pH of 7.2 and is extracted with an equal volume of chloroform (the partition coefficient of the un-ionised base into chloroform is 500).
   (ii) an acidic drug with a pKa 4.2 is extracted from a solution of pH 4.5 with an equal volume of chloroform (the partition coefficient of the un-ionised acid into chloroform is 300).

Answers: (i) 83.2%; (ii) 99.0%

6. Extracts containing benzylpenicillin were prepared for analysis in buffer at pH 6.5 at 25°C; the rate constant for the hydrolysis of benzylpenicillin under these conditions is 1.7 × 10^{-7} s. What is the maximum length of time the solutions can be stored before analysis so that no more than 1% decomposition occurs?

Answer: 16.4 h

(Continued)

Additional problems (Continued)

7. Determine the absolute configurations of the chiral centres in menthol and phenbutrazate. List the configurations of the pairs of enantiomeric diastereoisomers of menthol (Fig. 2.24).

Fig. 2.24

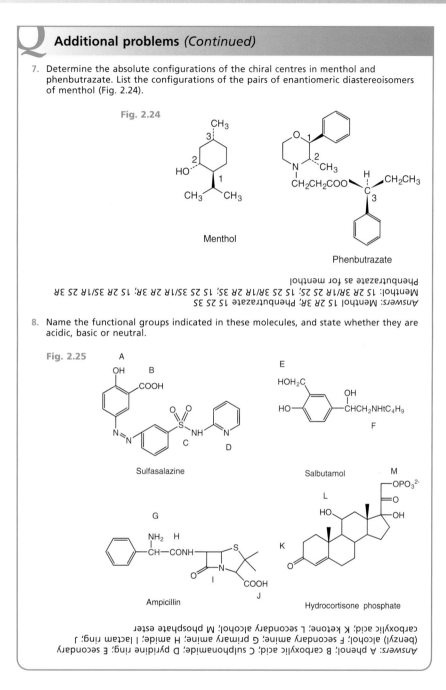

Menthol

Phenbutrazate

Answers: Menthol 1S 2R 3R; Phenbutrazate 1S 2S 3S
Menthol: 1S 2R 3R/1R 2S 3S; 1S 2S 3S/1R 2R 3R; 1S 2R 3S/1R 2S 3R; 1S 2S 3R/1R 2R 3S
Phenbutrazate as for menthol

8. Name the functional groups indicated in these molecules, and state whether they are acidic, basic or neutral.

Fig. 2.25

Sulfasalazine

Salbutamol

Ampicillin

Hydrocortisone phosphate

Answers: A phenol; B carboxylic acid; C sulphonamide; D pyridine ring; E secondary (benzyl) alcohol; F secondary amine; G primary amine; H amide; I lactam ring; J carboxylic acid; K ketone; L secondary alcohol; M phosphate ester

References

1. Stenlake JB. *Foundations of Molecular Pharmacology*. Athlone Press; 1979.
2. Florence AT, Attwood D. *Physicochemical Principals of Pharmacy*. 2nd ed. Macmillan Press; 1988.
3. Ariens EJ. *Trends Pharmacol Sci*. 1986;7:200-205.
4. Lehmann PA. *Trends Pharmacol Sci*. 1986;7:281-285.

Further reading

<http://www.sirius-analytical.com>
The website provides some additional information on pKa and partition coefficient determination.

Titrimetric and chemical analysis methods

3

KEYPOINTS

Principles

An analyte is chemically reacted with a standard solution of a reagent of precisely known concentration or with a concentration that can be precisely determined. The amount of a standard solution required to completely react with all of the sample is used to estimate the purity of the sample.

(Continued)

Introduction

Titrimetric methods are still widely used in pharmaceutical analysis because of their robustness, cheapness and capability for high precision. The only requirement of an analytical method that they lack is specificity. This chapter covers the theoretical basis of most of the commonly used methods; the practical aspects of titrations have been covered thoroughly by other textbooks.[1,2]

Instrumentation and reagents

Glassware

The manufacturers' tolerances for the volumes of a number of items of glassware are given in Chapter 1. The larger the volume measure, the smaller the tolerance percentage is of the nominal volume. Thus, for a Grade A 1 ml pipette the volume is within $\pm 0.7\%$ of the nominal volume, whereas for the 5 ml pipette the volume is within $\pm 0.3\%$ of the nominal volume. If greater accuracy than those guaranteed by the tolerances is required, then the glassware has to be calibrated by repeated weighing of the volume of water contained or delivered by the item of glassware. This exercise is also useful for judging how good one's ability to use a pipette is, since weighing of the volumes of water dispensed correctly several times from the same pipette should give weights that agree closely. (see Animation 3.1)

Primary standards and standard solutions

Primary standards are stable chemical compounds that are available in high purity and that can be used to standardise the standard solutions used in titrations. Titrants such as sodium hydroxide or hydrochloric acid cannot be considered as

Table 3.1 Primary standards and their uses

Primary standard	Uses
Potassium hydrogen phthalate	Standardisation of sodium hydroxide solution
Potassium hydrogen phthalate	Standardisation of acetous perchloric acid
Potassium iodate	Standardisation of sodium thiosulphate solution through generation of iodine
Anhydrous sodium carbonate	Standardisation of hydrochloric acid
Zinc metal	Standardisation of EDTA solution

EDTA, Ethylenediamine tetracetic acid.

primary standards since their purity is quite variable. So, for instance, sodium hydroxide standard solution may be standardised against potassium hydrogen phthalate, which is available in high purity. The standardised sodium hydroxide solution (secondary standard) may then be used to standardise a standard solution of hydrochloric acid. Table 3.1 lists some commonly used primary standards and their uses.

Direct acid/base titrations in the aqueous phase
Strong acid/strong base titrations

Figure 3.1 shows the titration curve obtained from the titration of a strong acid with a strong base. The pH remains low until just before the equivalence point, when it rises rapidly to a high value. In many titrations a coloured indicator is used, although electrochemical methods of end-point detection are also used. An indicator is a weak acid or base that changes colour between its ionised and un-ionised forms; the useful range for an indicator is 1 pH either side of its pKa value. For example, phenolphthalein (PP) pKa 9.4 (colour changes between pH 8.4 and pH 10.4) undergoes a structural rearrangement as a proton is removed from one of its phenol groups when the pH rises, and this causes the colour change (Fig. 3.2). Methyl orange (MO) pKa 3.7 (colour changes between pH 2.7 and pH 4.7) undergoes a similar pH-dependent structural change. Both these indicators fall within the range of the inflection of the strong acid/strong base titration curve.

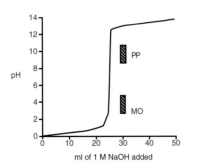

Fig. 3.1
The change in pH as 25 ml of 1 M HCl are titrated with 1 M NaOH.

Fig. 3.2
The structural rearrangement responsible for the colour change in phenolphthalein.

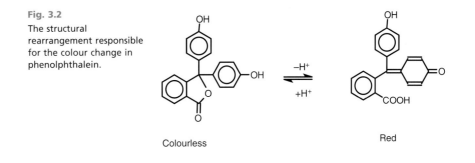

Colourless   Red

Phenolphthalein pKa 9.4

There are only a few direct strong acid/strong base titrations carried out in pharmacopoeial assays.

Strong acid/strong base titrations are used in pharmacopoeial assays of perchloric acid, hydrochloric acid, sulphuric acid and thiamine hydrochloride.

Weak acid/strong base and weak base/strong acid titrations (see Animation 3.2)

On addition of a small volume of the strong acid or strong base to a solution of the weak base or weak acid, the pH rises or falls rapidly to about 1 pH unit below or above the pKa value of the acid or base. Often a water-miscible organic solvent such as ethanol is used to dissolve the analyte prior to the addition of the aqueous titrant.

Figure 3.3 shows a plot of pH when 1 M NaOH is added to 25 ml of a 1 M solution of the weak acid aspirin.

In the case of aspirin, the choice of indicator is restricted by where the inflection in its titration curve lies; PP is suitable as an indicator whereas MO is not.

In the example of the titration of quinine with hydrochloric acid (Fig. 3.4), MO is a suitable indicator because it falls within the inflection of the titration curve whereas PP is not suitable.

Fig. 3.3
Titration curve for 25 ml of a 1.0 M solution of aspirin (pKa 3.5) titrated with 1.0 M NaOH.

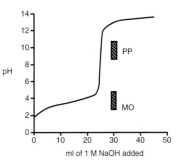

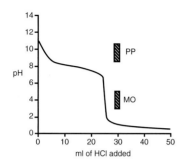

Fig. 3.4
25 ml of a 1.0 M solution of quinine (pKa 8.05) titrated with 1.0 M hydrochloric acid.

Some acids or bases can donate or accept more than one proton, i.e. 1 mole of analyte is equivalent to more than 1 mole of titrant. If the pKa values of any acidic or basic groups differ by more than *ca* 4, then the compound will have more than one inflection in its titration curve. Sodium carbonate is a salt of carbonic acid, and it can accept two protons. The pKa values of carbonate and bicarbonate are sufficiently different (pKa 10.32 and 6.38) for there to be two inflections in the titration curve. The two stages in the titration are:

$$CO_3^{2-} + H^+ \rightarrow HCO_3^-$$

$$HCO_3^- + H^+ \rightarrow H_2CO_3$$

Self-test 3.1

Which of these indicators could be used in the titration of aspirin and which could be used in the titration of quinine?

(i)   Bromophenol blue pKa 4.0
(ii) Methyl red pKa 5.1
(iii) Cresol red pKa 8.3
(iv) Chlorophenol blue pKa 6.0.

Answers: Aspirin: (iii) and (iv). Quinine: (i) and (ii)

In a titration of sodium carbonate, the first inflection is indicated by PP and the whole titration by MO (Fig. 3.5).

Self-test 3.2

A sample containing 25.14 g of neutral salts, glucose and a sodium carbonate/bicarbonate buffer was dissolved in 100 ml of water. A 25 ml aliquot of the resultant solution required 20.35 ml of 0.0987 M HCl when titrated to the PP end-point. A second 25 ml aliquot was titrated to the MO end-point and required 56.75 ml of the acid. Calculate the percentage of Na$_2$CO$_3$ (molecular weight 106) and NaHCO$_3$ (molecular weight 84) in the sample.

Answers: 3.39% and 2.12%, respectively

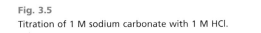

Fig. 3.5
Titration of 1 M sodium carbonate with 1 M HCl.

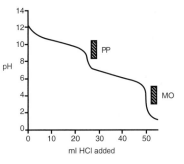

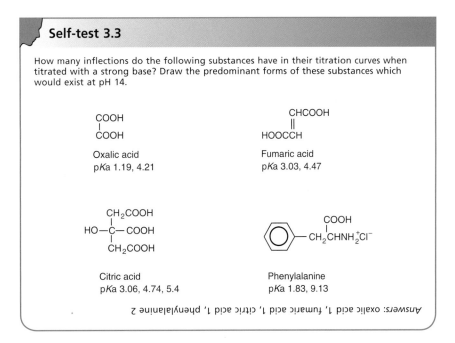

Self-test 3.3

How many inflections do the following substances have in their titration curves when titrated with a strong base? Draw the predominant forms of these substances which would exist at pH 14.

COOH
|
COOH

Oxalic acid
pKa 1.19, 4.21

CHCOOH
||
HOOCCH

Fumaric acid
pKa 3.03, 4.47

CH₂COOH
|
HO—C—COOH
|
CH₂COOH

Citric acid
pKa 3.06, 4.74, 5.4

COOH
|
CH₂CHNH₃⁺Cl⁻

Phenylalanine
pKa 1.83, 9.13

Answers: oxalic acid 1, fumaric acid 1, citric acid 1, phenylalanine 2

Weak acid/strong base titration is used in the pharmacopoeial assays of benzoic acid, citric acid, chlorambucil injection, mustine injection, nicotinic acid tablets and undecanoic acid.

Titrations of the salts of weak bases in mixed aqueous/non-aqueous media

Non-aqueous titrations, which are described below, are still used for the analysis of acids and salts of weak bases. However, in many instances it is simpler to titrate weak bases as their salts in a mixed non-aqueous/aqueous medium using potentiometric end-point detection. The protonated base behaves as a weak acid when titrated with sodium hydroxide.

$$RNH_3^+ + HO^- \rightarrow RNH_2 + H_2O$$

The advantage of adding a water-miscible solvent such as methanol to the titration is twofold. Firstly, the addition of the organic solvent effectively lowers

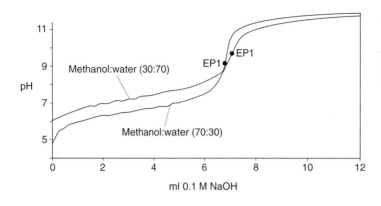

Fig. 3.6
Potentiometric titration of lidocaine
(lignocaine) hydrochloride with 0.1 M NaOH.
The samples were dissolved in methanol/
water (30:70, 50 ml) and methanol/water
(70:30, 50 ml).

the pKa value of the base, since the ionised form of the base is less stable in a mixed solvent system where the dielectric constant is lower, and, secondly, the organic solvent keeps the base in solution as it is converted to its free base form during the titration. An example of this can be seen for the titration of lidocaine (lignocaine) hydrochloride in methanol/water mixtures (Fig. 3.6), where the size of the inflection in the titration curve increases when moving from 30% methanol to 70% methanol. This is a very convenient procedure for many organic bases.

Indirect titrations in the aqueous phase

These can be of the strong acid/strong base, weak acid/strong base or weak base/ strong acid type. The more common examples are weak acid/strong base.

Estimation of esters by back titration

Excess of sodium hydroxide is added to the ester. The following reaction occurs:

$$RCOOR' + XSNaOH \rightarrow RCOONa + R'OH$$

The XSNaOH is back titrated with HCl using PP as an indicator.

This procedure is used in pharmacopoeial assays of benzyl benzoate, dimethyl phthalate, ethyl oleate, methyl salicylate, cetostearyl alcohol, emulsifying wax, castor oil, arachis oil, cod liver oil and coconut oil.

Saponification value (see Animation 3.3)

The assay of fixed oils provides a special case of ester hydrolysis since they are triesters of glycerol. The saponification value for a fixed oil is the number of mg of potassium hydroxide (KOH) equivalent to 1 g of oil. A high value means rancidity and a low value possible adulteration with mineral oil. Almost all edible oils have a saponification value between 188 and 196. Hydrolysis of the fixed oil is carried out with ethanolic KOH.

This procedure is used in the pharmacopoeial assays of castor oil, cod liver oil, cottonseed oil, almond oil and sesame seed oil.

Acid values are also determined for fixed oils. The acid value for a substance is the number of mg of KOH required to neutralise 1 g of the test substance when it is titrated with 0.1 M ethanolic KOH to a PP end-point. This value is quoted for many fixed oils in order to eliminate rancid oils, which contain large amounts of free fatty acid. Typically acid values for fixed oils are in the range of 1–2.

Calculation example 3.1

The following data were obtained for a sample of cod liver oil:

Weight of oil taken for analysis = 2.398 g

Ethanolic KOH (molecular weight 56.1) used in determination = 0.986 M

Amount of ethanolic KOH used for hydrolysis and in blank titration = 25 ml

Amount of 0.470 M HCl required to neutralise excess KOH = 35.2 ml

Amount of 0.470 M HCl required in the titration of blank = 52.3 ml

Calculation

Amount of KOH used initially = 52.3 × 0.47 = 24.6 mmole

Amount of HCl required to neutralise excess KOH = 35.20 × 0.470 = 16.5 mmole

Amount of KOH used in hydrolysis = 24.6 − 16.5 = 8.1 mmole × molecular weight = mg

Amount of KOH used in the hydrolysis = 8.1 × 56.1 = 454.0 mg

Amount of KOH/g of fixed oil used in the hydrolysis = 454/2.398 = 189.3 mg

Therefore saponification value = 189.3.

Self-test 3.4

Calculate the saponification value of a sample of castor oil from the following data:

- Weight of oil taken for analysis = 2.535 g
- Ethanolic KOH used in the hydrolysis = 1.03 M
- Amount of KOH used in hydrolysis = 25 ml
- Amount of 0.514 M HCl required to neutralise excess KOH = 34.2 ml
- Amount of 0.514 M HCl required in the titration of blank = 50.2 ml

Answer: 182

Estimation of alcohols and hydroxyl values by reaction with acetic anhydride (AA)

Alcohols can be determined by reaction with excess acetic anhydride (AA) (Fig. 3.7). This is a useful titrimetric method because the alcohol group is difficult to estimate by any other means.

Fig. 3.7
Estimation of benzyl alcohol by reaction with acetic anhydride.

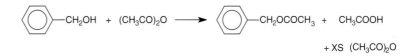

$$\bigcirc\!\!-CH_2OH + (CH_3CO)_2O \longrightarrow \bigcirc\!\!-CH_2OCOCH_3 + CH_3COOH$$

$$+ XS\ (CH_3CO)_2O$$

The excess AA and acetic acid may be back titrated with NaOH using PP as an indicator.

In a related assay, a hydroxyl value is determined for a fixed oil. A 1:3 mixture of AA in pyridine is used in the determination; the pyridine is present as a catalyst. The hydroxyl value may be defined as:

The number of mg of KOH required to neutralise a blank titration of the reagents – the number of mg KOH required to neutralise excess AA + acetic acid after reaction with 1 g of the test substance.

Calculation example 3.2

The following data were obtained for a sample of castor oil:

Weight of castor oil taken for analysis = 1.648 g

Volume of acetic anhydride used for the reaction = 5 ml

Molarity of ethanolic KOH used to neutralise the excess AA + acetic acid = 0.505 M

Volume of ethanolic KOH required to titrate 5 ml of reagent = 53.5 ml

Volume of ethanolic KOH required to neutralise excess AA + acetic acid after reaction with the castor oil = 44.6 ml

Number of mmoles of KOH used in the blank titration = 53.5 × 0.505 = 27.0

Number of mg of KOH used in the titration of the blank = 27.0 × 56.1 = 1515

Number of mmoles of KOH used in titration of AA + acetic acid = 44.6 × 0.505 = 22.5

Number of mg KOH used in titration of excess AA + acetic acid = 22.5 × 56.1 = 1262

Hydroxyl value = 1515 – 1262/1.648 = 154

To be completely accurate, the acid value for the fixed oil should be added to the hydroxyl value, since any free acid in the oil will titrate along with the excess reagents, giving a small overestimate. The acid value for castor oil is about 2.0, giving a hydroxyl value for the above sample of 156.

Reaction with acetic anhydride is used in pharmacopoeial assays of benzyl alcohol and dienestrol, and determination of hydroxyl values of castor oil, cetostearyl alcohol and cetomacrogol.

Non-aqueous titrations
Theory

Non-aqueous titration is the most common titrimetric procedure used in pharmacopoeial assays and serves a double purpose, as it is suitable for the titration of very weak acids and bases and provides a solvent in which organic compounds are soluble. The most commonly used procedure is the titration of organic bases with perchloric acid in acetic acid. These assays sometimes take some perfecting in terms of being able to judge the end-point precisely.

The theory is, very briefly, as follows: water behaves as both a weak acid and a weak base; thus, in an aqueous environment, it can compete effectively with very weak acids and bases with regard to proton donation and acceptance, as shown in Figure 3.8.

Fig. 3.8

Competition of water with weak acids and bases for proton acceptance and donation.

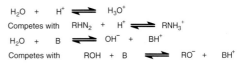

The effect of this is that the inflection in the titration curves for very weak acids and very weak bases is small, because they approach the pH limits in water of 14 and 0 respectively, thus making end-point detection more difficult. A general rule is that bases with pKa < 7 or acids with pKa > 7 cannot be determined accurately in aqueous solution. Various organic solvents may be used to replace water since they compete less effectively with the analyte for proton donation or acceptance.

Non-aqueous titration of weak bases

Acetic acid is a very weak proton acceptor and thus does not compete effectively with weak bases for protons. Only very strong acids will protonate acetic acid appreciably according to the equation shown below:

$$CH_3COOH + HA \rightleftharpoons CH_3COOH_2^+ + A^-$$

Perchloric acid is the strongest of the common acids in acetic acid solution, and the titration medium usually used for non-aqueous titration of bases is per-chloric acid in acetic acid. Addition of acetic anhydride, which hydrolyses to acetic acid, is used to remove water from aqueous perchloric acid. Weak bases compete very effectively with acetic acid for protons. Oracet blue, quinaldine red and crystal violet (very weak bases) are used as indicators in this type of titration. A typical analysis is shown in Figure 3.9 for L-3,4-dihydroxyphenylalanine (LDOPA).

When the base is in the form of a salt of a weak acid, removal of an anionic counter ion prior to titration is not necessary, e.g. for salts of bases with weak acids such as tartrate, acetate or succinate. However, when a base is in the form of a chloride or bromide salt, the counter ion has to be removed prior to titration. This is achieved by the addition of mercuric acetate; the liberated acetate is then titrated with acetous perchloric acid. This is illustrated in Figure 3.10 for the example of phenylephrine HCl.

Non-aqueous titration with acetous perchloric acid is used in the pharmaco-poeial assays of adrenaline, metronidazole, codeine, chlorhexidine acetate, chlor-promazine, amitriptyline HCl, propranolol HCl, lidocaine (lignocaine) HCl, and HCl and quaternary amine salts, such as neostigmine bromide and pancuronium bromide.

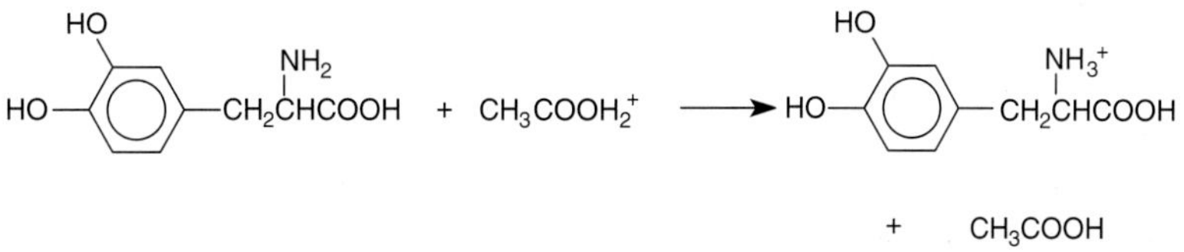

Fig. 3.9

Analysis of L-3,4-dihydroxyphenylalanine (LDOPA) by non-aqueous titration.

$$HO-\text{(ring)}-CH_2CHCOOH + CH_3COOH_2^+ \longrightarrow HO-\text{(ring)}-CH_2CHCOOH$$

$$+ \quad CH_3COOH$$

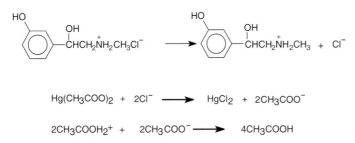

Fig. 3.10
The analysis of phenylephrine hydrochloride by non-aqueous titration.

$$Hg(CH_3COO)_2 + 2Cl^- \longrightarrow HgCl_2 + 2CH_3COO^-$$

$$2CH_3COOH_2^+ + 2CH_3COO^- \longrightarrow 4CH_3COOH$$

Non-aqueous titration of weak acids

For the non-aqueous titration of weak acids, a solvent such as an alcohol or an aprotic solvent is used, which does not compete strongly with the weak acid for proton donation. Typical titrants are lithium methoxide in methanol or tetrabutyl ammonium hydroxide in dimethylformamide. End-point detection may be carried out with thymol blue as an indicator or potentiometrically (see p. 81).

Non-aqueous titration of acidic groups is carried out in pharmacopoeial assays of barbiturates, uracils and sulphonamides.

Argentimetric titrations

Argentimetric titrations are based on the reaction:

$$AgNO_3 + Cl^- \rightarrow AgCl(s) + NO_3^-$$

Potassium chromate may be used as an indicator, producing a red colour with excess Ag^+ ion. More widely applicable is the method of back titration. Excess $AgNO_3$ is added to the sample containing chloride or bromide ions. The excess $AgNO_3$ is then titrated with ammonium thiocyanate, and ammonium ferrous sulphate is used as an indicator of excess SCN^-:

$$AgNO_3 + NH_4SCN \rightarrow AgSCN(s) + NH_4NO_3$$

Before the back titration can be carried out, the precipitated AgCl has to be filtered off or coated with diethylphthalate to prevent SCN^- causing dissociation of AgCl. Organically combined chlorine has to be liberated by hydrolysis with sodium hydroxide prior to titration. A halogen attached to an aromatic ring cannot be liberated by hydrolysis, and aromatic halides have to be burnt in an oxygen flask in order to release the halogen for titration.

Argentimetric titration is used in pharmacopoeial assays of sodium chloride and potassium chloride tablets, thiamine hydrochloride, mustine chloride and carbromal.

Compleximetric titrations

These titrations are used in the estimation of metal salts. Ethylenediamine tetracetic acid (EDTA) shown in Figure 3.11 is the usual titrant used. It forms stable 1:1 complexes with all metals except alkali metals such as sodium and potassium. The alkaline earth metals such as calcium and magnesium form complexes which are unstable at low pH values and are titrated in ammonium chloride buffer at pH 10. The general equation for the titration is:

$$M^{n+} + Na_2EDTA \rightarrow (MEDTA)^{n-4} + 2H^+$$

Fig. 3.11
Ethylenediamine tetraacetic acid (EDTA).

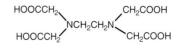

Ethylenediamine tetraacetic acid

The end-point of the reaction is detected using an indicator dye. The dye is added to the metal solution at the start of the titration and forms a coloured complex with a small amount of the metal. The first drop of excess EDTA causes this complex to break up, resulting in a colour change.

Titration with EDTA is used in the pharmacopoeial assays of bismuth subcarbonate, calcium acetate, calcium chloride, calcium gluconate, magnesium carbonate, magnesium hydroxide, magnesium trisilicate, bacitracin zinc, zinc chloride and zinc undecanoate.

Insoluble metal salts are estimated by back titration; the sample is heated with excess EDTA to form the soluble EDTA complex of the metal and then the excess EDTA is titrated with salt solutions containing Mg^{2+} or Zn^{2+} of known concentration.

Back titration with EDTA is used in the pharmacopoeial assays of aluminium glycinate, aluminium hydroxide, aluminium sulphate and calcium hydrogen phosphate.

Redox titrations

Redox titrations are based on the transfer of electrons between the titrant and the analyte. These types of titrations are usually followed by potentiometry, although dyes which change colour when oxidised by excess titrant may be used.

Theory

Reduction potential is a measure of how thermodynamically favourable it is for a compound to gain electrons. A high *positive* value for a reduction potential indicates that a compound is readily reduced and, consequently, is a strong oxidising agent, i.e. it removes electrons from substances with lower reduction potentials. The oxidised and reduced forms of a substance are known as a redox pair. Table 3.2 lists the standard reduction potentials for some typical redox pairs.

Table 3.2 Standard reduction potential (E_o) for some redox pairs relative to the standard hydrogen electrode potential 0

$Ce^{4+} + e$	$\rightarrow$	Ce^{3+}	1.61 V
$MnO_4^- + 5e + 8H^+$	$\rightarrow$	$Mn^{2+} + 4H_2O$	1.51 V
$Cl_2 + 2e$	$\rightarrow$	$2Cl^-$	1.36 V
$Br_2 + 2e$	$\rightarrow$	$2Br^-$	1.065 V
$Fe^{3+} + e$	$\rightarrow$	Fe^{2+}	0.771 V
$I_2 + 2e$	$\rightarrow$	$2I^-$	0.536 V
$Ag^{Cl} + e$	$\rightarrow$	$Ag^+ + Cl^-$	0.223 V
$2H^+ + 2e$	$\rightarrow$	H_2	0 V
$Fe^{2+} + 2e$	$\rightarrow$	Fe	−0.440 V
$Ca^{2+} + 2e$	$\rightarrow$	Ca	−2.888 V

A substance with a higher reduction potential will oxidise one with a lower reduction potential. The difference in potential between two substances is the reaction potential and is approximately the potential difference which would be measured if the substances comprised two halves of an electrical cell. For example, Cl_2 will oxidise Br^- according to the following equation:

$$Cl_2 + 2Br^- \rightarrow 2Cl^- + Br_2$$

Taking values from Table 3.2, the reaction potential is given by $1.36 - 1.065 = 0.29$ V.

For the reaction:

$$Ca + Cl_2 \rightarrow CaCl_2$$

The reaction potential is given by $1.36 - (-2.888) = 4.248$ V (i.e. a large difference and calcium burns in chlorine).

Self-test 3.5

Complete the equations where reaction is possible and indicate the reaction potential:

(i) $I_2 + 2Cl^-$ $\rightarrow$
(ii) $Br_2 + 2I^-$ $\rightarrow$
(iii) $Ce^{4+} + Fe^{2+}$ $\rightarrow$
(iv) $I_2 + Fe$ $\rightarrow$
(v) $Fe^{3+} + AgCl$ $\rightarrow$

Answers: (i) No reaction; (ii) 0.529 V; (iii) 0.839 V; (iv) 0.976 V; (v) No reaction (Ag is already in its Ag^+ form)

In the above examples we have ignored the effect of concentration of oxidant and reductant on E_o values; in fact, E (the observed electrode potential) is stable over a wide range of concentrations. The E-value for a solution containing a redox pair is governed by the Nernst equation:

$$E = E_o + 2RT/nF \ln[Ox]/[Red]$$

where [Ox] is the concentration of the oxidised form of a particular substance and [Red] is the concentration of the reduced form of a particular substance:

F = Faraday's constant
n = number of electrons transferred in the reaction

By substituting a value for the constant terms, this equation can also be written as:

$$E = E_o + 0.0591/n \log[Ox]/[Red]$$

where n is the number of electrons transferred during the reaction. It is clear that E is approximately equal to E_o except when there is a large difference between [Ox] and [Red].

Self-test 3.6

Calculate the E for the following redox pair when $Mn^{3+} = 0.5$ M and $Mn^{2+} = 0.01$ M (E_o $Mn^{3+}/Mn^{2+} = 1.51$ V).

Answer: 1.61 V

Fig. 3.12
Titration of 25 ml of 1 M Fe^{2+} with 1 M Ce^{4+}.

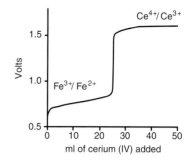

The titration curve for Fe^{2+} against Ce^{4+} is shown in Figure 3.12. This curve is for a titration carried out with a standard hydrogen electrode as the reference electrode.

Where a reference electrode has a reduction potential > 0, then the predicted reading of the potential for a redox pair is obtained by subtracting the reduction potential for the reference electrode, e.g. for an Ag/AgCl reference electrode, 0.223 V is subtracted.

Self-test 3.7

Using the values in Table 3.1, what would be the approximate potential measured for the Fe^{3+}/Fe^{2+} redox pair present in the first part of the titration shown in Figure 3.12 measured against?

(i) A standard hydrogen electrode
(ii) An Ag/AgCl electrode

Similarly, what would the approximate potential be for the Ce^{4+}/Ce^{3+} redox pair on the plateau after the end-point measured against?

(iii) A standard hydrogen electrode
(iv) An Ag/AgCl electrode

Answers: (i) 0.77 V; (ii) 0.55 V; (iii) 1.61 V; (iv) 1.39 V

In carrying out redox titrations, standard Ag/AgCl or Hg/Hg_2Cl_2 electrodes are used as a reference in conjunction with an inert redox electrode, e.g. platinum, which takes its potential from the particular redox pair in the solution in which it is immersed.

Redox titration is used in pharmacopoeial assays of ferrous salts, hydrogen peroxide, sodium perborate and benzoyl peroxide by titration with $KMnO_4$. In the case of $KMnO_4$ titrations, the end-point may be detected when the purple colour of the permanganate persists.

Iodometric titrations

There are a number of types of iodometric assays.

Direct titrations

Iodine is a moderately strong oxidising agent (see Table 3.1). During oxidation iodine is reduced as follows:

$$I_2 + 2e \rightleftharpoons 2I^-$$

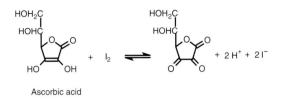

Fig. 3.13
Oxidation of ascorbic acid by iodine.

Ascorbic acid

It will oxidise substances with lower reduction potentials, e.g. the titration of ascorbic acid is carried out as shown in Figure 3.13.

The iodine solution used is standardised against sodium thiosulphate (see later). In addition, the end-point is detected using starch indicator, which produces a blue coloration with excess iodine.

Direct iodometric titration is used in pharmacopoeial assays of ascorbic acid, sodium stilbigluconate, dimercaprol injection and acetarsol.

Iodine displacement titrations

These titrations involve displacement of iodine from iodide by a stronger oxidising agent followed by titration of the displaced iodine with sodium thiosulphate. For example, the available chlorine in bleach is estimated as follows:

$$Cl_2 + 2I \rightleftharpoons 2Cl^- + I_2$$

The displaced iodine is then titrated with thiosulphate according to the following equation:

$$2S_2O_3^{2-} + I_2 \rightleftharpoons S_4O_6^{2-} + 2I^-$$

A different approach is used in the estimation of phenols. Bromine is generated by the reaction of potassium bromide with a defined volume of a standard solution of potassium bromate according to the following equation:

$$BrO_3^- + 5Br^- + 6H^- \rightarrow 3Br_2 + 3H_2O$$

The bromine generated is then reacted with the phenol, and 1 mole of phenol reacts with 3 moles of bromine (Fig. 3.14).

Excess bromine is used, and the bromine remaining after the above reaction is reacted with iodide as follows:

$$Br_2 + 2I^- \rightleftharpoons 2Br^- + I_2$$

The liberated iodine is then titrated with thiosulphate, thus quantifying the excess bromine.

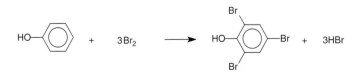

Fig. 3.14
Reaction of phenol with bromine.

Iodine displacement titrations are used in pharmacopoeial assays of liquefied phenol, methyl hydroxybenzoate, propyl hydroxybenzoate and phenidione.

Self-test 3.8

A sample of phenol glycerol injection was diluted with water and an aliquot was taken and reacted with excess bromine generated from potassium bromide and potassium bromate solutions. The excess bromine remaining after reaction was reacted with potassium iodide, and the liberated iodine was titrated with sodium thiosulphate. A blank titration was carried out, where the same quantity of bromine was generated as was used in the titration of the diluted injection; potassium iodide was then added and the liberated iodine was titrated with sodium thiosulphate. From the following data calculate the percentage of w/v of the phenol in the injection:

Weight of injection taken for analysis = 4.214 g.
The sample is diluted to 100 ml with water and then 25 ml of the solution is analysed.
The volume of 0.1015 M sodium thiosulphate required to titrate the excess bromine after reaction with the sample = 22.4 ml.
The volume of 0.1015 M sodium thiosulphate required to titrate the bromine blank = 48.9 ml.
Density of glycerol = 1.26.
The equations of the reactions are given above.

Answer: 5.04% w/v

Iodine-absorbing substances in penicillins

A major stability problem in penicillins is the hydrolysis of the lactam ring, as shown in Figure 3.15. Penicillins with an open lactam ring are inactive as antibiotics, since it is the reactive lactam ring which kills the bacteria.

When the lactam ring is open it will react with iodine. 1 mole of the ring-open form of penicillin will react with 8 equivalents of iodine; the intact lactam ring will not react. In this type of titration, excess iodine solution is added to a sample of the penicillin, and the iodine that is not consumed in the reaction is estimated by titration with sodium thiosulphate. The value obtained for the amount of hydrolysed penicillin in the sample should be no more than 5% of that obtained when all the penicillin in the same amount of sample is completely hydrolysed to the ring-open form and then reacted with iodine. Most of the pharmacopoeial monographs for penicillins indicate that this test should be carried out.

Ion pair titrations

This type of titration is widely used in the cosmetics and detergents industry since it is very useful for estimating surfactants, which often cannot be analysed by spectrophotometric methods because they lack chromophores. There are two types of titrations used.

Fig. 3.15
Hydrolysis of the lactam ring in penicillins.

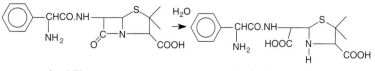

Ampicillin   Inactive ring-open form

Titrations using indicator dyes

A small amount of an anionic or cationic dye is added to an aqueous solution of the analyte, which is a lipophilic cationic or anionic compound. A small amount of coloured lipophilic ion pair is formed, and this is extracted into a small amount of chloroform, which becomes coloured by the ion pair. Titration of the lipophilic anion or cation is carried out with a lipophilic counter ion, e.g. benzethonium chloride or sodium dodecyl sulphate. At the end-point, excess of the titrant breaks up the coloured complex in the chloroform layer.

Ion pair titration using a coloured indicator complex is used in pharmacopoeial assays of dicyclamine elixir, procyclidine tablets, sodium dodecyl sulphate and cetrimide emulsifying ointment.

Titrations using iodide as a lipophilic anion

This procedure is more widely used in pharmacopoeial assays than the dye extraction procedure. Excess potassium iodide is added to an aqueous solution of the analyte, which is a lipophilic cation. A lipophilic ion pair is formed between the cation and the iodide ion and is then removed by extraction into an organic phase such as chloroform. The excess iodide remaining in the aqueous phase is then titrated in concentrated HCl (> 4 M) with potassium iodate. The iodate oxidises iodide to I^+, which immediately reacts with Cl^- to give ICl, resulting in the following equation:

$$KIO_3 + 2\,KI + 6\,HCl \rightarrow 3\,KCl + 3\,ICl + 3\,H_2O$$

A small amount of chloroform is used as an indicator and, in the presence of the reaction mixture, it becomes coloured purple by traces of iodine, which are present during titration. The purple colour disappears at the end-point, when the conversion of all I^- and I_2 into ICl is complete.

Ion pair formation with iodide followed by titration of excess iodide with iodate is utilised in pharmacopoeial assays of cetrimide, cetylpyridium bromide, domiphen bromide and benzalkonium chloride.

Diazotisation titrations

This type of titration is quite simple to carry out and is very useful for the analysis of sulphonamide antibiotics and aminobenzoic acid-derived local anaesthetics. Titration is carried out with acidified sodium nitrite, causing the primary aromatic amine function to be converted to a diazonium salt shown in Figure 3.16 for sulfacetamide.

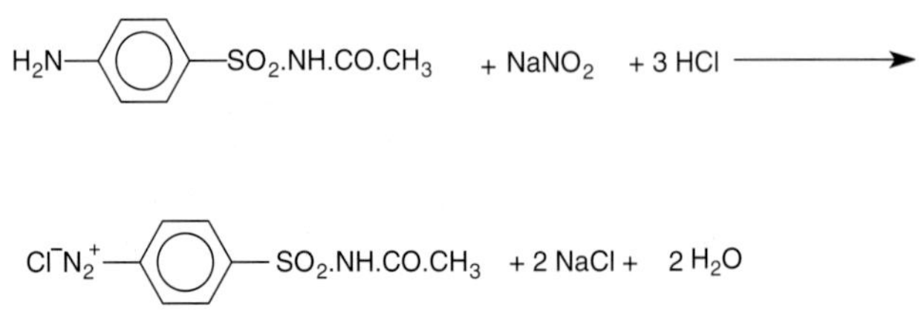

Fig. 3.16 Reaction of sulfacetamide with nitrous acid.

H_2N—⬡—$SO_2.NH.CO.CH_3$ $+ NaNO_2$ $+ 3\,HCl \longrightarrow$

$Cl^- N_2^+$—⬡—$SO_2.NH.CO.CH_3$ $+ 2\,NaCl +$ $2\,H_2O$

A small amount of iodide is included in the titration mixture. At the end-point the first drop of excess nitrous acid converts iodide to iodine, and this is detected using starch indicator.

Titration with nitrous acid is used in pharmacopoeial assays of benzocaine, dapsone, primaquine, procainamide, procaine, sulfacetamide, sulfadoxine, sulfamethizole, sulfapyridine and sulfathiazole.

Potentiometric titrations
Potentiometric end-point detection

All of the titrations discussed in the preceding sections can be carried out using a suitable electrode to measure the potential of the solution as the titration progresses. The advantage of making potentiometric measurements in order to detect end-points is that the measurements can be made in solutions which are coloured, unlike indicator-based end-point detection, and give unambiguous end-points where indicator colour changes are not clear or sudden. The disadvantage of potentiometric titrations is that they are relatively slow, since time has to be allowed for readings to stabilise, particularly near the end-point of the titration. However, potentiometric titrations can be automated, and potentiometric end-point detection is used in automatic titrators, where the titrant is pumped into the sample under microprocessor control. The electrode that is usually used to make the measurements in potentiometric titrations is the pH-sensitive glass indicator electrode. This electrode consists of a pH-sensitive glass membrane bulb which encloses a phosphate buffer solution containing potassium chloride solution and saturated with silver chloride. The solution is in contact with an internal reference electrode which consists of a silver wire. The circuit is completed by a second reference electrode, which in modern combination electrodes is a second silver/silver chloride electrode, which contacts the external solution via a porous junction (Fig. 3.17). The electrode monitors the variation in the potential difference, which is largely caused by the interaction of hydrogen ions with the outer surface of the pH-sensitive glass membrane.

The potential which develops on the inner and outer glass surfaces of the electrode is due to the following equilibria:

$$H^+ + Gl^- \rightleftharpoons H^+Gl^-$$

Outer membrane

$$H^+ + Gl^- \rightleftharpoons H^+Gl^-$$

Inner membrane

The number of Gl^- sites on the outer membrane increases with decreasing $[H^+]$, and thus its potential becomes increasingly negative with respect to the inner surface with increasing pH. The Nernst equation can be simplified and written in the following form for the glass electrode when the temperature is 20°C:

$$E = Ek - 0.0591\,pH$$

where E is the measured potential in volts and Ek is a constant composed of the sum of the various potential differences within the electrode, which do not vary appreciably. The combination electrode is constructed so that its potential is *ca* 0 V at pH 7.0. It can be seen from the equation above that E changes by 59.1 mV for each pH unit.

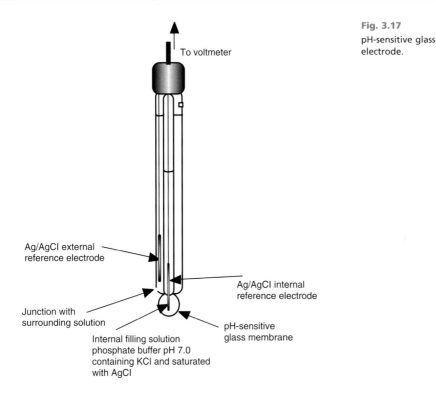

Fig. 3.17
pH-sensitive glass
electrode.

Self-test 3.9

Assuming an indicator electrode is constructed so that $E = 0$ V at pH 7.0, calculate what its potential would be at: (i) pH 1; (ii) pH 14.

Answers: (i) + 0.36 V; (ii) −0.41 V

When potentiometric titration is carried out, the volume of titrant added is plotted against the measured potential. Since the electrode takes time to equilibrate, the volume of titrant required to reach the end-point is first calculated and a volume of titrant is added to within *ca* 1 ml of the end-point. Then the titrant is added in 0.1 ml amounts until the steep inflection in the titration curve is passed. The end-point of the titration is the point where the slope of the titration curve is at its maximum. Thus, if dE/dV is plotted for the titration, the maximum of the plot gives the end-point. The end-point can also be determined from the mid-point of the inflection in the titration curve or from the tabulated data (Table 3.3). Figure 3.18 shows a curve for the titration of 2 mmoles of aspirin with 0.1 M NaOH. The end-point corresponds to the mid-point of the inflection or, if the tabulated data are examined, it can be taken to be the mid-point between the two volumes, where dE/dV is greatest, i.e. at 20.05 ml between 20 and 20.1 ml. The

Table 3.3 Potential difference values obtained for titration of 2 mmoles of aspirin (pKa 3.5) against 0.1 M NaOH

Ml of 0.1 M NaOH added	Potential mV
14	185
16	172
18	151
19	132
19.1	129
19.2	126
19.3	122
19.4	119
19.5	113
19.6	107
19.7	100
19.8	89
19.9	71
20	−44
20.1	−177
20.2	−195
20.3	−206
20.4	−212
21	−236
23	−266

Fig. 3.18
Titration of 20 mmoles of aspirin (pKa 3.5) with 0.1 M NaOH. The end-point corresponds to the mid-point of the inflection.

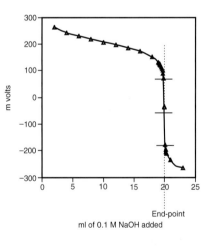

actual end-point for exactly 2 mmoles of aspirin titrated with 0.1 M NaOH should be 20 ml; addition of 0.1 ml aliquots toward the end-point means that the end-point is only accurate to within ± 0.05 ml.

Use of potentiometric titration to determine pKa values (see Animation 3.4)

Potentiometric titration provides the principal method for determining pKa values, and it is best applied to substances with pKa values < 11. For example, the pKa of benzoic acid can be determined as follows: a 0.01 M solution of benzoic acid (50 ml) is titrated with 0.1 M KOH. The KOH is added in 0.5 ml increments; it would be expected that 5 ml of 0.1 M KOH would be required to neutralise the benzoic acid. The pH of the titration is monitored with a glass electrode and the pH of the mixture after 2.5 ml of 0.1 M KOH has been added will equal the p*K*a value of benzoic acid, since:

$$pKa = pH - \log \frac{[C_6H_5COOK]}{[C_6H_5COOK]}$$

The p*K*a value may be checked after addition of each 0.5 ml, since the concentrations of acid and salt are known at each point on the titration curve. The slight increase in volume due to the addition of the 0.1 M KOH may be ignored. For a base, the Henderson–Hasselbalch equation is written as given in Chapter 2, page 29. Automatic titrator software will evaluate the titration curve and report half-neutralisation points. Figure 3.19 shows a potentiometric titration curve for the amino acid glycine which has two p*K*a values.

Self-test 3.10

50 ml of a 0.01 M solution of the base diphenhydramine is titrated with 0.1 M HCl, and the pH is monitored with a glass electrode. After 3 ml of 0.1 M HCl has been added the pH of the solution is 8.82. What is the p*K*a of diphenhydramine?

Answer: 9.0

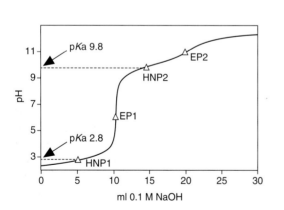

Fig. 3.19
Determination of the p*K*a values for glycine using potentiometric titration.

Karl Fischer titration (coulometric end-point detection)

The Karl Fischer titration is a specialised type of coulometric titration. Coulometry in itself is a useful technique but is not used as a mainstream technique for pharmaceutical analysis. Essentially, coulometry measures the amount of charge that has to be passed through a solution of analyte in order to reduce or oxidise it. The amount of charge required can be equated to the number of moles of analyte present in solution, since, according to Faraday's law, in the case where one molecule reacts with one electron, 1 mole of analyte will react with 96 485 coulombs of electricity, where coulombs = amps × s. In the case of the Karl Fischer titration, the end-point detection is based on the following reaction:

$$I_2 + 2e \rightarrow 2I^-$$

A pair of platinum electrodes that provide variable potential, so that a constant current is supplied to the titration cell, detect the end-point. When excess iodine is produced at the end-point, the resistance of the cell falls. Up to the end-point, the reaction at the cathode of the electrode pair is:

$$CH_3OH + e \rightarrow CH_3O^- + 1/2H_2(g)$$

At the end-point it is the excess iodine that is reduced, which requires less voltage than the reaction shown above; this causes the steep drop in potential at the end-point.

The Karl Fischer reagent consists of a mixture of anhydrous methanol, an anhydrous base (the base was originally pyridine, but bases such as imidazole or diethanolamine are more commonly used now), iodine and sulphur dioxide. It is important for the reliability of the titration that it remains buffered within the optimal pH range of 4–7. Various other inert co-solvents may be used in the preparation of the reagent. The reaction that occurs in the presence of water with pyridine as the basic component, shown below, looks complicated, but essentially the reaction involves the reduction of iodine to iodide by sulphur dioxide, which itself is oxidised to sulphur trioxide.

$$H_2O + I_2 + SO_2 + 3C_5H_5N + CH_3OH \rightarrow 2C_5H_5HI + C_5H_5NH.SO_4CH_3$$

A variety of automated Karl Fischer systems are available (www.metrohm.com). The apparatus used basically consists of a titration vessel of about 60 ml capacity fitted with two platinum electrodes, a nitrogen inlet tube, burette and a vent tube protected by a suitable desiccant. The substance being examined is introduced through an inlet tube, and the sample is stirred during the titration with a magnetic stirrer. The potential is adjusted so that a current of 10 μA passes between the platinum electrodes. At the end of the reaction a steep fall in potential indicates the presence of excess iodine in solution. Karl Fischer volumetric titration can be used to determine water between *ca* 10 μg and several hundred mg. Figure 3.20 shows an automated Karl Fischer titration apparatus.

Coulometric titration is an alternative to volumetric titration. In this case, the instrument used generates iodine from iodide at a platinum anode; any water present in the sample solution immediately converts the iodine back to iodide until the end-point is reached. The end-point is detected as in the volumetric titration, using a pair of platinum electrodes, in addition to the anode that is used to generate the iodine *in situ*. In this case, the amount of water present is determined from the number of coulombs required to generate iodine (2 coulombs are

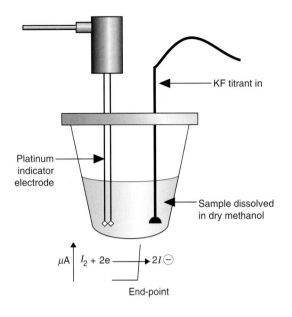

Fig. 3.20
Karl Fischer titrator apparatus.

KF titrant in

Platinum indicator electrode

Sample dissolved in dry methanol

μA $I_2 + 2e \longrightarrow 2I \ominus$

End-point

equivalent to 1 mole of water) up to the end-point. The coulometric apparatus is best used for low levels of water, down to 10 μg per sample.

Automation of wet chemical methods
Automatic titration (Fig. 3.21)

Titrations can be automated and controlled by a microprocessor. The titrant is delivered via an automatic burette, and the end-point is detected potentiometrically with a glass combination electrode. Alternatively, if ions other than hydrogen are being measured, another ion-selective electrode may be used. The

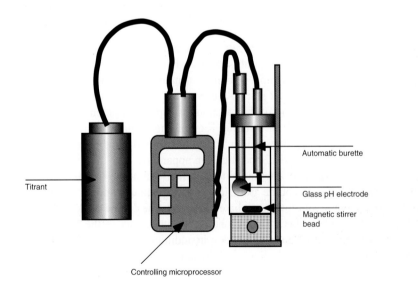

Fig. 3.21
Automatic titration apparatus.

Automatic burette

Titrant

Glass pH electrode

Magnetic stirrer bead

Controlling microprocessor

apparatus is microprocessor controlled and can be programmed to run in various modes:

(i)   The rate of delivery of the titrant can be controlled according to rate of change of potential, so it is added more slowly as the rate of change in potential increases, i.e. as the end-point is approached.
(ii) For titrations which take time to equilibrate as the titrant is added, the instrument can be programmed to delay after each incremental addition until the potential becomes stable.
(iii) The detection of the end-point can be pre-set at a fixed potential.

The microprocessor control also enables the instrument to be set to calculate pKa values directly from the pH profile it obtains by titration of a sample. A sample changer can be incorporated, so that several samples can be automatically titrated.

Flow injection analysis

Flow injection analysis (FIA) represents a refinement of wet chemical methods. The basis of the technique is that the sample is injected into a continuously flowing stream of reagent. The sample reacts with the reagent, and this reaction is measured with a detector. The range of detectors available is the same as that which is used in conjunction with HPLC (Ch. 12, p. 322) except that there is no chromatographic separation involved. Thus the technique is not as selective as chromatographic methods, and its selectivity is dependent on the specificity of the reaction between the analyte and the reagent or the property used for detecting it. A simple schematic diagram of a flow injection analysis system is shown in Figure 3.22. The basic setup may be modified to include several manifolds that allow the introduction of the sample followed by additional reagents. The advantages of the technique are its cheapness and rapidity.

A precise volume of sample (1–100 μl) is injected and passed through the incubation coil, which is of sufficient length to allow the sample to disperse in the reagent but not long enough for the sample to become diluted so much that the integrity of the plug of sample is lost. The detector response is dependent on the degree of dispersion of the sample. A typical flow of the reagent + analyte is as shown in Figure 3.23.

The parameters which have to be optimised include:

(i)   The length and internal diameter of the incubation coil
(ii) The flow rate
(iii) The volume of sample injected
(iv) The concentration of sample and reagents used.

Fig. 3.22
A simple flow injection analysis system.

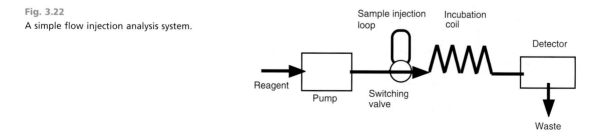

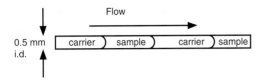

Fig. 3.23
Segmented flow in flow injection analysis (FIA).

Since a number of factors are involved in the optimisation, some time is required to develop the method. However, when set up the method can replace titrations, and replicate analyses can be conducted very quickly with minimal consumption of reagents.

As in chromatography, the ideal peak shape obtained in FIA should be Gaussian, although in practice the ideal shape may not have time to develop. The mathematics governing the dispersion processes have been developed thoroughly, and the process is largely analogous to the dispersion occurring in capillary gas chromatography, where longitudinal diffusion is the major factor governing band broadening.

Figure 3.24 illustrates an application of FIA to the Karl Fischer titration. The consumption of the reagent by water is detected spectrophotometrically by monitoring the stream of reagent at 615 nm. The absorbance due to the iodine in the reagent is removed by its reaction with water, which causes formation of iodide and thus negative absorbance is measured.

Applications of FIA in pharmaceutical analysis
Determination of chloroxine

The antibiotic chloroxine was determined utilising the formation of a complex between the drug and Al^{3+} in an FIA system. The complex was determined by measurement of fluorescence with 399 nm as the excitation wavelength

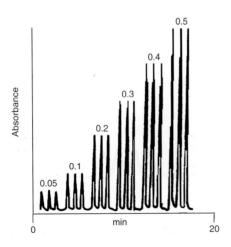

Fig. 3.24
Calibration of Karl Fischer flow injection analysis (FIA) method for determination of residual in water in pharmaceuticals. The analyte was methanol containing 0.05, 0.1, 0.2, 0.4 and 0.5% w/v water.

and 496 nm as the emission wavelength. In order to ensure solubility of the complex in the aqueous reagents, a surfactant was included in the reagent mixture. The precision of the method was greater than that obtained using a laborious batch method for measuring samples manually using a fluorescence spectrophotometer.[3]

Determination of captopril

An FIA method for the determination of captopril was based on the oxidation of the thiol group in the molecule by Ce^{4+}. This reaction results in the emission of light (chemiluminescence), which can be measured. In this example the dye rhodamine G was used to enhance the emission of light by the reaction. The method developed was rapid and precise.[4]

Determination of non-steroidal anti-inflammatory drugs

Diclofenac sodium, famotidine and ketorolac were analysed utilising their formation of a coloured charge transfer complex with 2,4 dichloro-6-nitrophenol. The complexes were detected by UV/visible spectrophotometry at 450 nm. The method was not affected by the presence of common excipients in the formulations analysed. The precision and accuracy of the method were comparable to those of HPLC methods used to analyse the same samples.[5]

Determination of promethazine

The generation of a coloured product upon the oxidation of promethazine with Ce^{4+} was used in the development of an FIA method. Promethazine in tablet form could be analysed by this method with a precision of $\pm$ 1% and at a rate of 122 samples per h.[6] In a similar method, promazine was oxidised by passing through a short column containing MnO_2, and then the oxidation product was measured.[7]

Determination of chlorocresol

Chlorocresol is a preservative commonly used in injections and its determination often involves the use of laborious extraction procedures in order to separate it from formulation components, followed by spectrophotometric measurement. An FIA method for chlorocresol was developed by utilising its reaction with nitrous acid to form a coloured nitro compound. The method was accurate to 99.5% of the true value of chlorocresol in a formulation, and a precision of $\pm$ 1% was achieved.[8]

Limit test for heavy metals

Many pharmacopoeial monographs contain a limit test for heavy metals. Sometimes the metal is specified, e.g. lead, but often the test is more general. Pharmacopoeial tests often involve precipitation of the metals as their sulphides. An FIA method was developed based upon complex formation between heavy metals and diethyldithiocarbamate (DDC). Figure 3.25 shows the FIA system used for this analysis and illustrates how relatively simple components can be assembled to carry out a complex analytical task. The analysis was achieved

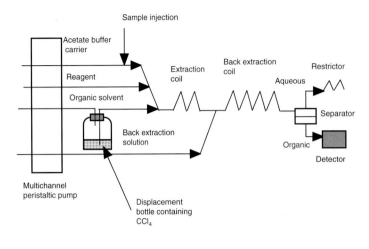

Fig. 3.25
Flow injection analysis (FIA) system used to analyse heavy metal residues by extraction of their complexes with DDC into carbon tetrachloride.

by using a segmented flow system where alternate segments of buffer solution + reagent and carbon tetrachloride were produced. In the first extraction coil, the heavy metals in the sample are extracted as their complexes, along with some excess complexing agent, into carbon tetrachloride. In the second extraction coil, the excess reagent in the organic layer is back extracted by the borax solution, which is mixed into the carrier stream. The flow was then passed into a phase separator, which only allowed the organic solvent to flow through to the detector.[9]

Use of segmented flow in determination of partition coefficients

A system similar to the one described above was used for the determination of partition coefficients. An FIA system with segmented flow was devised so that the partitioning of a drug between aqueous buffer and chloroform could be measured. The aqueous and organic phases were separated using a phase separator. The system could be set up to measure the concentration of the drug in either the organic or the aqueous phase. Such a system enables rapid repeat determinations of partition coefficient at various pH values with minimal sample consumption.[10]

Automated dissolution testing

FIA was used to optimise sampling from a tablet dissolution apparatus in order to determine the rate of release of iron (II) from a sustained release formulation. The dissolution medium was automatically sampled at 30-minute intervals, and the 100 μl aliquots of medium were mixed with the iron-complexing agent ferrozine, diluted and then passed into a spectrophotometric detector. The system was microprocessor controlled, thus enabling unattended sampling of the dissolution medium for a prolonged period.[11]

Additional problems

1. 0.4681 g of the acidic (monobasic) drug ibuprofen (molecular weight 206.3) is dissolved in 50 ml of methanol, and 0.4 ml of phenolphthalein solution is added. The sample is titrated with 0.1005 M sodium hydroxide until a pink colour is obtained. A blank titration is carried out.

Results

Volume of NaOH required to titrate the blank = 0.050 ml
Volume of NaOH required to titrate the sample = 22.75 ml

Calculate the % purity of the ibuprofen.

Answer: 100.5%

2. 0.1563 g of phenylephrine hydrochloride (molecular weight 203.7) was dissolved in a mixture of 0.5 ml of 0.1001 M hydrochloric acid and 80 ml of ethanol. A potentiometric titration was carried out using 0.1032 M ethanolic sodium hydroxide.

Results

Two end-points obtained were at 0.48 ml and 7.78 ml.
Calculate the % purity of the phenylephrine HCl.

Answer: 98.2%

3. 4.079 g of glutaraldehyde (molecular weight 100.1) solution (weight per ml 1.132 g) was mixed with 100 ml of a 7% w/v solution of hydroxylamine hydrochloride solution and allowed to stand for 30 minutes. The solution was titrated with 1.004 M sodium hydroxide using bromothymol blue as an indicator. The equation for the reaction with hydroxylamine is given below.

$$OHCCH_2CH_2CHO + 2HONH_2.HCl \rightarrow HONHCCH_2CH_2CH_2CHNOH + 2HCl$$

The volume of NaOH required = 41.63 ml.
Calculate the % w/w and the % w/v of glutaraldehyde in the solution.

Answer: 51.3% w/v, 58.1% w/w

4. 2.054 g of macrogol monostearate (average molecular weight 706.5) was added to a 200 ml flask and 25 ml of an ethanolic solution of potassium hydroxide (molecular weight 56.1, *ca* 0.5 M) was added. The sample was heated under a reflux condenser for 1 hour. The excess of alkali was then titrated with 0.5016 M hydrochloric acid using phenolphthalein solution as an indicator. The operation was repeated without the macrogol monostearate.

Results

Volume of HCl required to titrate the excess alkali = 18.35 ml
Volume of HCl required to titrate the blank = 24.03 ml

Calculate the saponification value for the macrogol stearate. How would the value of *n* given in the formula below affect the saponification value?

$$H - (OCH_2CH_2)_n OCOC_{17}H_{35}$$

Answer: 77.8

5. 1.507 g of macrogol lauryl ether was placed in a 150 ml acetylation flask fitted with an air condenser, and 5 ml of acetic anhydride in pyridine (1:3) solution was added. The sample was heated for 1 hour in a water bath, then removed, and 5 ml of water was added through the top of the condenser. The flask was shaken and replaced in the water bath for 10 minutes, removed and allowed to cool. The sample was titrated with 0.5034 M ethanolic potassium hydroxide (molecular weight 56.1) using phenolphthalein as an indicator. The process was repeated without addition of the macrogol.

(Continued)

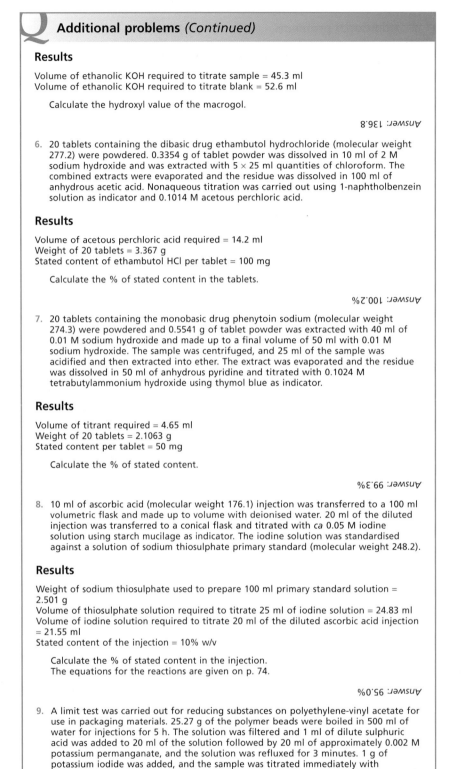

Additional problems (Continued)

Results

Volume of ethanolic KOH required to titrate sample = 45.3 ml
Volume of ethanolic KOH required to titrate blank = 52.6 ml

Calculate the hydroxyl value of the macrogol.

Answer: 136.8

6. 20 tablets containing the dibasic drug ethambutol hydrochloride (molecular weight 277.2) were powdered. 0.3354 g of tablet powder was dissolved in 10 ml of 2 M sodium hydroxide and was extracted with 5 × 25 ml quantities of chloroform. The combined extracts were evaporated and the residue was dissolved in 100 ml of anhydrous acetic acid. Nonaqueous titration was carried out using 1-naphtholbenzein solution as indicator and 0.1014 M acetous perchloric acid.

Results

Volume of acetous perchloric acid required = 14.2 ml
Weight of 20 tablets = 3.367 g
Stated content of ethambutol HCl per tablet = 100 mg

Calculate the % of stated content in the tablets.

Answer: 100.2%

7. 20 tablets containing the monobasic drug phenytoin sodium (molecular weight 274.3) were powdered and 0.5541 g of tablet powder was extracted with 40 ml of 0.01 M sodium hydroxide and made up to a final volume of 50 ml with 0.01 M sodium hydroxide. The sample was centrifuged, and 25 ml of the sample was acidified and then extracted into ether. The extract was evaporated and the residue was dissolved in 50 ml of anhydrous pyridine and titrated with 0.1024 M tetrabutylammonium hydroxide using thymol blue as indicator.

Results

Volume of titrant required = 4.65 ml
Weight of 20 tablets = 2.1063 g
Stated content per tablet = 50 mg

Calculate the % of stated content.

Answer: 99.3%

8. 10 ml of ascorbic acid (molecular weight 176.1) injection was transferred to a 100 ml volumetric flask and made up to volume with deionised water. 20 ml of the diluted injection was transferred to a conical flask and titrated with *ca* 0.05 M iodine solution using starch mucilage as indicator. The iodine solution was standardised against a solution of sodium thiosulphate primary standard (molecular weight 248.2).

Results

Weight of sodium thiosulphate used to prepare 100 ml primary standard solution = 2.501 g
Volume of thiosulphate solution required to titrate 25 ml of iodine solution = 24.83 ml
Volume of iodine solution required to titrate 20 ml of the diluted ascorbic acid injection = 21.55 ml
Stated content of the injection = 10% w/v

Calculate the % of stated content in the injection.
The equations for the reactions are given on p. 74.

Answer: 95.0%

9. A limit test was carried out for reducing substances on polyethylene-vinyl acetate for use in packaging materials. 25.27 g of the polymer beads were boiled in 500 ml of water for injections for 5 h. The solution was filtered and 1 ml of dilute sulphuric acid was added to 20 ml of the solution followed by 20 ml of approximately 0.002 M potassium permanganate, and the solution was refluxed for 3 minutes. 1 g of potassium iodide was added, and the sample was titrated immediately with

(Continued)

Q Additional problems *(Continued)*

0.01046 M sodium thiosulphate, using starch solution as indicator. A blank titration was carried out using 20 ml of water in place of the extract from the polymer. To pass the limit test, the difference between the titration volumes should not be more than 0.5 ml. The equation for reaction of iodide with potassium permanganate is as follows:

$$2KMnO_4 + 10KI + 8H_2SO_4 \rightarrow 5I_2 + 6K_2SO_4 + 2MnSO_4 + 8H_2O$$

Results

Volume of thiosulphate required for the blank titration = 19.23 ml
Volume of thiosulphate required to titrate the aqueous extract from the polymer = 18.85 ml

Calculate the mmoles of $KMnO_4$ equivalent to the reducing substances extracted from 1 g of the polymer beads.

Answer: 0.000786 mmoles

References

1. Beckett AH, Stenlake JB. *Practical Pharmaceutical Chemistry Part One*. 4th ed. London: Athlone Press; 1988.
2. Skoog DA, West DM. *Fundamentals of Analytical Chemistry*. 4th ed. Philadelphia: Sanders College Publishing; 1986.
3. Pérez-Ruiz T, Martinez-Lozano C, Tomás V, Carpene J. Fluorimetric determination of chloroxine using manual and flow-injection methods. *J Pharm Biomed Anal*. 1996;14:1505-1511.
4. Zhang ZD, Baeyens WRG, Zhang XR, Vander Weken G. Chemiluminescence flow-injection analysis of captopril applying a sensitized rhodamine 6G method. *J Pharm Biomed Anal*. 1996;14:939-945.
5. Kamath BV, Shivram K, Shah AC. Determination of diclofenac sodium, famotidine and ketorolac tromethamine by flow injection analysis using dichloronitrophenol. *J Pharm Biomed Anal*. 1994;12:343-346.
6. Calatayud JM, Sancho TG. Spectrophotometric determination of promethazine by flow injection analysis and oxidation by CeIV. *J Pharm Biomed Anal*. 1992;10:37-42.
7. Kojlo A, Puzanowska-Tarasiewicz H, Calatatud JM. Analytical application of the binary and ternary complexes of 2,10-disubstituted phenothiazines. *J Pharm Biomed Anal*. 1992;10:785-788.
8. Bloomfield MN, Prebble KA. The determination of the preservative, chlorocresol, in a pharmaceutical formulation by flow injection analysis. *J Pharm Biomed Anal*. 1992;10:775-778.
9. Danielsson L-G, Huazhang Z. FIA-extraction applied to the limit test for heavy metals. *J Pharm Biomed Anal*. 1989;7:937-945.
10. Danielsson L-G, Nord L, Yu-Hui Z. Rapid determination of conditional partition constants in an FIA system. *J Pharm Biomed Anal*. 1992;10:405-412.
11. Georgiou CA, Valsami GN, Macheras PE, Koupparis MA. Automated flow-injection technique for use in dissolution studies of sustained-release formulations: application to iron(II) formulations. *J Pharm Biomed Anal*. 1994;12:635-641.

Further reading

Felix FS, Angnes L. Fast and accurate analysis of drugs using amperometry associated with flow injection analysis. *J Pharm Sci*. 2010;99:4784-4804.

Lara FJ, Garcia-Campana AM, Aaron JJ. Analytical applications of photoinduced chemiluminescence in flow systems – A review. *Anal Chim Acta*. 2010;679:17-30.

Mach H, Bhambhani A, Meyer BK, et al. The use of flow cytometry for the detection of subvisible particles in therapeutic protein formulations. *J Pharm Sci*. 2011;100:1671-1678.

www.metrohm.com.

Contains a range of information on automatic titration.

Ultraviolet and visible spectroscopy

4

KEYPOINTS

Principles

Radiation in the wavelength range 200–700 nm is passed through a solution of a compound. The electrons in the bonds within the molecule become excited so that they occupy a higher quantum state and in the process absorb some of the energy passing through the solution. The more loosely held the electrons are within the bonds of the molecule, the longer the wavelength (lower the energy) of the radiation absorbed.

Applications in pharmaceutical analysis

- A robust, workhorse method for the quantification of drugs in formulations where there is no interference from excipients.
- Determination of the pKa values of some drugs.
- Determination of partition coefficients and solubilities of drugs.
- Used to determine the release of drugs from formulations with time, e.g. in dissolution testing.
- Can be used to monitor the reaction kinetics of drug degradation.
- The UV spectrum of a drug is often used as one of a number of pharmacopoeial identity checks.

(Continued)

Strengths

- An easy-to-use, cheap and robust method offering good precision for making quantitative measurements of drugs in formulations.
- Routine method for determining some of the physico-chemical properties of drugs, which need to be known for the purposes of formulation.
- Some of the problems of the basic method can be solved by the use of derivative spectra.

Limitations

- Only moderately selective. The selectivity of the method depends on the chromophore of the individual drugs, e.g a coloured drug with an extended chromophore is more distinctive than a drug with a simple benzene ring chromophore.
- Not readily applicable to the analysis of mixtures.

Introduction

The interaction between radiation and matter is a fascinating area in its own right. Most drug molecules absorb radiation in the ultraviolet region of the spectrum, although some are coloured and thus absorb radiation in the visible region, e.g. a substance with a blue colour absorbs radiation in the red region of the spectrum. The absorption of UV/visible radiation occurs through the excitation of electrons within the molecular structure to a higher energy state; Figure 4.1 illustrates the nature of the transitions taking place. These transitions occur from the bottom vibrational state in the electronic ground state of the molecule to any one of a number of vibrational levels in the electronic excited state. The transition from a single ground state energy to one of a number of excited states gives width to UV spectra. Figure 4.1 shows a UV spectrum in which individual bands for different Vo to Vn transitions can be seen. Vibrational fine structure can be seen, although the bands overlap extensively; the vibrational bands themselves have width due to rotational transitions that are intermediate in energy between each vibrational transition. The relative energy of electronic:vibrational:rotational transitions is 100:1:0.01. In most molecules the vibrational behaviour is complex and the degree of overlap of the different energies of the vibrational transitions is too great for vibrational fine structure to be observed.

Fig. 4.1
Excitation of an electron from the ground to the excited electronic state.

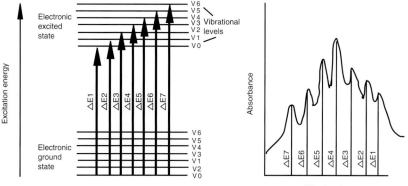

Factors governing absorption of radiation in the UV/visible region (see Animation 4.1 and Animation 4.2)

Radiation in the UV/visible region is absorbed through excitation of the electrons involved in the bonds between the atoms making up the molecule so that the electron cloud holding the atoms together redistributes itself and the orbitals occupied by the bonding electrons no longer overlap. Short wavelength UV radiation < 150 nm (> 8.3 eV) can cause the strongest bonds in organic molecules to break and thus is very damaging to living organisms. It is the weaker bonds in molecules that are of more interest to analysts because they can be excited by longer wavelength UV radiation > 200 nm (> 6.2 eV), which is at a longer wavelength than the region in which air and common solvents absorb. Examining a very simple organic molecule such as ethylene (Fig. 4.2) it can be seen that it contains two types of carbon–carbon bonds, a strong σ bond formed by extensive overlap of the sp^2 orbitals of the two carbons and a weaker π bond formed by partial overlap of the p orbitals of the carbon atoms. The σ bond would become excited and break when exposed to radiation at *ca* 150 nm. The weaker π bond requires less energetic radiation at *ca* 180 nm to produce the π^* excited state shown in Figure 4.2. This excitation can occur without the molecule falling apart since the σ orbitals remain unexcited by the longer wavelength radiation at 180 nm. However, a single double bond is still not useful as a chromophore for determining analytes by UV spectrophotometry since it is still in the region where air and solvents absorb. (see Animation 4.3)

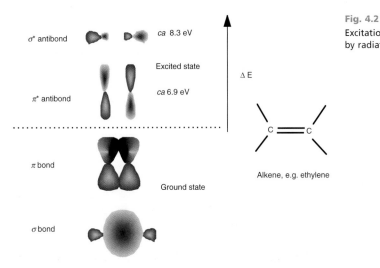

σ* antibond — *ca* 8.3 eV

Excited state

π* antibond — *ca* 6.9 eV

ΔE

π bond

Ground state

σ bond

Alkene, e.g. ethylene

Fig. 4.2
Excitation of the carbon–carbon bonds in ethylene by radiation in the short wavelength UV region.

If more double bonds are present in a structure in conjugation (i.e. two or more double bonds in a series separated by a single bond), absorption takes place at longer wavelengths and with greater intensity, as detailed in Table 4.1 for a series of polyenes. The *A* (1%, 1 cm) value, which is described later, gives a measure of the intensity of absorption. The type of linear conjugated system which is present in polyenes is not very common in drug molecules.

Such extended systems of double bonds are known as *chromophores*. The most common chromophore found in drug molecules is a benzene ring

Table 4.1 Longest wavelength maxima and absorption intensities of some polyenes

Polyene	λ max	A (1%, 1 cm)
$CH_3(CH=CH)_3CH_3$	275	2800
$CH_3(CH=CH)_4CH_3$	310	6300
$CH_3(CH=CH)_5CH_3$	342	9000
$CH_3(CH=CH)_6CH_3$	380	9800

Table 4.2 The UV absorption characteristics of some chromophores based on the benzene ring

Chromophore	Longest wavelength λ max	A (1%, 1 cm)
Benzene	255 nm	28
Benzoic acid	273	85
Cinnamic acid	273	1420
Protriptyline $(CH_2)_3NHCH_3$	292	530
Phenol	270 nm ⇌ 287 nm → Bathochromic	72 ⇌ 271 → Hyperchromic
Aniline	255 nm ⇌ 286 nm → Bathochromic	16 ⇌ 179 → Hyperchromic

(Table 4.2). Benzene itself has its λ max at a much shorter wavelength than a linear triene such as hexatriene (λ max 275 nm), and its strongest absorbance is at the wavelength of absorption of an isolated double bond at 180 nm. It also has a strong absorption band at 204 nm. This is due to the symmetry of benzene; it is not possible to have an excited state involving all three bonds in benzene because this would mean that the dipole (polarisation of the chromophore), a two-dimensional concept which is created in the excited state, would be symmetrical and thus would have to exist in three dimensions rather than two. There is a weak absorption in the benzene spectrum close to the λ max for hexatriene, and this can occur because vibration of the benzene ring in a particular direction can distort its symmetry and thus allow all three double bonds to be involved in an excited state. If the symmetry of the benzene ring is lowered by substitution, the bands in the benzene spectrum undergo a bathochromic shift – a shift to longer wavelength. Substitution can involve either extension of the chromophore or attachment of an auxochrome (a group containing one or more lone pair of electrons) to the ring or both. Table 4.2 summarises the absorption bands found in some simple aromatic systems, and these chromophore/auxochrome systems provide the basis for absorption of UV radiation by many drugs. The hydroxyl group and amino group auxochromes are affected by pH (see Animation 4.4), undergoing bathochromic (moving to a longer wavelength) and hyperchromic (absorbing more strongly) shifts when a proton is removed under alkaline conditions, releasing an extra lone pair of electrons. The effect is most marked for aromatic amine groups. The absorption spectrum of a drug molecule is due to the particular combination of auxochromes and chromophores present in its structure.

Beer–Lambert Law

Figure 4.3 shows the absorption of radiation by a solution containing a UV-absorbing compound.

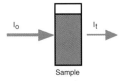

Fig. 4.3
Absorption of light by a solution.

The measurement of light absorption by a solution of molecules is governed by the Beer–Lambert Law, which is written as follows:

$$\log I_o / I_t = A = \varepsilon bc$$

where I_o is the intensity of incident radiation; I_t is the intensity of transmitted radiation; A is known as the absorbance and is a measure of the amount of light absorbed by the sample; ε is a constant known as the molar extinction coefficient and is the absorbance of a 1 M solution of the analyte; b is the pathlength of the cell in cm, usually 1 cm and c is the concentration of the analyte in moles litre^{-1}.

Self-test 4.1

Calculate the percentage of the incident radiation absorbed by a sample with an absorbance of (i) 2; (ii) 0.1.

Answers: (i) 99.0%; (ii) 20.6%

In pharmaceutical products, concentrations and amounts are usually expressed in grams or milligrams rather than in moles and, thus, for the purposes of the analysis of these products, the Beer–Lambert equation is written in the following form:

$$A = A\,(1\%, 1\,\text{cm})\, bc$$

where A is the measured absorbance; A (1%, 1 cm) is the absorbance of a 1% w/v (1 g/100 ml) solution in a 1 cm cell; b is the pathlength in cm (usually 1 cm) and c is the concentration of the sample in g/100 ml. Since measurements are usually made in a 1 cm cell, the equation can be written:

$$\left[c = \frac{A}{A(1\%, 1\,\text{cm})} \right]$$

which gives the concentration of the analyte in g/100 ml.

BP monographs often quote a standard A (1%, 1 cm) value for a drug, which is to be used in its quantitation.

Self-test 4.2

What are the concentrations of the following solutions of drugs in g/100 ml and mg/100 ml?

(i) Carbimazole, A (1%, 1 cm) value = 557 at 291 nm, measured absorbance = 0.557 at 291 nm.

(ii) Hydrocortisone sodium phosphate, A (1%, 1 cm) value = 333 at 248 nm, measured absorbance = 0.666 at 248 nm.

(iii) Isoprenaline, A (1%, 1 cm) value = 100 at 280 nm, measured absorbance = 0.500 at 280 nm.

Answers: (i) Carbimazole 0.001 g/100 ml, 1 mg/100 ml; (ii) Hydrocortisone sodium phosphate 0.002 g/100 ml, 2 mg/100 ml; (iii) Isoprenaline 0.005 g/100 ml, 5 mg/100 ml

---

Instrumentation

A simple diagram of a UV/visible spectrophotometer is shown in Figure 4.4. The components include:

(i) *The light sources* – a deuterium lamp for the UV region from 190 to 350 nm and a quartz halogen or tungsten lamp for the visible region from 350 to 900 nm.

(ii) *The monochromator* – used to disperse the light into its constituent wavelengths, which are further selected by the slit. The monochromator is rotated so that a range of wavelengths is passed through the sample as the instrument scans across the spectrum.

(iii) *The optics* – may be designed to split the light beam so that the beam passes through two sample compartments, and, in such a double-beam instrument, a blank solution can then be used in one compartment to correct the reading or spectrum of the sample. The blank is most commonly the solvent in which the sample is dissolved.

Fig. 4.4
Schematic diagram of a UV/visible spectrophotometer.

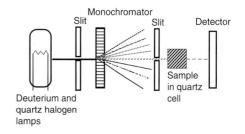

Diode array instruments

A photomultiplier tube is used for detection in older types of UV/visible instruments, but, increasingly, photodiodes are used as detectors in spectrophotometers. A diode array consists of a series of photodiode detectors positioned side by side on a silicon crystal. The array typically contains between 200 and 1000 elements, depending on the instrument. The scan cycle is *ca* 100 ms, compared with the minute or more required to obtain a spectrum with a traditional scanning instrument. Light is passed through a polychromator, which disperses it so that it falls on the diode array, which measures the whole range of the spectrum at once. This type of instrumentation is useful in, for instance, the dissolution testing of multicomponent formulations where it is possible to select wavelengths that are specific for the different analytes of interest.

Instrument calibration

Pharmacopoeial monographs usually rely on standard A (1%, 1 cm) values in order to calculate the concentration of drugs in extracts from formulations. In order to use a standard value, the instrument used to make the measurement must be properly calibrated with respect to its wavelength and absorption scales. In addition, checks for stray light and spectral resolution are run. These checks are now often built into the software of UV instruments so that they can be run automatically, to ensure that the instrument meets good manufacturing practice requirements. Some of the practical aspects of UV/visible spectrophotometry are described in Box 4.1.

Box 4.1 Practical aspects of UV/visible spectrophotometry

- Care should be taken to avoid touching the optical surfaces of sample cells with the fingers since fingerprints can cause significant absorbance. The optical surfaces of the cell can be wiped carefully with tissue.
- The precision of the pathlength of cells is important. Tolerances for cells of good quality are ± 0.01 mm for pathlength. For maximum quantitative accuracy, the same cell should be used for measurement of both the standard and the sample. The cell should always face in the same direction in a cell holder to ensure that any cell optical effects are identical for both blank and sample measurements.
- Distilled water is the ideal solvent but is not suitable for many organic compounds. Methanol and ethanol are next best, but they cannot be used below a wavelength of 210 nm.
- The solvent used to dissolve the sample, concentration, pH, and temperature can affect the position and intensity of absorption bands of molecules. These factors should be controlled as far as possible. Expansion of organic solvent with temperature can cause a change in the reading, as can evaporation; thus sample cells should have tops, particularly if an organic solvent is being used.
- Ideally absorbances measured should be in the range 0.4–1.0 to avoid being outside the linear range of the instrument.
- Scattering gives an apparent increase in absorbance and is caused by particles suspended in solution. It is important that the sample solutions are free from particles.

Calibration of absorbance scale

The British Pharmacopoeia (BP) uses potassium dichromate solution to calibrate the absorbance scale of a UV spectrophotometer; the A (1%, 1 cm) values at specified wavelengths have to lie within the ranges specified by the BP. The spectrum of a 0.006% w/v solution of potassium dichromate in 0.005 M H_2SO_4 is shown in Figure 4.5. The absorbance scale calibration wavelengths, with corresponding A (1%, 1 cm) values for 0.006% w/v potassium dichromate solution, that are specified by the BP are as follows: 235 nm (122.9–126.2), 257 nm (142.4–145.7), 313 nm (47.0–50.3), 350 nm (104.9–108.2).

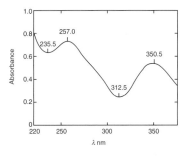

Fig. 4.5

The UV spectrum of 0.006% w/v potassium dichromate solution between 220 and 350 nm.

Calibration of wavelength scale

The wavelength scale of a UV/visible spectrophotometer is checked by determining the specified wavelength maxima of a 5% w/v solution of holmium perchlorate. Figure 4.6 shows the spectrum of holmium perchlorate; the tolerances for calibration wavelengths specified by the BP are 241.15 ± 1 nm, 287.15 ± 1 nm and 361.5 ± 1 nm.

The wavelength scale may also be calibrated according to the spectral lines of deuterium or mercury discharge lamps, and such tests may be built into some instruments.

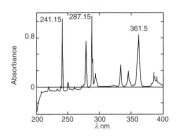

Fig. 4.6

The absorbance maxima of a 5% w/v solution of holmium perchlorate between 200 and 400 nm.

Determination of instrumental resolution

The resolving power of an instrument is controlled by its slit width settings. For some pharmacopoeial tests a certain resolution is specified. The resolving power of an instrument can be assessed by using a 0.02% w/v solution of toluene in hexane. The BP specifies that the ratio of the absorbance for this solution at 269 nm to that at 266 nm should be at least 1.5.

Determination of stray light

Stray light is light which falls on the detector within a UV instrument without having passed through the sample. It can arise either from light scattering within the instrument or by entry of light into the instrument from outside. It gives a false low-absorbance reading for the sample since it appears as though the sample is absorbing less light than it actually is. This is most serious where the sample has a high absorbance, e.g. at an absorbance of 2 the sample is absorbing most of the light passing through it and thus it would only require very low-intensity stray light to lower the reading substantially. Stray light is checked by measuring the absorbance of a 1.2% solution of KCl in water against a water blank at a wavelength of 200 nm. If the absorbance of the sample is < 2, then stray light is present and the instrument needs to be serviced.

UV spectra of some representative drug molecules

Steroid enones

The chromophores of most drugs are based on a modification of the benzene ring chromophore. One large class of drugs that does not fit into this category is steroidal androgens and corticosteroids. The spectra of hydrocortisone and betamethasone are shown in Figure 4.7. These spectra are common to many steroids, and all have absorbance maxima of similar intensity, at around 240 nm. The extra double bond in betamethasone as compared with hydrocortisone does not make a great difference to the wavelength of maximum absorption since it does not extend the original chromophore linearly. However, the shape of the absorption band for betamethasone is quite different from that for hydrocortisone. Such differences in the spectra can be employed in qualitative identity tests; these are used particularly in conjunction with high-pressure liquid chromatography (HPLC) identification checks where the method of detection is by diode array UV spectrophotometry (Ch. 12, p. 322).

Table 4.3 summarises the absorption data for some steroid structures and illustrates the effect of molecular weight on the A (1%, 1 cm) value. The strength of the enone chromophore is similar for all the steroids since the A (1%, 1 cm) value is based on the absorption of a 1% w/v solution; it will thus decrease as the molecular weight of the steroid increases. This is, of course, true for all molecules.

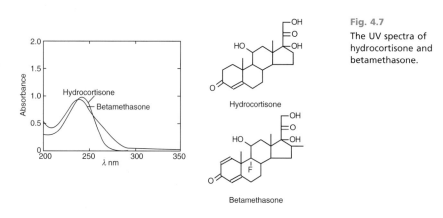

Fig. 4.7
The UV spectra of hydrocortisone and betamethasone.

Table 4.3 Absorption maxima for some corticosteroids			
Steroid	Molecular weight	λ max	A (1%, 1 cm) value
Hydrocortisone	362.5	240	435
Betamethasone	392.5	240	390
Clobetasone butyrate	479.0	236	330
Betamethasone sodium phosphate	516.4	241	296

Ephedrine: the benzoid chromophore

Figure 4.8 shows the UV absorption spectrum of a 100 mg/100 ml solution of ephedrine. Ephedrine has the simplest type of benzene ring chromophore, which

Fig. 4.8
The UV spectrum of ephedrine, a simple benzoid spectrum.

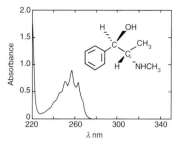

has a spectrum similar to that of benzene with a weak symmetry forbidden band *ca* 260 nm with an *A* (1%, 1 cm) value of 12. Like benzene its most intense absorption maximum is below 200 nm. There are no polar groups attached to or involved in the chromophore, so its vibrational fine structure is preserved because the chromophore does not interact strongly with the solvent.

Drugs having a chromophore like that of ephedrine include diphenhydramine, amphetamine, ibuprofen and dextropropoxyphene.

Ketoprofen: extended benzene chromophore

The spectrum of ketoprofen is shown in Figure 4.9. In this case, the simple benzoid chromophore has been extended by four double bonds, and thus the symmetry of the benzene ring has been altered. In addition, the strong absorbance band present in benzene at 204 nm has undergone a bathochromic shift, giving a λ max for ketoprofen at 262 nm having an *A* (1%, 1 cm) value of 647.

Other drugs which have an extended benzoid chromophore include cyproheptadine, dimethindine, protriptyline, zimeldine.

Fig. 4.9
UV absorption spectrum of ketoprofen.

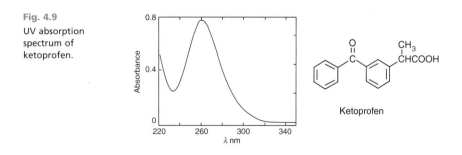

Ketoprofen

Procaine: amino group auxochrome

Figure 4.10 shows the UV absorption spectra of a solution of procaine in 0.1 M HCl and 0.1 M NaOH. In procaine, the benzene chromophore has been extended by the addition of a C=O group, and, under acidic conditions, as in Figure 4.10, the molecule has an absorption at 279 nm with an *A* (1%, 1 cm) value of 100. In addition to the extended chromophore, the molecule also contains an auxochrome in the form of an amino group, which under basic conditions has a lone pair of electrons that can interact with the chromophore producing a bathochromic shift.

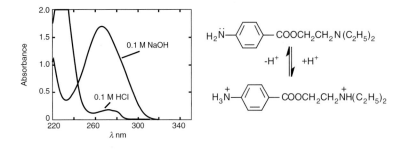

Fig. 4.10
UV spectrum of procaine under acidic and basic conditions.

Under acidic conditions, the amine group is protonated and does not function as an auxochrome, but when the proton is removed from this group under basic conditions a bathochromic shift is produced and an absorption with λ max at 270 nm with an A (1%, 1 cm) value of 1000 appears.

Drugs with a chromophore such as that of procaine include procainamide and proxymetacaine. It should be noted that local anaesthetics such as bupivacaine and lidocaine (lignocaine) do not fall into this category since they are aromatic amides and the lone pair on the nitrogen atom is not fully available due to electron withdrawal by the adjacent carbonyl group.

Phenylephrine: hydroxyl group auxochrome

The chromophore of phenylephrine is not extended but its structure includes a phenolic hydroxyl group. The phenolic group functions as an auxochrome under both acidic and alkaline conditions. Under acidic conditions it has two lone pairs of electrons, which can interact with the benzene ring, and under basic conditions it has three. Figure 4.11 shows the bathochromic and hyperchromic shift in the spectrum of phenylephrine that occurs when 0.1 M NaOH is used as a solvent instead of 0.1 M HCl. Under acidic conditions the λ max is at 273 and has an A (1%, 1 cm) value of 110, and under alkaline conditions the λ max is at 292 nm and has an A (1%, 1 cm) value of 182.

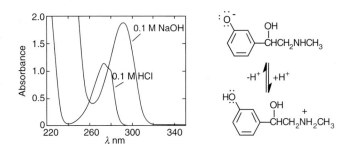

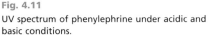

Fig. 4.11
UV spectrum of phenylephrine under acidic and basic conditions.

The types of shifts observed for procaine and phenylephrine can be exploited in order to achieve analysis of mixtures. Two examples of this are given later in the chapter.

Self-test 4.3

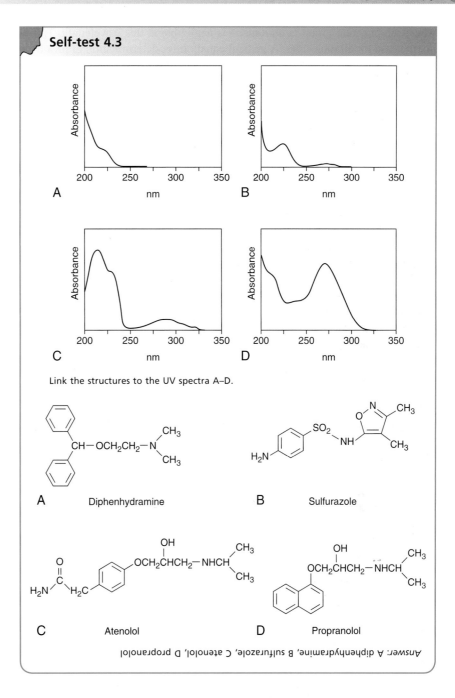

Link the structures to the UV spectra A–D.

A Diphenhydramine

B Sulfurazole

C Atenolol

D Propranolol

Answer: A diphenhydramine, B sulfurazole, C atenolol, D propranolol

Use of UV/visible spectrophotometry to determine pKa values

Where a pH-dependent UV shift is produced, it is possible to use it to determine the pKa of the ionisable group responsible for the shift. In the case of phenylephrine, the pKa value of the phenolic group can be determined conveniently from the absorbance at 292 nm, since the absorbance of the molecular species where the phenolic group is un-ionised is negligible at this wavelength. This is not the case for all molecules. A general equation for determination of pKa from absorbance measurement at a particular wavelength is given below.

The following equation can be used for an acid (for a base the log term is subtracted) where increasing pH produces a bathochromic/hyperchromic shift:

$$pKa = pH + \log \frac{Ai - A}{A - Au}$$

where A is the measured absorbance in a buffer of known pH at the wavelength selected for analysis; Ai is the absorbance of the fully ionised species and Au is the absorbance of the un-ionised species.

The wavelength used for analysis is one where there is the greatest difference between the ionised and un-ionised species. An approximate knowledge of the pKa value is required to select a suitable pH value, within ± 1 of the pKa value, for measurement of A. For accurate determination, measurement is made at a number of closely spaced pH values.

It should be noted that if the acid or base undergoes a shift to lower absorbance and shorter wavelength with increasing pH, the log term above is subtracted; this situation is less common in drug molecules.

Calculation example 4.1

The absorbance of a fixed concentration of phenylephrine at 292 nm is found to be 1.224 in 0.1 M NaOH and 0.02 in 0.1 M HCl. Its absorbance in buffer at pH 8.5 is found to be 0.349. Calculate the pKa value of its acidic phenolic hydroxyl group.

$$pKa = 8.5 + \log \frac{1.224 - 0.349}{0.349 - 0.02} = 8.5 + 0.402 = 8.902.$$

Self-test 4.4

Calculate the pKa value of the weakly basic aromatic amine in procaine from the data given below. Absorbance of a fixed concentration of procaine in 1 M HCl at 296 nm = 0.031; absorbance in 0.1 M NaOH = 1.363; absorbance in buffer at pH 2.6 = 0.837.

Answer: 2.41

Applications of UV/visible spectroscopy to pharmaceutical quantitative analysis

Pharmacopoeial methods rely heavily on simple analysis by UV/visible spectro-photometry to determine active ingredients in formulations. These methods are usually based on the use of a standard A (1%, 1 cm) value for the active ingredient being assayed, and this relies on the UV spectrophotometer being accurately calibrated as described earlier in the chapter. Such methods also presume that there is no interference from excipients (preservatives, colourants, etc.) present in formulations and that the sample is free of suspended matter, which would cause light scattering.

Assay examples

Furosemide (frusemide) in tablet form

A typical example of a straightforward tablet assay is the analysis of furosemide (frusemide) tablets:

(i)   Tablet powder containing *ca* 0.25 g of furosemide (frusemide) is shaken with 300 ml of 0.1 M NaOH to extract the acidic furosemide (frusemide).
(ii) The extract is then made up to 500 ml with 0.1 M NaOH.
(iii) A portion of the extract is filtered and 5 ml of the filtrate is made up to 250 ml with 0.1 M NaOH.
(iv) The absorbance of the diluted extract is measured at 271 nm.
(v)   The *A* (1%, 1 cm) value at 271 is 580 in basic solution.

From the data below calculate the % of stated content in a sample of furosemide (frusemide) tablets:

- Stated content per tablet: 40 mg of furosemide (frusemide)
- Weight of 20 tablets: 1.656 g
- Weight of tablet powder taken for assay: 0.5195 g
- Absorbance reading: 0.596 (see Calculation example 4.2).

Calculation example 4.2

Expected content in tablet powder taken: $\dfrac{0.5195}{1.656} \times 40 \times 20 = 251.0$ mg

Dilution factor: 5 – 250 ml = 50

Concentration in diluted tablet extract: $\dfrac{0.596}{580} = 0.001028$ g/100 ml $= 1.028$ mg $= 100$ ml

Concentration in original tablet extract: $1.028 \times 50 = 51.40$ mg/100 ml

Volume of original extract: 500 ml

Therefore, amount of furosemide (frusemide) in original extract: $51.40 \times 5 = 257.0$

Percentage of stated content: $\dfrac{257.0}{251.0} \times 100 = 102.4\%$

Assay of cyclizine lactate in an injection

The steps in this assay are more difficult to follow since a number of extractions take place prior to preparing the final dilution, in order to remove excipients:

(i)   Dilute 5 ml of injection to 100 ml with 1 M sulphuric acid.
(ii) Add 2 g of sodium chloride to 20 ml of this solution and shake with two 50 ml quantities of ether.
(iii) Add 20 ml of 5 M sodium hydroxide and extract with three 50 ml quantities of ether.

(iv) Combine the ether extracts and then wash with two 10 ml quantities of a saturated solution of sodium chloride.

(v) Extract the ether layer with two 25 ml quantities of 0.05 M sulphuric acid and then with two 10 ml quantities of water.

(vi) Combine the acidic and aqueous extracts and dilute to 100 ml with water.

(vii) Dilute 5 ml of this solution to 200 ml with 0.05 M sulphuric acid and measure the absorbance of the resulting solution at 225 nm.

Calculate the percentage of w/v of cyclizine lactate in the injection from the following information:

- A (1%, 1 cm) of cyclizine lactate at 225 nm = 331
- Volume of injection assayed = 5 ml
- Measured absorbance = 0.413
- Measurements were made in a 1 cm cell.

Self-test 4.5

Calculate the percentage of stated content of promazine hydrochloride in promazine tablets from the following information:

(i) Tablet powder containing *ca* 80 mg of promazine hydrochloride is ground to a paste with 10 ml of 2 M HCl.

(ii) The paste is then diluted with 200 ml of water, shaken for 15 min and finally made up to 500 ml.

(iii) A portion of the extract is filtered.

(iv) 5 ml of the filtrate is taken and diluted to 100 ml with 0.1 M HCl.

(v) The absorbance is read at a wavelength of 251 nm:

- A (1%, 1 cm) value of promazine.HCl at 251 nm = 935
- Stated content of promazine.HCl per tablet = 50 mg
- Weight of 20 tablets = 1.667 g
- Weight of tablet powder taken for assay = 0.1356 g
- Absorbance reading = 0.755.

Answer: Percentage of stated content = 99.3

Calculation example 4.3

The first dilution is 5 ml to 100 ml ($\times$ 20). Then 20 ml of this dilution is taken and extracted with ether to remove excipients; the cyclizine remains in the acidic water layer since it is a base. After extraction with ether, the acidic layer is basified and the cyclizine is extracted into ether; it is then back extracted into 0.1 M sulphuric acid and made up to 100 ml; thus the dilution factor in the second step is 20 to 100 ml ($\times$ 5). Finally, a third dilution is carried out, in which 5 ml of the second dilution is diluted to 200 ml ($\times$ 40):

Total dilution: $20 \times 5 \times 40 = 4000$

For the diluted injection concentration: $\dfrac{0.413}{331} = 0.001248$ g/100 ml

Concentration in original solution: $0.001248 \times 4000 = 4.992$ g/100 ml

Concentration of injection = 4.992% w/v

Self-test 4.6

Determine the concentration of the following injections: *Isoxsuprine injection* is diluted as follows:

(i) Diluted 10 ml of injection to 100 ml and then 10 ml of the dilution to 100 ml:

- Absorbance reading at 274 nm = 0.387
- A (1%, 1 cm) value at 274 nm = 73.

Haloperidol injection:

(i) Add 15 ml of 1 M HCl to 5 ml of injection.
(ii) Extract three times with ether, washing the ether extracts with 10 ml of water.
(iii) Combine the aqueous layers and dilute to 100 ml.
(iv) Take 10 ml of the diluted aqueous solution and dilute to 100 ml.

- Absorbance reading at 245 nm = 0.873
- A (1%, 1 cm) value at 245 nm = 346.

Answers: Isoxsuprine injection = 0.530% w/v; haloperidol injection = 0.505 % w/v

Assay of penicillins by derivatisation (Fig. 4.12)

The BP utilises formation of a derivative in order to quantify penicillins in formulations. Some penicillins do not have distinctive chromophores; a further problem with these molecules is that when they are in suspensions they are not readily extracted away from excipients, since they are quite insoluble in organic solvents which are immiscible with water. Using the formation of a complex with the mercuric ion in the presence of imidazole as a catalyst, a derivative of the penicillin structure is produced, which has an absorption maximum between 325 and 345 nm. In the assay, comparison with pure standard for the particular penicillin is carried out rather than relying on a standard A (1%, 1 cm) value. This assay is used by the BP for analysis of preparations containing ampicillin, amoxicillin, carbenicillin, cloxacillin, flucloxacillin and phenoxymethylpenicillin. The assay is not used for the closely related cefalexins.

Fig. 4.12
Reaction of penicillins with mercury imidazole reagent.

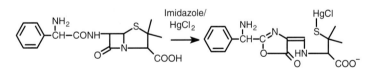

Ampicillin

λ max *ca* 325 nm

Calculation example 4.4

Cloxacillin injection is assayed using the mercury–imidazole reaction in comparison with a cloxacillin standard. The sample and standard were both diluted in 500 ml of water, and then 25 ml was taken from each of the solutions and was made up to 100 ml. 2 ml of the sample and standard solutions were then reacted with mercury–imidazole reagent. From the data below calculate the amount of cloxacillin per vial:

Weight of the content of 10 vials = 2.653 g

Weight of injection powder used for assay = 0.1114 g

(Continued)

Calculation example 4.4 *(Continued)*

Weight of cloxacillin sodium standard used in calibration solution = 0.1015 g

Absorbance of sample solution = 0.111

Absorbance of standard solution = 0.106

In this calculation the dilutions can be ignored since:

$$\text{Weight of cloxacillin in sample} = \frac{\text{Absorbance sample}}{\text{Absorbance of standard}} \times \text{weight of standard}$$

$$\text{Weight of cloxacillin in sample:} \frac{0.111}{0.106} \times 0.1015 = 0.1063 \text{ g}$$

$$\text{Contents of 1 vial:} \frac{2.653}{10} = 0.2653 \text{ g}$$

$$\text{Amount of cloxacillin in 1 vial:} \frac{0.2653}{0.1114} \times 0.1063 = 0.2532 \text{ g}$$

Assay of adrenaline in lidocaine (lignocaine) adrenaline injection

Adrenaline is present as a vasoconstrictor in some local anaesthetic injections in a much smaller amount than the local anaesthetic itself, which obscures the absorption of adrenaline in the UV region. The selectivity of UV/visible spectroscopy for the analysis of adrenaline can be increased by complex formation, which occurs between iron (II) and molecules containing a catechol group (Fig. 4.13). These complexes are purple in colour and absorb at *ca* 540 nm, at much longer wavelengths than, for instance, local anaesthetics, which do not form such complexes. The adrenaline in the injection is quantified against a standard solution of adrenaline.

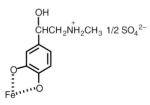

Adrenaline iron (II) complex

Fig. 4.13

The complex formed between adrenaline and iron, which is used to analyse adrenaline at low levels in an injection.

Self-test 4.7

Adrenaline in bupivacaine/adrenaline injection is assayed by complex formation with iron (II). 20 ml of the injection is mixed with 0.2 ml of reagent and 2 ml of buffer and a reading is taken in a 4 cm pathlength cell. A reading of a solution containing 5.21 µg/ml of adrenaline is taken under the same conditions. The following results were obtained:

- Absorbance of sample = 0.173
- Absorbance of standard solution = 0.181

Calculate the percentage of w/v of adrenaline in the injection.

Answer: 0.0005% w/v

Difference spectrophotometry

In difference spectroscopy, a component in a mixture is analysed by carrying out a reaction which is selective for the analyte. This could be simply bringing about a shift in wavelength through adjustment of the pH of the solution in which the analyte is dissolved or a chemical reaction such as oxidation or reduction. In the following example the selective alkaline shift of aspirin is used to determine it in a preparation also containing dextropropoxyphene, naphthalene sulphonic acid and caffeine. Caffeine, dextropropoxyphene and the naphthalene sulphonic acid anion do not undergo appreciable alkaline shifts whereas aspirin does. Figure 4.14A shows the spectrum of the extract from tablets in 0.1 M HCl – in fact there is relatively minor interference at the wavelength used for the determination of aspirin but by using the sample in HCl in place of a blank in the reference cell one can be sure that interference from the excipients is eliminated. Figure 4.14B shows the difference spectrum with the capsule extract in 0.1 M HCl in the reference cell and the capsule extract in 0.1 M NaOH in the sample cell. The absorbance at 299 nm is thus wholly due to aspirin. The problem remains of how to quantify the analyte in such a sample. This can be readily carried out using standard additions, which involves adding a known amount of aspirin standard to the sample and comparing the absorbance of the original sample extract with the absorbance of the spiked sample.

Fig. 4.14
UV difference spectrum used in the quantification of aspirin in dextropropoxyphene capsules.

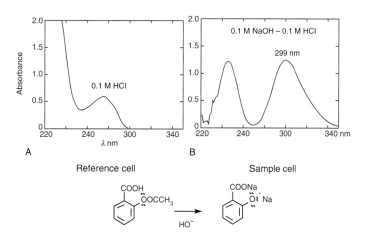

Analysis of aspirin in dextropropoxyphene compound tablets

Analysis was carried out by difference spectrophotometry. A one-point standard calibration for the determination of aspirin in dextropropoxyphene compound capsules was prepared by adding a known amount of aspirin to the sample from a standard stock solution. Stated content in the capsules: aspirin 250 mg, dextropropoxyphene napsylate 100 mg and caffeine 30 mg:

(i) 5 ml of the solution of sample in methanol is diluted to 500 ml with 0.1 M HCl: reference solution 1.

(ii) 5 ml of the solution of sample in methanol is diluted to 500 ml with 0.1 M NaOH.

(iii) 5 ml of sample solution and 5 ml of aspirin standard solution were mixed and diluted to 500 ml with 0.1 M HCl: reference solution 2.

(iv) 5 ml of the solution of sample in methanol and 5 ml of aspirin standard solution were mixed and then diluted to 500 ml with 0.1 NaOH.

Readings were taken at 299 nm of the sample solutions with and without standard addition against reference solutions 2 and 1, respectively. The following data were obtained:

- Weight of contents of 20 capsules = 10.556 g
- Weight of capsule content analysed = 0.1025 g
- Capsule contents were dissolved in methanol and adjusted to 100 ml
- Concentration of aspirin standard solution = 50.4 mg/100 ml
- Absorbance of sample at 299 nm in 0.1 M NaOH without standard addition = 0.488
- Absorbance of sample at 299 nm in 0.1 M NaOH with standard addition = 0.974.

Calculation example 4.5

In dilution (iii) aspirin standard solution is diluted 5 ml to 500 ml ($\times$ 100).

Concentration of aspirin standard in standard addition solution: $\dfrac{50.4}{100} = 0.504$ mg $= 100$ ml

The difference between the absorbance with standard addition and that without represents the absorbance due to a 0.504 mg/100 ml solution of aspirin.

Absorbance difference: $0.974 - 0.488 = 0.486$

Therefore, concentration of aspirin in the sample solution: $\dfrac{0.488}{0.486} \times 0.504 = 0.506$ mg/100 ml

Dilution factor for sample = 5 ml to 500 ml ($\times$ 100)

Concentration of aspirin in undiluted sample solution: $0.506 \times 100 = 50.6$ mg/100 ml

Volume of initial extract = 100 ml

Therefore, amount of aspirin extracted from the capsule powder = 50.6 mg.

Amount expected in capsule powder analysed: $250 \times 20 \times \dfrac{0.1025}{10.556} = 48.6$ mg

Therefore, percentage of stated content: $\dfrac{50.6}{48.6} \times 100 = 104.1$

Derivative spectra

Derivative spectra can be used to clarify absorption bands in more complex UV spectra. The technique is used extensively in the rapidly developing field of near-infrared spectrophotometry (see Ch. 5) and can also be applied in the determination of the purity of chromatographic peaks when they are monitored by diode array detection. The main effect of derivatisation is to remove underlying broad absorption bands where there is only a gradual change in slope. The first derivative spectrum is obtained by plotting, for instance, the slopes of 2 nm segments of the spectrum, and this results, as shown for a Gaussian band in Figure 4.15, in a spectrum where the slope is zero at the maximum of the peak and the slope is maximum at approximately half the peak height. In the second derivative spectrum the slopes of adjacent 2 nm segments are compared, and this gives the points of maximum curvature of the spectrum. The rate of curvature of a spectrum has its greatest negative value at its maximum and the greatest rates of curvature are observed for narrow absorption bands. Figure 4.15 shows the first, second, third and fourth derivatives of a Gaussian band.

Fig. 4.15
Derivatives of a Gaussian absorption band.

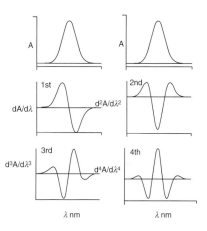

As would be expected, the first-order spectrum of pseudoephedrine, shown in Figure 4.16, gives maxima at the points where the slope is at a maximum in the zero-order spectrum. In addition, the second-order spectrum gives minima corresponding to the maxima in the zero-order spectrum, i.e. where the negative curvature of the spectrum is at its maximum.

By examining the UV spectrum of an elixir containing pseudoephedrine, dextromethorphan and triprolidine (30 mg, 10 mg and 1.25 mg, respectively) shown in Figure 4.17, it can be seen that the pseudoephedrine spectrum lies on top of a large background due to dextromethorphan and triprolidine, which have much stronger chromophores than pseudoephedrine. However, the underlying slope of the absorption curve due to contributions from dextromethorphan and triprolidine is shallow. The steepest underlying increase is due to dextromethorphan, which reaches a maximum at 278 nm. When the second derivative spectrum is examined, it can be seen that the only peaks derive from pseudoephedrine and, even where the dextromethorphan makes its maximum contribution at 278 nm, there is little absorption in the second derivative spectrum. Thus it would be possible to use the height of the pseudoephedrine peak to determine the amount of pseudoephedrine in the elixir with suitable calibration, e.g. standard additions of pseudoephedrine to the sample extract.

The signal:noise ratio is poorer in the second derivative spectrum because, through dividing the spectrum into segments in order to calculate the derivative, the underlying noise is less efficiently averaged out, which occurs when the spectrum is scanned in much narrower segments.

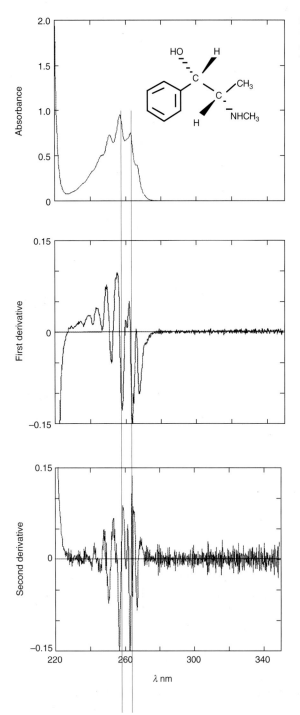

Fig. 4.16
UV spectrum of pseudoephedrine with its first and second derivative spectra. The minima correspond to the maxima in the absorbance spectrum.

Fig. 4.17
(A) UV spectrum of an extract elixir containing pseudoephedrine, dextromethorphan and triprolidine. (B) Second derivative spectrum of the extract. Note that the absorbance maximum of dextromethorphan disappears.

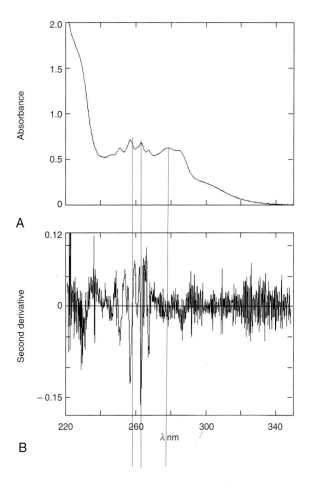

A

B

Applications of UV/visible spectroscopy in preformulation and formulation

UV/visible spectrophotometry is a standard method for determining the physico-chemical properties of drug molecules prior to formulation and for measuring their release from formulations. The type of properties which can be usefully determined by the UV method are listed as follows.

Partition coefficient

The partition coefficient of a drug between water and an organic solvent may be determined by shaking the organic solvent and the water layer together and determining the amount of drug in either the aqueous or organic layer by UV spectrophotometry. If buffers of different pH values are used, the variation of partition coefficient with pH may be determined, and this provides another means of determining the pKa value of a drug.

Solubility

The solubility of a drug in, for instance, water may be simply determined by shaking the excess of the drug in water or buffer until equilibrium is reached and then using UV spectrophotometry to determine the concentration of the drug that has gone into solution. Another method for determining solubility, where an ionisable group is present in the drug, is to dissolve varying concentrations of the salt of the drug in water and then add excess acid to a solution of the salt of an acidic drug or excess base to a solution of the salt of a basic drug, thus converting the drugs into their un-ionised forms. When the solubility of the un-ionised drug in water is exceeded, a cloudy solution will result and UV spectrophotometry can be used to determine its degree of turbidity by light scattering, which can be measured at almost any wavelength, e.g. 250 nm.

Release of a drug from a formulation

UV spectrophotometry is used routinely to monitor in vitro release of active ingredients from formulations. For simple formulations the drug is simply monitored at its λ max. In the example shown in Figure 4.18, the rate release of pseudoephedrine from a controlled release formulation was monitored.[1] The release of the drug was followed by monitoring its release into distilled water using a UV spectrophotometer set at 206 nm. In the example given in Figure 4.18, the particle size of the ethylcellulose used in the formulation affected the rate of release.

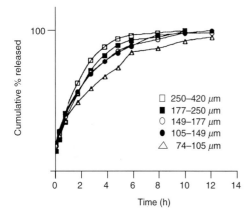

Fig. 4.18
Release of pseudoephedrine from a controlled release formulation.
Reproduced with permission from Kaitikaneni PR, Upadrashta SM, Neau SN, Mitra AK. Ethylcellulose matrix controlled release tablets of a water-soluble drug. Int J Pharm 1995;123:119-125.

If UV-absorbing excipients were present in such a formulation, the UV wavelength used for monitoring release would need to be selected carefully, or HPLC coupled to UV detection might be used. For such studies the sampling of the dissolution medium may be fully automated so that the medium is filtered and pumped through to the UV spectrophotometer at set time intervals in order to take a reading.

Q Additional problems

1. The BP assay for orciprenaline tablets is described below.
Weigh and powder 20 tablets. Shake a quantity of the powder containing 80 mg of orciprenaline sulphate with 50 ml of 0.01 M hydrochloric acid, filter and add sufficient 0.01 M hydrochloric acid to the filtrate to produce 100 ml. Dilute 10 ml to 100 ml with 0.01 M hydrochloric acid, and measure the absorbance of the resulting solution at the maximum at 276 nm. Calculate the content of orciprenaline sulphate taking 72.3 as the value of *A* (1%, 1 cm) at 276 nm.

The following information was obtained during the assay:

Weight of 20 tablets = 2.5534 g
Weight of tablet powder assayed = 0.5266 g
Absorbance reading = 0.5878
Stated content per tablet = 20 mg.

Calculate the % of the stated content of the orciprenaline sulphate in the tablets.

Answer: 98.56%

2. Calculate the content of methoxamine hydrochloride in an injection from the following information:
The assay was carried out by diluting 1 ml of the injection to 100 ml with water and 20 ml of the diluted injection was then diluted to 100 ml. An absorbance reading of the final dilution was taken at 290 nm with a UV spectrophotometer:

Absorbance of diluted injection solution = 0.542
A 1% 1 cm value of methoxamine hydrochloride at 290 nm = 137.

Answer: 1.978% w/v

3. Weigh and powder 20 tablets. Shake a quantity of the powder containing 20 mg of propranolol hydrochloride with 20 ml of water for 10 minutes. Add 50 ml of methanol, shake for a further 10 minutes add to produce 100 ml and filter. Dilute 10 ml of the filtrate to 50 ml with methanol and measure the absorbance of the resulting solution at the maximum at 290 nm. The assay of propranolol hydrochloride was carried out as described above. Using the following data calculate the % of stated content in the tablets:

Stated content per tablet = 10 mg
Weight of 20 tablets = 3.6351 g
Weight of powder taken for assay = 0.3967 g
A (1% 1 cm) at the maximum at 290 nm = 210
Absorbance reading obtained at 290 nm = 0.913.

Answer: 99.59%

4. Weigh and powder 20 tablets. Shake a quantity of the powder containing 20 mg of warfarin sodium with 250 ml of 0.01 M sodium hydroxide for 15 minutes and filter. To 20 ml of the filtrate add 0.15 ml of hydrochloric acid, and extract with three 15 ml quantities of chloroform. Extract the combined chloroform layers with three 20 ml quantities of 0.01 M sodium hydroxide. Dilute the combined aqueous layers to 100 ml with 0.01 M sodium hydroxide, filter and measure the absorbance of the resulting solution at the maximum at 307 nm. The assay of warfarin sodium was carried out as described above. From the data below calculate the % of stated content in the tablets:

Stated content per tablet = 3 mg
Weight of 20 tablets = 4.415 g
Weight of tablet powder assayed = 1.457 g
A (1%,1 cm) at the maximum at 307 nm = 431
Absorbance reading of diluted tablet extract at 307 nm = 0.6913.

Answer: 101.3%

5. Shake a quantity of cream containing about 7.5 mg of acyclovir with 50 ml of 0.5 M sulphuric acid. Shake well with 50 ml of ethyl acetate, allow to separate and collect the lower aqueous layer. Wash the organic layer with 20 ml of 0.5 M sulphuric acid, and dilute the combined washings and the aqueous layer to 100 ml with 0.5 M sulphuric acid. Mix well and filter. Discard the first few ml of filtrate and to 10 ml of the filtrate add water to produce 50 ml. Measure the absorbance of the resulting

(Continued)

Q **Additional problems** *(Continued)*

solution at the maximum at 255 nm. Using the data below calculate the %w/w of acyclovir in the cream:

Weight of cream analysed = 0.1564 g
Absorbance reading of diluted sample = 0.863
A (1%,1 cm) value at 255 nm = 562.

Answer: 4.91 %w/w

Reference

1. Kaitikaneni PR, Upadrashta SM, Neau SN, Mitra AK. Ethylcellulose matrix controlled release tablets of a water-soluble drug. *Int J Pharm*. 1995;123:119-125.

Further reading

Beckett AH, Stenlake JB. *Practical Pharmaceutical Chemistry, Part 2*. 4th ed. London: Athlone Press; 1988.

Clark BJ, Frost T, Russell MA. *Techniques in Visible and Ultraviolet Spectrometry*, Vol. 4. London: Chapman and Hall; 1993.

Rojas FS, Ojeda CB. Recent development in derivative ultraviolet/visible absorption spectrophotometry: 2004-2008. *Anal Chim Acta*. 2009;635:22-44.

www.spectroscopynow.com

The best web resource for spectroscopy. Contains useful links to tutorial materials and journals.

www.agilent.com

Many examples of applications of UV/visible spectroscopy and descriptions of instruments.

www.unicam.co.uk/com/cda/home

A wide range of instruments are made by this company.

www.anachem.umu.se/jumpstation.htm

Contains links to websites on different analytical techniques.

www.webanalytes.com

Contains links to websites providing information on different analytical techniques.

5 Infrared spectrophotometry

KEYPOINTS

Principles

- Electromagnetic radiation ranging between 400 cm^{-1} and 4000 cm^{-1} (2500 and 20 000 nm) is passed through a sample and is absorbed by the bonds of the molecules in the sample, causing them to stretch or bend. The wavelength of the radiation absorbed is characteristic of the bond absorbing it.

Applications

- A qualitative fingerprint check for the identity of raw material used in manufacture and for identifying drugs.
- Used in synthetic chemistry as a preliminary check for compound identity, particularly for the presence or absence of a carbonyl group, which is difficult to check by any other method.
- Can be used to characterise samples in the solid and semi-solid states such as creams and tablets.
- Used as a fingerprint test for films, coatings and packaging plastics.
- Can be used to detect polymorphs of drugs (polymorphs are different crystal forms of a molecule that have different physical properties such as solubility and melting point, which may be important in the manufacturing process and bioavailability).

(Continued)

> **KEYPOINTS** *(Continued)*
>
> **Strengths**
> - Provides a complex fingerprint which is unique to the compound being examined.
> - Computer control of instruments means that matching of the spectrum of a compound to its standard fingerprint can now be readily carried out.
>
> **Limitations**
> - Rarely used as a quantitative technique because of relative difficulty in sample preparation and the complexity of spectra.
> - Usually can only detect gross impurities in samples.
> - Sample preparation requires a degree of skill, particularly when potassium bromide (KBr) discs are being prepared.
> - The technique is lacking in robustness since sample handling can have an effect on the spectrum obtained, and thus care has to be taken in sample processing.

Introduction

The infrared region can be divided up as shown in Table 5.1.

Table 5.1 Infrared ranges

Ranges	Far infrared	Middle infrared	Near infrared
Wavelength range	50–1000 μm	2.5–50 μm	0.8–2.5 μm
Wave number range	200–10 cm^{-1}	4000–200 cm^{-1}	12500–4000 cm^{-1}
Energy range	0.025–0.0012 eV	0.5–0.025 eV	1.55–0.5 eV

The middle-infrared region is commonly used for structural confirmation, but near-infrared spectrophotometry, which has been used for very many years to control products such as flour and animal feed, is finding increasing applications in quality control in the pharmaceutical industry. For the purposes of explaining infrared spectroscopy, a molecule is viewed as being joined by bonds which behave like springs. If the simple molecule HCl is examined in the gas phase, it can be seen that it has an absorbance maximum at *ca* 2900 cm^{-1}, which results from the transition between the bottom vibrational state V_0 and the first excited state V_1 (Fig. 5.1). The spacing of the lower vibrational levels in IR spectrophotometry is equal, so even if the V_1–V_2 transition occurred, the energy absorption would be the same as for V_0–V_1. Quantum mechanics does not allow a V_0–V_2

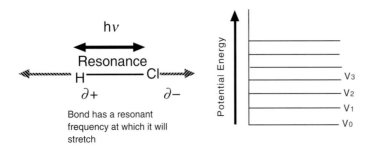

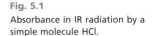

Fig. 5.1
Absorbance in IR radiation by a simple molecule HCl.

Fig. 5.2
Vibration modes of a methylene group.

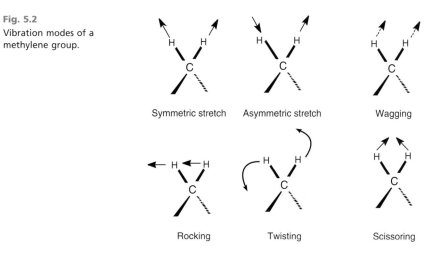

Symmetric stretch   Asymmetric stretch   Wagging

Rocking   Twisting   Scissoring

transition, although these types of transitions over 2 or 3 levels occur weakly and give rise to near-infrared spectra.

In order for the electrical component in electromagnetic radiation to interact with a bond, the bond must have a dipole. Thus symmetrical bonds, such as those in O_2 or N_2, do not absorb infrared radiation. However, the majority of organic molecules have plenty of asymmetry. Even in small organic molecules the modes of vibration are complex. This is illustrated by the vibrational modes which can occur in a methylene group, shown in Figure 5.2. The large number of bonds in polyatomic molecules means that the data obtained by IR analysis is extremely complex and provides a unique 'fingerprint' identity for the molecule. Quite a lot of structural information can be obtained from an IR spectrum, but even with modern instrumentation it is not possible to completely 'unscramble' the complex absorbance patterns present in IR spectra.

Factors determining intensity and energy level of absorption in IR spectra

Intensity of absorption

The intensity with which a bond absorbs radiation depends on its dipole moment. Thus the order of intensity of absorption for the following C–X bonds is:

$$CO > CCl > CN > CCOH > CCH$$

Similarly:

$$OH > NH > CH$$

The intensity depends on the relative electronegativity of the atoms involved in the bond.

Self-test 5.1

Predict the order of intensity of absorption of the following bonds:

(i)	(ii)	(iii)	(iv)	(v)	(vi)
C–OH	C=NH	C=C–H	C=C–OH	C–F	C=S

Answer: (v); (i); (ii); (iv); (vi); (iii)

The intensity of the stretching of carbon–carbon double bonds is increased when they are conjugated to a polar double bond, and such bonds in the A ring of the corticosteroids are quite prominent (e.g. see Fig. 5.12).

The order of intensity is as follows:

$$CCCO > CCCC > CCC—$$

Energy level of absorption

The equation which determines the energy level of vibration of a bond is shown below:

$$Evib \propto \sqrt{\frac{k}{\mu}}$$

k is a constant related to the strength of the bond, e.g. double bonds are stronger than single bonds and therefore absorb at a higher energy than single bonds. μ is related to the ratio of the masses of the atoms joined by the bond.

$$\mu = \frac{m_1 m_2}{m_1 + m_2}$$

e.g. for O–H bonds, $\mu = \frac{16 \times 1}{17} = 0.94$; for C–O bonds, $\mu = \frac{12 \times 16}{28} = 6.86$

where m_1 and m_2 are the masses of the atoms involved in the bond.

According to the μ term, the highest energy bonds are the X–H (OH, NH, CH). The order of energy absorption for some common bonds is as follows, which reflects μ and the strength of the bonds:

$$OH > NH > CH > CN > CC > CO > CC > CO > CC > CF > CCl$$

Instrumentation

Two types of instruments are commonly used for obtaining IR spectra: dispersive instruments, which use a monochromator to select each wavenumber in turn in order to monitor its intensity after the radiation has passed through the sample, and Fourier transform instruments, which use an interferometer. The latter generates a radiation source in which individual wavenumbers can be monitored within a *ca* 1 s pulse of radiation without dispersion being required. In recent years, Fourier transform instruments have become very common. A simple diagram of the layout of a continuous wave instrument is shown in Figure 5.3. The actual

Fig. 5.3
Schematic diagram of a continuous wave IR instrument.

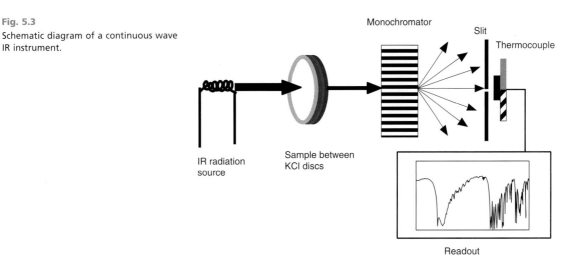

arrangement of the optics is much more complicated than this, but the diagram shows the essential component parts for a dispersive IR instrument. The filament used is made of metal oxides, e.g. zirconium, yttrium and thorium oxides, and is heated to incandescence in air. The sample is contained in various ways within discs or cells made of alkali metal halides. Once the light has passed through the sample, it is dispersed so that an individual wavenumber or small number of wavenumbers can be monitored in turn by the detector across the range of the spectrum.

In a Fourier transform IR instrument (see Animation 5.1), the principles are the same except that the monochromator is replaced by an interferometer. An interferometer uses a moving mirror to displace part of the radiation produced by a source (Fig. 5.4), thus producing an interferogram, which can be transformed using an equation called the 'Fourier transform' in order to extract the spectrum from a series of overlapping frequencies. The advantage of this technique is that a full spectral scan can be acquired in about 1 s, compared with the 2–3 min required for a dispersive instrument to acquire a spectrum. Also, because the instrument is attached to a computer, several spectral scans can be taken and averaged in order to improve the signal : noise ratio for the spectrum.

Fig. 5.4
Michelson interferometer used in FT–IR instruments.

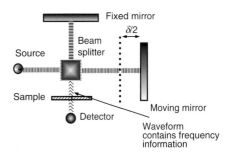

Instrument calibration

In order to ensure that instruments conform with BP specifications, the wavelength scale of the instrument is checked by obtaining an IR spectrum of polystyrene film (shown in Figure 5.5). Some of the bands used to check the accuracy of the wavelength scale of an IR spectrophotometer are shown in Figure 5.5. The permitted tolerances for variation in the wavelengths of absorption are mainly ± 0.3 nm. Two of the bands at 907 cm^{-1}, 1028 cm^{-1}, 1495 cm^{-1} or 1601 cm^{-1} (usually 1028 and 1601 cm^{-1}) are overlain onto standard BP spectra to indicate that the spectra have been obtained on a correctly calibrated instrument. In addition to specifying tolerances for the wavelength scale, the BP specifies the degree of resolution which the instrument must be capable of achieving, e.g. the maximum at 2849.5 cm^{-1} and the minimum at 2870 cm^{-1} should have a valley between them of $> 18\%$ transmittance. In Figure 5.5 the valley between the minimum and maximum at these two wavelengths is *ca* 25% transmittance. In addition, the difference between the percentage transmittance at the transmission maximum at 1589 cm^{-1} and the transmission minimum at 1583 cm^{-1} should be greater than 12.

Sample preparation

Traditionally three modes of sample preparation have been used prior to IR analysis:

(i)   The sample is run as a film sandwiched between two NaCl or potassium chloride (KCl) discs. For this method the sample must be a liquid, in which case it can be run without preparation, or must be ground to a paste in a liquid matrix, usually liquid paraffin (Fig. 5.6). In this case the liquid paraffin (Nujol) contributes some peaks to the spectrum at *ca* 3000 cm^{-1} and *ca* 1400–1500 cm^{-1}. However, sample preparation is relatively simple and this procedure is used where a chemist just wants a quick identification of certain structural features in a molecule. This procedure is also used to identify different crystal forms (polymorphs) of a drug because the pressures used to prepare KBr discs can cause polymorph interconversion.

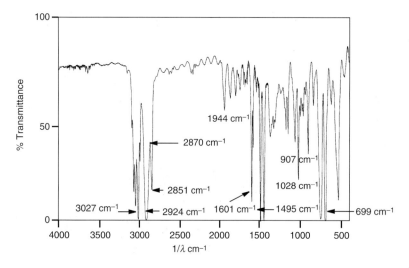

Fig. 5.5
IR spectrum of polystyrene film used to check instrument calibration.

Fig. 5.6
Preparation of samples as discs and mulls.

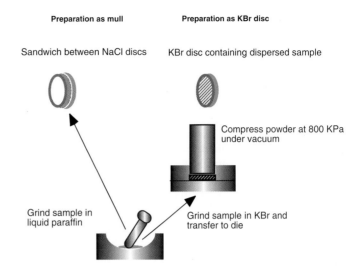

Preparation as mull

Sandwich between NaCl discs

Grind sample in
liquid paraffin

Preparation as KBr disc

KBr disc containing dispersed sample

Compress powder at 800 KPa
under vacuum

Grind sample in KBr and
transfer to die

(ii) The sample is ground to a powder with KBr or KCl. KBr is usually used unless a hydrochloride salt is being analysed, in which KCl is used to avoid halogen exchange. On a weight-for-weight basis, the weight of the sample used is about 1% of the weight of KBr used. About 200 mg of the finely ground powder are transferred to a die block and the sample is then compressed into a disc under vacuum by subjecting it to a pressure of 800 kPa (Fig. 5.6). This is the procedure used in pharmacopoeial methods to prepare a drug for analysis by IR.

(iii) IR spectra of liquids or solutions in an organic solvent, commonly chloroform, may be obtained by putting the liquid into a short pathlength cell with a width of *ca* 1 mm. Cells are constructed from sodium or potassium chlorides, and obviously aqueous samples cannot be used.

(iv) A more recent development in sample preparation is the use of diffuse reflectance (Fig. 5.7). Diffuse reflectance is a readily observed phenomenon. When light is reflected off a matt surface, the light observed is of the same intensity no matter what the angle of observation. Samples

Fig. 5.7
A simple diagram of a diffuse
reflectance system.

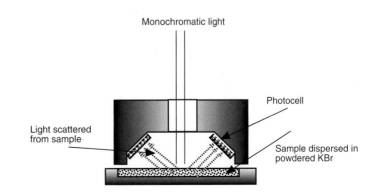

Monochromatic light

Photocell

Light scattered
from sample

Sample dispersed in
powdered KBr

for diffuse reflectance are treated in the same way as those prepared for KBr disc formation except that, instead of being compressed, the fine powder is loaded into a small metal cup, which is placed in the path of the sample beam. The incident radiation is reflected from the base of the cup and, during its passage through the powdered sample and back, absorption of radiation takes place, yielding an infrared spectrum which is very similar to that obtained from the KBr disc method. In fact, the spectrum produced is an absorbance spectrum rather than a transmittance spectrum, but it can be readily converted into a transmittance spectrum if the instrument is attached to a computer. The diffuse reflectance technique is widely used in near-infrared spectrophotometry and it can also be used to examine films and coatings if they are put onto a reflective background. It is also a useful technique for examining polymorphs since the sample can be prepared for analysis with minimal grinding and compression, which can cause interconversion of polymorphs.

(v)   Attenuated total reflectance (ATR) is another recent development in sample handling (Fig. 5.8). In this case the sample may be run in a gel or cream, and this method may be used to characterise both formulation matrices and their interactions with the drugs present in them. If the active ingredient is relatively concentrated and if a blank of the matrix is run using the same technique it may be subtracted from the sample to yield a spectrum of the active ingredient. ATR also provides another technique which can be used for the characterisation of polymorphs.

Self-test 5.2

Suggest methods for analysis of the following samples by IR spectrophotometry:

(i)   Pethidine.hydrochloride.
(ii)   Pethidine free base (liquid).
(iii) A cream containing 2% w/w salicylic acid.
(iv) A polymorphic form of a drug.
(v)   A plastic to be used in packaging.

Answers: (i) KCl disc or diffuse reflectance infrared Fourier transform (DRIFT) in KCl powder; (ii) Analysed as a liquid film between two NaCl discs; (iii) Analysis by ATR; (iv) Preparation as a Nujol mull to avoid interconversion of polymorphs or using DRIFT; (v) A sample of the film is inserted into the IR instrument

---

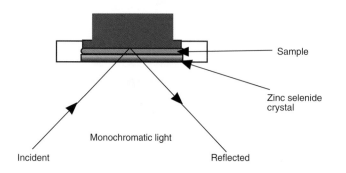

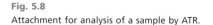

Fig. 5.8
Attachment for analysis of a sample by ATR.

Sample

Zinc selenide crystal

Monochromatic light

Incident   Reflected

Application of IR spectrophotometry in structure elucidation

As indicated earlier, the extent to which IR spectrophotometry can be used to elucidate structures is limited. The information given in Figure 5.9 is confined to the more easily recognisable bands in the IR spectra of molecules; this is to discourage the notion that IR is a technique used for extensive structure elucidation – in pharmaceutical analysis it is a fingerprint technique. The most readily assigned absorptions are usually at > 1500 cm^{-1}. The bands 1500 cm^{-1} are in the fingerprint region of the spectrum where the absorption is very complex, and it is difficult to be confident in the assignment of absorptions to particular functional groups. Fuller tables of the bands in the fingerprint region are given elsewhere,[1] and the present treatment is focused largely on the bands > 1500 cm^{-1}. Some additional important bands are listed in table 5.2.

Fig. 5.9

The major absorptions which can be observed in drug molecules. stg. = strong absorption; md. = medium absorption; wk. = weak absorption; brd. = broad; shp. = sharp; conj. = conjugated; v.brd. = very broad; A–F additional notes below.

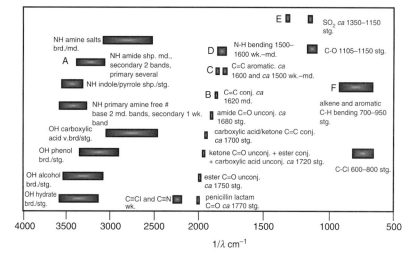

Table 5.2	Additional comments on IR bands in Figure 5.9
Band	**Comment**
A	Restricted rotation about N–CO bond produces diastereomers, giving two bands in the case of secondary amides; see spectrum of phenoxymethyl penicillin (Fig. 5.14)
B	C=C unconjugated gives a very weak absorption but, when conjugated, the C=C bond gives a much stronger absorption, found typically in many steroids
C	C=C aromatic: the band at 1600 cm^{-1} may be weak unless the aromatic ring is substituted with polar substituents, e.g. a phenol, aromatic ether or aromatic amine free base
D	N–H bend is often obscured by stronger aromatic C=C stretching bands
E	SO$_2$ bands: although this absorption is in the fingerprint region, these bands are quite prominent in sulphonamides
F	C–H bending in many cases is not very distinctive in drug molecules because of the complexity of the fingerprint region

Examples of IR spectra of drug molecules

Some examples of interpretations are given in Figures 5.10–5.14 and Tables 5.3–5.6. In the examples, only limited interpretation of the fingerprint region is attempted since assignments in this region are often not certain. Even above 1500 cm^{-1} it is sometimes difficult to assign bands; thus IR is not a primary structure elucidation technique.

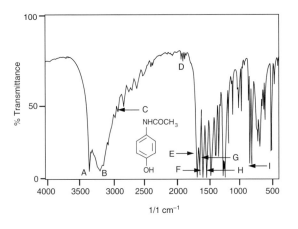

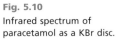

Fig. 5.10
Infrared spectrum of paracetamol as a KBr disc.

Table 5.3 Interpretation of the IR spectrum of paracetamol		
Wavenumber	**Assignment**	**Comments**
A 3360 cm^{-1}	N–H amide stretch	This band can be seen quite clearly although it is on top of the broad OH stretch
B 3000–3500 cm^{-1}	Phenolic OH stretch	Very broad due to strong hydrogen bonding and thus obscures other bands in this region
C *ca* 3000 cm^{-1}	C–H stretching	Not clear due to underlying OH absorption
D 1840–1940 cm^{-1}	Aromatic overtone region	Quite clear fingerprint but does not reflect 2 band pattern proposed for *p*-di-substitution[2]
E 1650 cm^{-1}	C=O amide stretch	C=O stretching in amides occurs at a low wavenumber compared to other unconjugated C=O groups
F 1608 cm^{-1}	Aromatic C=C stretch	This band is strong since the aromatic ring has polar substituents which increase the dipole moment of the C=C bonds in the ring
G 1568 cm^{-1}	N–H amide bending	Strong absorption in this case but this is not always so
H 1510 cm^{-1}	Aromatic C=C stretch	Evidence of a doublet due to interaction with ring substituents
I 810 cm^{-1}	=C–H bending	Possibly aromatic C–H bending but the fingerprint region is too complex to be completely confident of the assignment

Fig. 5.11
The infrared spectrum of aspirin as a KBr disc (see Animation 5.2).

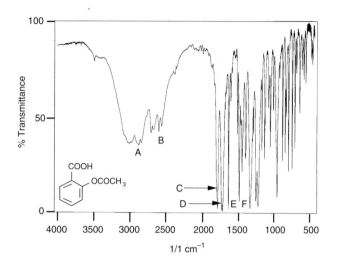

Table 5.4 Interpretation of the IR spectrum of aspirin

Wavenumber	Assignment	Comments
A 2400–3300 cm^{-1}	Carboxylic OH stretch	Very broad and complex due to strong hydrogen bonding. The broad band obscures other bands in this region
B *ca* 3000 cm^{-1}	C–H stretching	Not clear due to underlying OH absorption
C 1757 cm^{-1}	C=O ester stretch	Owing the acetyl group, which is an unconjugated aliphatic ester
D 1690 cm^{-1}	C=O conjugated carboxylic acid stretch	C=O of the acid is conjugated to the aromatic ring
E 1608 cm^{-1}	Aromatic C=C stretch	These bands are intense since the ring is substituted with polar groups
F 1460 cm^{-1}	Aromatic C=C stretch	

Table 5.5 Interpretation of the IR spectrum of dexamethasone

Wavenumber	Assignment	Comments
A 3140–3600 cm^{-1}	Alcoholic OH stretch	Broad due to hydrogen bonding
B 2750–3122 cm^{-1}	C–H stretch	Complex region due to the large hydrocarbon skeleton of steroid
C 1705 cm^{-1}	C=O unconjugated ketone stretch	Ketone at 20-position C=O stretch, generally lower than an ester C=O stretch
D 1655 cm^{-1}	C=O conjugated ketone stretch	Ketone at 3-position
E 1615 cm^{-1}	C=C conjugated	Strengthened by being conjugated to a C=O group. Tri-substituted C=C absorbs at a higher wave-number than di-substituted
F 1600 cm^{-1}	C=C conjugated	Strengthened by being conjugated to a C=O group. Di-substituted C=C absorbs at lower wavenumber than tri-substituted

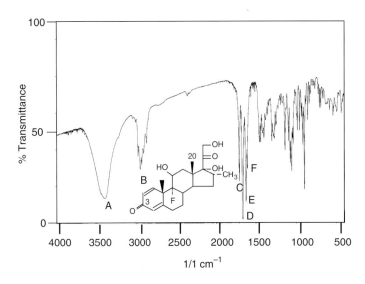

Fig. 5.12
The infrared spectrum of dexamethasone obtained as a KBr disc. Corticosteroids provide some of the best examples for the assignment of IR bands because of the prominence of the bands in their spectra above 1500 cm⁻¹. (see Animation 5.3)

The spectrum of dexamethasone obtained by the DRIFT technique is shown in Figure 5.13 and is very similar to that obtained using a KBr disc. However, the proportion of dexamethasone powdered with KBr and used to obtain the DRIFT spectrum was 10 times that used to prepare the KBr disc, which yielded the spectrum shown in Figure 5.12. As discussed earlier in this chapter, the use of DRIFT has some advantages over the preparation of a KBr disc.

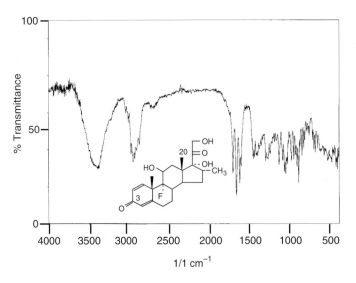

Fig. 5.13
IR spectrum of dexamethasone obtained using the DRIFT technique.

Fig. 5.14

IR spectrum of phenoxymethyl penicillin potassium obtained as a KBr disc.

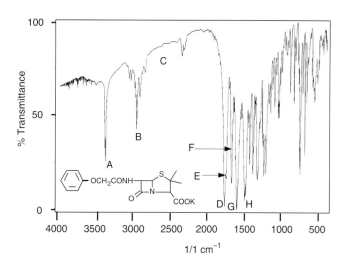

Table 5.6 Interpretation of IR spectrum of phenoxymethyl penicillin potassium

Wavenumber	Assignment	Comments
A 3360 cm^{-1}	N–H amide stretch	Two bands indicating restricted rotation about the N–CO bond, resulting in stereoisomers
B 2900–3100 cm^{-1}	C–H stretch	Aliphatic and aromatic C–H stretching
C 2400–*ca* 3000 cm^{-1}		OH stretch absent since the carboxylic acid is in the form of its potassium salt
D 1765 cm^{-1}	C=O lactam ring stretch	High energy C=O stretch typical of a lactam ring
E 1744 cm^{-1}	C=O carboxylic acid stretch	Salt, thus absence of H bonding means the stretch is of higher energy than in an acid. Compare with esters
F 1690 cm^{-1}	C=O amide stretch	
G 1610 cm^{-1}	C=C stretch	Aromatic ring stretch, broad band possibly obscuring amide N–H bend
H 1505 cm^{-1} and 1495 cm^{-1}	C=C stretch	Aromatic ring

IR spectrophotometry as a fingerprint technique
Preparation of samples for fingerprint determination

The majority of samples prepared for fingerprint determination in order to determine their degree of conformity with BP standards are prepared as KBr or KCl discs. The instructions with regard to sample preparation stipulate that 1–2 mg of the substance being investigated should be ground with 0.3–0.4 g of KBr or KCl. The KBr or KCl should be free from moisture. The mixture should be compressed at 800 kPa, and discs should be discarded if they do not appear uniform. Any disc having a transmittance < 75% at 2000 cm^{-1} in the absence of a specific absorption band should be discarded.

Self-test 5.3

Assign the bands A–E indicated in the spectrum of hydrocortisone.

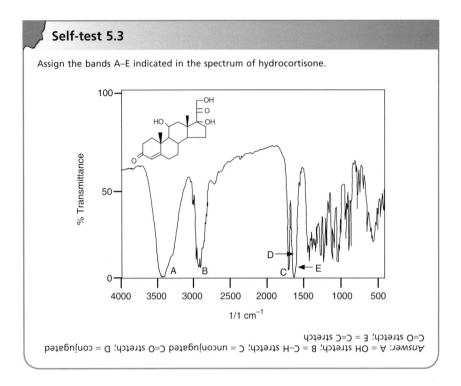

The instrument used to measure the IR spectrum should be calibrated using a polystyrene film. Formulations are usually extracted with a specified solvent, and it is stipulated that adequate spectra will be obtained only if excipients in the formulation are adequately removed. For pure substances, if difficulty is encountered with obtaining a fingerprint match to the BP spectrum of a reference standard for the substance being examined, the analysis should be repeated where the substance being investigated and the reference standard have been recrystallised from the same solvent. As can be seen in Figure 5.15, even closely related

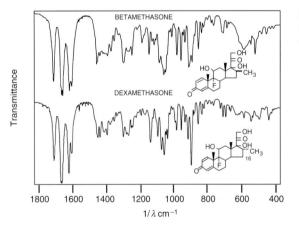

Fig. 5.15

Comparison of the fingerprint regions of dexamethasone and betamethasone.

compounds give different IR spectra in the fingerprint region. Dexamethasone and betamethasone only differ in their stereochemistry at the 16 position on the steroid skeleton. However, this small difference is great enough to result in a different fingerprint spectrum for the two compounds. There are even slight differences in the absorptions of the bands due to C=C stretching at 1620 cm^{-1}.

Self-test 5.4

Compare the fingerprint regions of the following spectra with the spectrum of paracetamol given in Figure 5.10. Which spectrum is due to paracetamol? Suggest what the structure of the unknown compound might be.

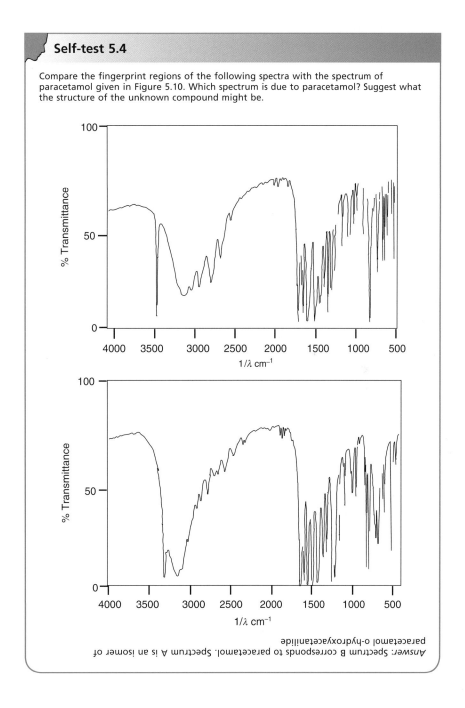

Answer: Spectrum B corresponds to paracetamol. Spectrum A is an isomer of paracetamol o-hydroxyacetanilide

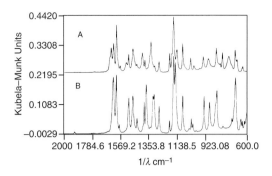

Fig. 5.16
Fingerprint regions of two polymorphs (A & B) of sulfamethoxazole. Spectra obtained by DRIFT. *(Reproduced with permission from Hartauer KJ, Miller ES, Guillory JK.* Int J Pharm. *1992;85:163-174.)*

Infrared spectrophotometry as a method for identifying polymorphs

IR spectrophotometry, along with differential scanning calorimetry and X-ray powder diffraction, provides a method for characterising polymorphic forms of drugs. The existence of polymorphs, different crystalline forms of a substance, has an important bearing on drug bioavailability, the chemical processing of the material during manufacture and patent lifetime. Until recently the standard method of sample preparation for characterising polymorphs by IR was by using a Nujol mull to prepare the sample. However, the DRIFT technique has an advantage since it does not introduce the interfering peaks which are present in Nujol and which may obscure areas of interest in the fingerprint region of the spectrum. In addition, low polarity samples may be soluble in Nujol, thus causing their polymorphs to break down. Figure 5.16 shows the spectra of the fingerprint region of two polymorphs of sulfamethoxazole prepared by powdering the samples with KBr and then analysing using DRIFT.[3] The units on the *y*-axis are Kubela–Munk units, which are an expression of the data obtained by DRIFT. These can be mathematically converted into transmittance or absorbance if required.

Near-infrared analysis (NIRA)

KEYPOINTS

Principles
- Electromagnetic radiation in between 1000 and 2500 nm is weakly absorbed by the X–H bonds of molecules, causing them to stretch. The wavelength of the radiation absorbed is characteristic of the bond absorbing it

Applications
- Quantitative analysis of multiple components in a sample and in pack quantification of drugs in formulations
- Fingerprint check for the identity of a drug and quality control of complex excipients such as lactose and cellulose used in formulation

(Continued)

- Determination of physico-chemical properties of drugs and excipients such as particle size, water content and polymorphism
- Determination of the physical properties of formulations such as blend uniformity and particle size

Strengths

- NIR radiation has good penetration properties and thus minimal sample preparation is required and thick sample layers can be used to compensate for the weakness of NIR absorption
- Intense radiation sources can be used since they can be protected by quartz envelopes, unlike middle-IR sources
- Has the potential to replace chromatography as a method for more rapid analysis of multicomponent samples

Limitations

- Extensive method development is required before the technique can be used as a truly rapid analysis technique. Development of a method requires a specialist operator with computing knowledge
- Instruments are expensive compared with middle-IR instruments

Introduction

The near-infrared region of the spectrum is generally defined as the wavelength range from 700 nm to about 2500 nm. The absorption bands in this region of the spectrum are due to overtones and combinations of fundamental mid-IR vibration bands. Quantum mechanical selection rules forbid transitions over more than one energy level. However, molecules do not behave as ideal oscillators, and anharmonic vibration enables overtone bands to occur at two, three, four times, etc. the energy level of the fundamental bands of the mid-IR region. Such overtone bands are *ca* 1000 times weaker than the bands seen in the mid-infrared region. Most of the useful bands in this region are overtones of X–H stretching. The NIRA technique was developed in the 1950s, but the paucity of structural information which could be obtained from it caused it to be neglected until the 1980s, when applications for it were found in the agricultural and textile industries. The strength of NIRA lies in the quantitative information which it can yield and its ability to identify constituents in multicomponent samples. The applications in quantitative analyses arrived with the ready availability of advanced computing facilities and this is the weakness of the technique, i.e. extensive software development has to take place before the spectral measurements yield useful information. However, it might be anticipated that increasingly sophisticated software will become available. NIRA has the potential to produce great savings in sample preparation and analysis and lends itself very well to process control. The technique is largely used in the DRIFT mode.

Examples of NIRA applications

Extensive use has been made of NIRA in agriculture, where it has been used to determine the protein, fibre, water and triglyceride contents of feedstuffs and the quality of crops. By training the computer to recognise the near-infrared (NIR) spectra of the major components making up a crop, the individual components can be monitored in the crop itself. The components that can be measured by

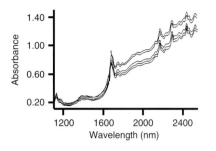

Fig. 5.17
NIRA of USP aspirin samples with decreasing particle size. *(Reproduced with permission from Ciurczak EW. Appl Spectrosc Rev. 1987;23:147-163.)*

NIRA often cannot be measured by the usual spectroscopic methods. The fundamental work done in the quality control of agricultural products can be readily extended to the quality control of pharmaceutical formulations.

Determination of particle size in United States Pharmacopoeia (USP) grade aspirin

It has been found that there is a linear relationship between NIR absorption and particle size. NIRA can provide a rapid means for determining particle size. Figure 5.17 shows the effect of particle size on the NIR spectra of USP grade aspirin;[4] the absorbance of the sample increases with decreasing particle size. Particle size is an important factor to be controlled in formulation and manufacture, and NIRA provides a rapid means for its determination. In order to validate such a technique it would have to be calibrated against one of the existing methods for particle size determination.

Determination of blend uniformity

NIRA provides an excellent method for the direct monitoring of the uniformity of blends when drugs are being formulated. Figure 5.18 shows the effect of blending time on the uniformity of a sample containing hydrochlorothiazide, lactose,

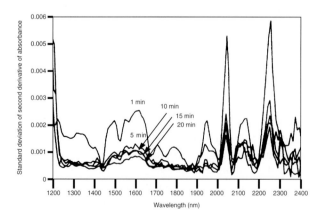

Fig. 5.18
The effect of differences in blend time on the uniformity of a formulation containing lactose and hydrochlorothiazide. *(Reproduced with permission from Wargo DJ, Drennen JK. J Pharm Biomed Anal. 1996;14:1415-1423.)*

magnesium stearate and croscarmellose sodium.[5] The most notable variations in absorbance intensity in the spectrum of the blend occur at 2030 nm and 2240 nm. Absorbance at these wavelengths can be attributed to hydrochlorothiazide and lactose, respectively. The more complete the blend, the less the standard deviations of the absorbances at these wavelengths obtained when several batches sampled at the same time point are compared. As would be expected, the standard deviations shown in Figure 5.17 decrease with blend time, but the decrease is less marked after 10 min. In this study it was found that blending for more than 20 min caused a loss in uniformity due to an alteration in the flow properties of the powder, resulting from a change in the distribution of the magnesium stearate. NIR probes can be inserted directly into blenders to monitor mixing.

Determination of active ingredients in multicomponent dosage forms

NIRA has been used to analyse multicomponent tablets, e.g. aspirin/caffeine/butalbarbital, and can examine such tablets in a pass/fail manner.[6] The tablets fail when the ingredients fall outside the specified range as shown in Figure 5.19, which is derived by the monitoring of two wavelengths in the NIR spectrum of the formulation. This might appear simple, but a great deal of development work was carried out in order to determine which wavelengths to monitor in order give the best discrimination.

In-pack determination of active ingredients

In clinical trials of a new drug it is important to ensure that the tablets have been packed and coded correctly. Figure 5.20 shows the absorbance of tablets monitored at a wavelength which can be correlated with the content of active ingredient.[7] It was possible to distinguish between tablets containing 0, 5, 10, 15 and 20% of the active ingredient. It was also possible to adapt the method to determination of the active ingredient of the tablets 'in pack' using a fibreoptic probe, although the precision was not quite as good as that obtained from the unpackaged tablets.

Determination of polymorphs

NIRA provides a non-destructive alternative to differential scanning calorimetry for the determination of polymorphic forms of drugs, e.g. the polymorphic forms of caffeine.[4] NIRA has also been used to determine optical purity. While the pure

Fig. 5.19

Application of NIRA to control of the ingredients in tablets containing three components. *(Reproduced with permission from Ciurczak EW, Maldacker T. Spectroscopy. 1986;1:36-39.)*

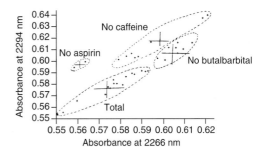

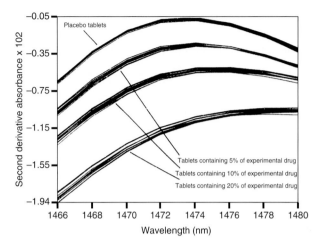

Fig. 5.20
Determination of the amount of active ingredient in tablets by direct use of NIRA. *(Reproduced with permission from Dempster MA, Jones JA, Last IR, MacDonald BF, Prebble KA. J Pharm Biomed Anal. 1993;11(12):1087-1092.)*

opposite enantiomers of a substance have identical NIR spectra, mixing two enantiomers together causes a change in the spectrum. Thus there is potential for determining the percentage of each enantiomer in an enantiomeric mixture and hence for the control of enantiomeric impurities.[4]

Moisture determination

Moisture determination by NIRA continues to be an area of interest. In a recent paper the determination of water in the anti-fungal compound caspofungin acetate was demonstrated.[8] The method used the chemometric method of partial least squares (PLS) analysis of the second derivative spectrum in order to develop a quantitative method for water in the samples. The NIRA method was validated against Karl Fischer titration. The water affects the whole spectral region between 950 and 1650 nm, and thus a method examining the effects of increasing levels of water on the whole spectral region was found to be robust. The PLS method uses broad bands of wavelengths to construct a calibration model. The statistical concepts are quite difficult to understand; however, a recent book[9] provides an excellent introduction to chemometrics, which is a subject of increasing importance in analytical chemistry.

Process control of components in a shampoo

NIRA was studied as a technique for process control in the manufacture of shampoo.[10] The formulation contained detergent, solids, water and glycerol. In order to carry out the process control, samples of shampoo were taken at various points in the production process. NIR reflectance spectra were obtained for 75 samples over the range 1100–2500 nm. A multiple step-up linear regression analysis was performed at nine wavelengths. This type of statistical test consists of multiple correlations of absorbances at different wavelengths with the concentration of the ingredients of the shampoo determined by classical methods. Correlation coefficients of 0.99 were obtained for water, solids and detergent, with a rather lower correlation for glycerol, which at 1% in the matrix was close to the limits of detection. The technique was deemed suitable for flow-through monitoring. The computer monitoring of the process by NIRA could be used to control actuators and valves within the chemical processing plant.

Additional problems

1. Four steroids (i), (ii), (iii) and (iv) correspond to the structures below (Fig. 5.21). The steroids are analysed by IR as KBr discs. The principal bands in their spectra between 1500 cm^{-1} and 4000 cm^{-1} are given below. Determine which of the structures given below correspond to (i), (ii), (iii) and (iv).
   (i) Steroid *ca* 3000 cm^{-1}, 1710 cm^{-1}, 1670 cm^{-1}, 1620 cm^{-1}.
   (ii) Steroid 3460 cm^{-1} (broad band), *ca* 3000 cm^{-1}, 1710 cm^{-1}, 1660 cm^{-1}, 1620 cm^{-1}, 1610 cm^{-1}.
   (iii) Steroid 2900–3500 cm^{-1} (very broad band obscuring other bands in this region), 1605 cm^{-1}, 1580 cm^{-1}, 1500 cm^{-1}.
   (iv) Steroid 3400 cm^{-1} (broad band), *ca* 3000 cm^{-1}, 1670 cm^{-1}, 1605 cm^{-1}.

Fig. 5.21

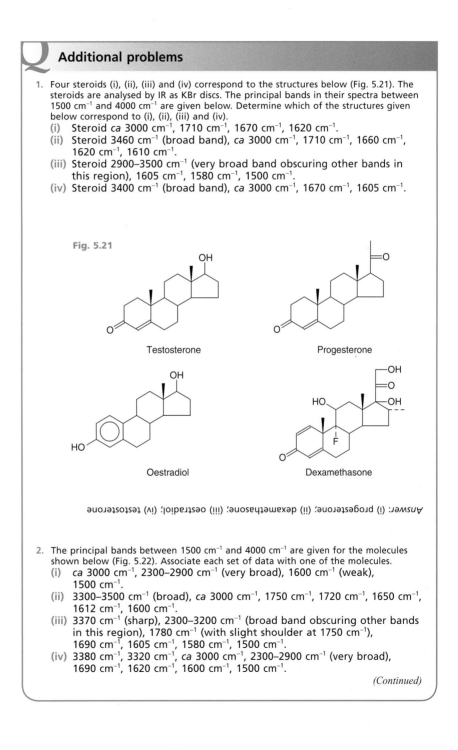

Testosterone

Progesterone

Oestradiol

Dexamethasone

Answer: (i) progesterone; (ii) dexamethasone; (iii) oestradiol; (iv) testosterone

2. The principal bands between 1500 cm^{-1} and 4000 cm^{-1} are given for the molecules shown below (Fig. 5.22). Associate each set of data with one of the molecules.
   (i) *ca* 3000 cm^{-1}, 2300–2900 cm^{-1} (very broad), 1600 cm^{-1} (weak), 1500 cm^{-1}.
   (ii) 3300–3500 cm^{-1} (broad), *ca* 3000 cm^{-1}, 1750 cm^{-1}, 1720 cm^{-1}, 1650 cm^{-1}, 1612 cm^{-1}, 1600 cm^{-1}.
   (iii) 3370 cm^{-1} (sharp), 2300–3200 cm^{-1} (broad band obscuring other bands in this region), 1780 cm^{-1} (with slight shoulder at 1750 cm^{-1}), 1690 cm^{-1}, 1605 cm^{-1}, 1580 cm^{-1}, 1500 cm^{-1}.
   (iv) 3380 cm^{-1}, 3320 cm^{-1}, *ca* 3000 cm^{-1}, 2300–2900 cm^{-1} (very broad), 1690 cm^{-1}, 1620 cm^{-1}, 1600 cm^{-1}, 1500 cm^{-1}.

(Continued)

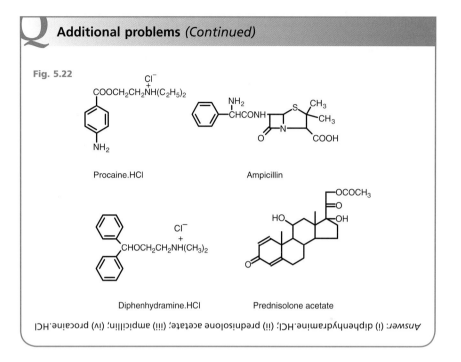

Additional problems *(Continued)*

Fig. 5.22

Procaine.HCl

Ampicillin

Diphenhydramine.HCl

Prednisolone acetate

Answer: (i) diphenhydramine.HCl; (ii) prednisolone acetate; (iii) ampicillin; (iv) procaine.HCl

References

1. Williams DH, Fleming I. *Spectroscopic Methods in Organic Chemistry*. 4th ed. London: McGraw-Hill; 1989.
2. Schrimer RE. *Modern Methods of Pharmaceutical Analysis*, Vol. 1. Boca Raton: CRC Press; 1991.
3. Hartauer KJ, Miller ES, Guillory JK. *Int J Pharm*. 1992;85:163-174.
4. Ciurczak EW. *Appl Spectrosc Rev*. 1987;23:147-163.
5. Wargo DJ, Drennen JK. *J Pharm Biomed Anal*. 1996;14:1415-1423.
6. Ciurczak EW, Maldacker T. *Spectroscopy*. 1986;1:36-39.
7. Dempster MA, Jones JA, Last IR, MacDonald BF, Prebble KA. *J Pharm Biomed Anal*. 1993;11(12):1087-1092.
8. Dunko A, Dovletoglou A. *J Pharm Biomed Anal*. 2002;28:145-154.
9. Brereton RE. *Chemometrics. Data Analysis for the Laboratory and Chemical Plant*. New York: Wiley; 2003.
10. Walling PL, Dabney JM. *J Soc Cosmet Chem*. 1988;39:191-199.

Further reading

Bunaciu AA, Aboul-Enein HY, Fleschin S. Application of Fourier transform infrared spectrophotometry in pharmaceutical drugs analysis. *Appl Spectrosc Rev*. 2010;45:206-219.

Bunaciu AA, Aboul-Enein HY, Fleschin S. Recent applications of Fourier transform infrared spectrophotometry in herbal medicine analysis. *Appl Spectrosc Rev*. 2011;46:251-260.

Karande AD, Heng PWS, Liew CV. In-line quantification of micronized drug and excipients in tablets by near infrared (NIR) spectroscopy: real time monitoring of tabletting process. *Int J Pharm*. 2010;396:63-74.

Komsta L, Czarnik-Matusewicz H, Szostak R, et al. Chemometric detection of acetaminophen in pharmaceuticals by infrared spectroscopy combined with pattern recognition techniques: comparison of attenuated total reflectance-FTIR and Raman spectroscopy. *J AOAC Int*. 2011;94:743-749.

Mantanus J, Ziemons E, Lebrun P, et al. Active content determination of non-coated pharmaceutical pellets by near infrared spectroscopy: method development, validation and reliability evaluation. *Talanta*. 2010;80:1750-1757.

Sasic S. Parallel imaging of active pharmaceutical ingredients in some tablets and blends on Raman and near-infrared mapping and imaging platforms. *Anal Methods*. 2011;3:806-813.

www.spectroscopynow.com

Good coverage of IR, NIR spectroscopy and also chemometrics.

http://www.ijvs.com/index.html

Website of electronic journal on vibrational spectroscopy. Useful articles both introductory and advanced. Strong focus on Raman spectroscopy.

http://www.spectroscopyeurope.com/

European Journal on Spectroscopy. Subscription to electronic journal is free.

Additional reading

Socrates G. *Infrared Characteristic Group Frequencies: Tables and Charts*. 2nd ed. Wiley Interscience; 1994.

Griffiths P, De Haseth JA. *Fourier Transform Infrared Spectrometry*. Wiley Interscience; 1986.

Murray I, Cowe IA. *Making Light Work: Advances in Near Infrared Spectroscopy*. Wiley Interscience; 1992.

Siesler HW. *Near-infrared Spectroscopy*. Wiley-VCH; 2002.

Journal of Near Infrared Spectroscopy.

Atomic spectrophotometry

Atomic emission spectrophotometry (AES)

KEYPOINTS

Principles

Atoms are thermally excited so that they emit light and the radiation emitted is measured.

Applications in pharmaceutical analysis

- Quantification of alkali metals in alkali metal salts, infusion and dialysis solutions.
- Determination of metallic impurities in some of the other inorganic salts used in preparing these solutions.

Strengths

- Flame photometry provides a robust, cheap and selective method based on relatively simple instrumentation for quantitative analysis of some metals.

Limitations

- Only applicable to the determination of alkali and some alkaline earth metals.

Introduction

Atomic emission spectroscopy plays an important role in the control of sodium, potassium and lithium in a number of raw materials and formulations.

Atoms contain various energy states, as illustrated in Figure 6.1 for the sodium atom. The normal unexcited state is the ground state. Sodium contains one

Fig. 6.1
Electronic transitions within a sodium atom giving rise to the main bands in its emission spectrum.

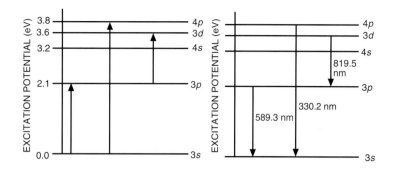

electron in its outer ($3p$) orbital, and, if energy is gained by the atom, this electron may be excited to a higher state and then subsequently lose its excess energy by falling back to a lower energy orbital. Thus, when a sodium salt is heated in a flame, the outer electrons in the volatilised atoms are excited and then return to the ground state with emission of energy, which appears, for example, as yellow light (wavelength 589.3 nm). The major line in the sodium emission spectrum (see Animation 6.1) is due to an electron falling from the $3p$ excited state to the $3s$ ground state; the atomic emission spectrum of sodium contains two other major lines, at 819.5 nm and 330.2 nm, due to the transitions shown in Figure 6.1. Atomic emission lines are very narrow (< 0.01 nm). Only a limited number of elements are sufficiently excited by thermal energy for AES measurements to be carried out. Common elements with emission lines suitable for utilisation in their quantitation are Ca, Ba, Na, Li and K.

Instrumentation

An atomic emission spectrophotometer (Fig. 6.2) (see Animation 6.3) is composed of the following components:

(i) **Flame.** The sample containing the metal is volatilised in a natural gas/compressed air flame at 2000°C. A higher temperature (2500°C) may be obtained using air/acetylene and is required for analysis of Mg by AES.

(ii) **Monochromator/Filter.** The radiation emitted by the excited atoms is passed through a filter, or a monochromator in more expensive instruments. Thus a narrow band of emitted radiation is selected and interfering sources of radiation such as the flame and other components in the sample are screened out.

Fig. 6.2
Schematic diagram of an atomic emission spectrophotometer.

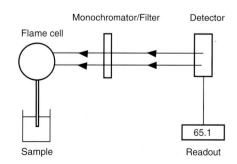

(iii) **Detector.** The intensity of the selected radiation is then measured using a photosensitive cell.

Examples of quantitation by AES

In order to measure a sample by AES, a calibration curve is constructed by aspirating solutions of known concentration into the flame.

Assay of sodium and potassium ions in an i.v. infusion

Standard solutions of sodium chloride (NaCl) and potassium chloride (KCl) in water were prepared and diluted appropriately to give a calibration curve across the working range across the range of the instrument (*ca* 0.05–1 mg/100 ml). The assay was then carried out by diluting the infusion until its concentration was close to that at the mid-point of the calibration series. Water is used as a blank. The following results were obtained:

(i) • Weight of NaCl used to prepare standard solution = 0.5092 g
   • Weight of KCl used to prepare standard solution = 0.1691 g. Both standards were transferred to the same 1000 ml volumetric flask and diluted to 1000 ml.

(ii) Dilutions were carried out on standards:
   • *Step 1*: 20 ml of the standard solution was transferred to a 100 ml volumetric flask and was diluted to 100 ml (diluted standard solution)
   • *Step 2*: A calibration series was prepared by transferring the following volumes of diluted standard solutions to 100 ml volumetric flasks 0, 5, 10, 15 and 25 ml.

(iii) The infusion solution was diluted as follows:
   • *Step 1*: 5 ml to 250 ml
   • *Step 2*: 10 ml to 100 ml.

(iv) The instrument was used with a sodium filter to establish the sodium calibration curve and then the sodium in the sample. The instrument was switched to a potassium filter in order to determine the potassium calibration curve and the potassium in the sample. Table 6.1 shows the readings obtained for sodium (Na) and potassium (K) in the calibration solutions as well as the concentrations of Na and K in the calibration solutions (calculated below). Calculate the concentrations of Na and K in the infusion solution in mmoles/l. Atomic weights: Na = 23; K = 39.1; Cl = 35.5.

Table 6.1 Data used in Calculation example 6.1

Amount of Na mg/100 ml	Flame photometry reading	Amount of K mg/100 ml	Flame photometry reading
0	0	0	0
0.2002	20.7	0.08923	22.4
0.4004	41.0	0.1785	41.2
0.6006	60.6	0.2677	61.2
0.8008	80.3	0.3569	80.3
1.010	100	0.4462	100

Calculation example 6.1

0.5092 g of NaCl/l is equivalent to $0.5092 \times \dfrac{23}{58.5} = 0.2002$ g of Na/l $= 200.2$ mg/l.

$= 20.02$ mg/100 ml.

0.1691 g of KCl is equivalent to $0.1691 \times \dfrac{39.1}{74.1} = 0.08923$ g of K/l $= 89.23$ mg/l.

$= 8.923$ mg/100 ml.

Dilutions of standards

Step 1: 20 to 100 ml ($\times$ 5).

Step 2: Point 1 $= 5$ to 100 ($\times$ 20).

Total dilution $= 5 \times 20 = 100$.

Concentrations in solution used for point 1.

$$\text{Na} = \frac{20.02}{100} = 0.2002 \text{ mg/100 ml} \quad \text{K} = \frac{8.923}{100} = 0.08923 \text{ mg/100 ml}.$$

The rest of the points in the calibration series are simply $\times$ 2, $\times$ 3, $\times$ 4 and $\times$ 5. These values give the concentrations in Table 6.1.

The equations of the lines obtained for the above data were:

For Na, $y = 99.0 \times + 0.722$.

For K, $y = 222 \times + 1.3$.

Reading of diluted sample for Na $= 70.2$. Reading of diluted sample for K $= 70.6$.

Dilution of sample

Step 1: 5 to 250 ml ($\times$ 50).

Step 2: 10 ml to 100 ml ($\times$ 10), total dilution $50 \times 10 = 500$.

Concentration of Na in infusion

Substituting into the equation of the line for Na.

$$\text{Concentration of Na in diluted sample} = \frac{70.2 - 0.772}{99.0} = 0.701 \text{ mg/100 ml}.$$

Dilution factor $= \times 500$.

Concentration of Na in infusion $= 0.701 \times 500 = 351$ mg/100 ml $= 3510$ mg/l.

$$= \frac{3510}{23} = 153 \text{ mmoles/l}.$$

Self-test 6.1

From the data given in Calculation example 6.1, calculate the concentration of K in the infusion.

Answer: 39.9 mmoles/l

Self-test 6.2

From the following data calculate the potassium content per tablet in effervescent KCl bicarbonate tablets.

- Weight of 20 tablets = 35.6751 g
- Weight of tablet powder taken for assay = 0.1338 g

The sample is dissolved in 500 ml of water and then 5 ml of the sample solution is taken and diluted to 100 ml.

- Weight of KCl used to prepare standard = 0.1912 g

The standard was dissolved in 100 ml of water and 5 ml of the standard solution was diluted to 250 ml.
The diluted standard solution was used to prepare a calibration series by transferring 0, 5, 10, 15, 20 and 25 ml to 100 ml volumetric flasks and making up to volume.
The following readings were obtained for the calibration series: 0, 20.3, 40.1, 60.3, 80.1 and 100.

- Reading obtained for potassium in the diluted sample solution = 73.9.

Answer: (From a computer-fitted calibration curve) K 496.2 mg per tablet

Interferences in AES analysis (see Animation 6.3)
Ionisation

At high flame temperatures, atoms such as K may completely lose an electron, thus reducing the observed emission from the sample:

$$K \underset{+e}{\overset{-e}{\rightleftharpoons}} K^+$$

Ionisation is an equilibrium and may be shifted to the left by addition of another readily ionised element to the sample, which produces electrons. The emission lines from the added metal are unlikely to interfere because AE lines are very narrow, and thus there will be no overlap, e.g. strontium chloride solution is added in order to suppress the ionisation of K in the BP assay of effervescent KCl tablets.

Viscosity

Organic substances in a sample can either increase or decrease the rate at which it is drawn into the flame relative to a standard solution by increasing or decreasing the viscosity, e.g. sucrose decreases the rate, thus giving a false low reading, while ethanol increases the rate, thus giving a false high reading.

Anionic interference

Anions such as sulphate and phosphate form involatile salts with metal ions and reduce the reading of the sample solution. These anions may be removed by the addition of lanthanum chloride, which precipitates them out and replaces them with the chloride anion.

Assays based on the method of standard additions

The method of standard additions can be used with many analytical techniques where interference from the matrix has to be eliminated and is of general use in residue or trace analysis. Essentially the technique involves addition of increasing volumes of a standard solution to a fixed volume of the sample to form a calibration series. An advantage of the technique is that, since several aliquots of sample are analysed in order to produce the calibration series, the method gives a measure of the precision of the assay. For example, five identical aliquots of sample solution are mixed with increasing volumes of a standard solution. If x is the amount of metal ion in the sample solution, the amounts of metal ion added should be *ca* 0, 0.5x, 1.5x, 2.0x and 2.5x. The calibration curve obtained will look something like that shown in Figure 6.3. The concentration of the metal in the sample is given by the distance between the origin and where the graph intersects the *x*-axis, i.e. the point where $y = 0$ in the equation of the line.

Fig. 6.3
A standard additions curve.

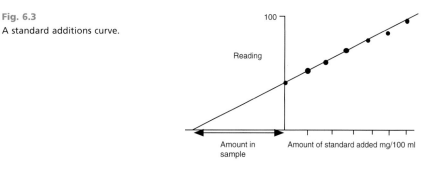

Assay for KCl, NaCl and glucose i.v. infusion

Analysis of the infusion was carried out using the method of standard additions, and the data below was obtained. From the tabulated data given below, plot a curve and determine percentage of w/v of NaCl and KCl in the infusion.

(i)   The following standard stock solutions were prepared in order to calibrate the instrument for sodium and potassium:
  • NaCl (0.2351 g) was dissolved in de-ionised water and the solution was made up to 1000 ml.
  • KCl (0.3114 g) was dissolved in de-ionised water, and the solution was made up to 1000 ml.

(ii) An aliquot (20 ml) of each stock solution was transferred to the same 100 ml volumetric flask, and the volume was adjusted to 100 ml with de-ionised water (diluted stock solution).

(iii) The sample of i.v. infusion was diluted by transferring 5 ml to a 100 ml volumetric flask and making up to volume with de-ionised water.

(iv) A calibration curve was prepared by transferring, in each case, 5 ml of diluted sample solution plus varying amounts of diluted stock solution to a 100 ml volumetric flask as indicated in Table 6.2 and then making up to 100 ml with de-ionised water.

Table 6.2 Results obtained from additions of Na and K

Volume of sample solution added	Volume of diluted stock solution added	Final volume	Reading of Na	Reading for K
5	0	100	26.1	30.1
5	5	100	39.3	45.2
5	10	100	54.2	58.8
5	15	100	69.2	73.1
5	20	100	84.1	87.0
5	25	100	100	100

Calculation example 6.2

Dilutions of standards

Initial concentration of NaCl = 0.2531 g/l = 253.1 mg/l = 25.31 mg/100 ml.

Dilution 1: 20 to 100 ml ($\times$ 5).

Dilution 2: Point 1 on calibration curve = 5 to 100 ml ($\times$ 20).

Total dilution = 5 $\times$ 20 = 100.

Concentrations in solution used for point 1.

$$NaCl = \frac{25.31}{100} = 0.2531 \text{ mg/100 ml.}$$

The rest of the points are simply $\times$ 2, $\times$ 3, $\times$ 4 and $\times$ 5, this value giving the following concentrations of added NaCl in the calibration series: 0.2531, 0.5062, 0.7593, 1.012 and 1.266 mg/100 ml.

The data were used to plot a calibration curve for NaCl.

Equation of line obtained for NaCl: $y = 58.57x + 25.09$.

When $y = 0$, the negative x value = concentration of NaCl in the diluted sample.

$$\text{Concentration of NaCl in diluted sample} = \frac{25.09}{58.57} = 0.4284 \text{ mg/100 ml.}$$

Dilutions of sample were 5 to 100 ml ($\times$ 20) then 5 to 100 ml ($\times$ 20) = $\times$ 400.

Concentration of NaCl in sample = 171.4 mg/100 ml = 0.1714 g/100 ml = 0.1714% w/v.

Self-test 6.3

From the data given above, calculate the percentage of w/v of KCl in the sample.

Answer: From computer fitting of calibration curve KCl = 0.2742% w/v

AES is used in pharmacopoeial assays of (1) Na in albumin solution and plasma protein solution; (2) K, Na and barium (Ba) in calcium acetate used to prepare dialysis solutions; (3) Ca in adsorbed vaccines (e.g. diphtheria and tetanus). It is also used to determine sodium and potassium concentrations in urine.

Atomic absorption spectrophotometry (AAS)

> **KEYPOINTS**
>
> **Principles**
>
> Atoms of a metal are volatilised in a flame and their absorption of a narrow band of radiation produced by a hollow cathode lamp, coated with the particular metal being determined, is measured.
>
> **Applications in pharmaceutical analysis**
> * Determination of metal residues remaining from the manufacturing process in drugs.
>
> **Strengths**
> * More sensitive than AES. A highly specific method of analysis useful in some aspects of quality control.
>
> **Limitations**
> * Only applicable to metallic elements.
> * Each element requires a different hollow cathode lamp for its determination.

Introduction

For many atoms the energy difference between their ground state orbital and the excited state is too great for thermal excitation of a significant number of electrons to take place. Where energy differences are too great to get an emission reading, AAS may be used. Metal atoms are volatilised in a flame and radiation is passed through the flame. In this case, the volatilised atoms, which are mainly in their ground state and thus not emitting energy, will absorb radiation with an energy corresponding to the difference between their ground state and the excited state (Fig. 6.4). The number of atoms in the ground state which are available for excitation is much greater than the small fraction that become excited and emit energy in AES. Thus AAS is a much more sensitive technique than AES. Since the width of absorption or emission lines in atomic spectra is extremely narrow, the only source of light where significant absorption can be observed, after it passes through the sample, is where the light is produced by excitation of the atoms of the element being analysed. The lamp used is called a 'hollow cathode lamp' and the cathode is coated with the metal which is to be analysed. For example, in the analysis of zinc (Zn), a Zn-coated cathode is used and the excitation of the Zn atoms produces a narrow band of radiation at 214 nm, which can

Fig. 6.4
Excitation of Zn by absorption of the radiation produced by a Zn-coated hollow cathode lamp.

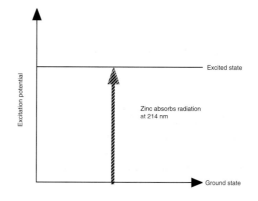

be efficiently absorbed by the atoms in the flame. The disadvantage of this is that the lamp has to be changed every time a different element is being analysed and only one element can be analysed at a time. Modern instruments have about 12 lamps mounted on a carousel, which may be automatically rotated into line with the flame and improve the speed of multi-element analyses. Further information on the technique can be found in the additional reading.

Instrumentation

An atomic absorption spectrophotometer (Fig. 6.5) consists of the following components:

(i) *Light source.* A hollow cathode lamp coated with the element being analysed.

(ii) *Flame.* The flame is usually air/acetylene, providing a temperature *ca* 2500°C. Nitrous oxide/acetylene may be used to produce temperatures up to 3000°C, which are required to volatilise salts of elements such as aluminium or calcium.

(iii) *Monochromator.* The monochromator is used to narrow down the width of the band of radiation being examined and is thus set to monitor the wavelength being emitted by the hollow cathode lamp. This cuts out interference by radiation emitted from the flame, from the filler gas in the hollow cathode lamp and from other elements in the sample.

(iv) *Detector.* The detector is a photosensitive cell.

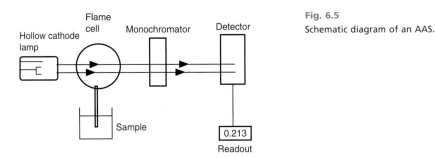

Fig. 6.5
Schematic diagram of an AAS.

Examples of assays using AAS (see Animation 6.4)

AAS is used principally in limit tests for metals in drugs prior to their incorporation into formulations. The sample is generally dissolved in 0.1 M nitric acid to avoid formation of metal hydroxides from heavy metals, which are relatively involatile and suppress the AAS reading.

Assay of calcium and magnesium in haemodialysis fluid

The calcium (Ca) and magnesium (Mg) in a haemodialysis solution were analysed using atomic absorption spectrophotometry as follows:

(i) Standard solutions containing Ca at a concentration of 10.7 mg/100 ml of water and containing Mg at a concentration of 11.4 mg/100 ml of water were diluted as follows:

(ii) Dilution: 10 ml of both solutions were transferred to the same 100 ml volumetric flask and diluted to 100 ml (diluted standard solution).

(iii) The calibration series was prepared by diluting the diluted standard solution with water as indicated in Table 6.3.

Note:

- The dialysis solution was diluted from 5 to 250 ml before analysis of Ca
- Atomic absorption reading obtained for Ca = 0.343
- The dialysis solution was diluted from 10 to 100 ml before analysis of Mg
- Atomic absorption reading obtained for Mg = 0.554
- Ca atomic weight = 40
- Mg atomic weight = 24
- Calculate the concentration of Ca in the dialysis solution in mmol l^{-1}.

Calculation example 6.3

Concentration of Ca standard solution = 10.7 mg/100 ml.

Initially both solutions were diluted 10 to 100 ml ($\times$ 10).

Thus the concentration of Ca in the diluted standard solution = 1.07 mg/100 ml.

For point 2 on the calibration curve, 5 ml of the diluted standard solution was diluted to 100 ml ($\times$ 20).

$$\text{Concentration of Ca used for point } 2 = \frac{1.07}{20} = 0.0535 \text{ mg/100 ml.}$$

Points 3, 4, 5 and 6 are $\times$ 2, $\times$ 3, $\times$ 4 and $\times$ 5, this value giving the following concentrations: 0.107, 0.165, 0.2140 and 0.2675 mg/100 ml.

In conjunction with the absorption readings these values were used to plot a calibration curve for Ca. The equation obtained for the calibration line was:

$y = 2.664\, x - 0.007$.

Reading for Ca in the diluted dialysis solution = 0.343.

From the equation for the calibration line, the concentration of Ca in the diluted dialysis solution = 0.1314 mg/100 ml.

The dialysis solution was diluted 5 to 250 ml ($\times$ 50) for Ca analysis.

Therefore concentration of Ca in the undiluted dialysis solution =

$$6.57 \text{ mg/100 ml} = 65.7 \text{ mg/l} = \frac{65.7}{40} \text{ mmoles/l} = 1.643 \text{ mmoles/l.}$$

Table 6.3 Data obtained from assay of Ca and Mg by AAS

Volume taken for dilution (ml)	Final volume (ml)	Readings for Ca dilution series	Readings for Mg dilution series
0	100	0.002	0.005
5	100	0.154	0.168
10	100	0.310	0.341
15	100	0.379	0.519
20	100	0.619	0.685
25	100	0.772	0.835

Self-test 6.4

From the data given above, calculate the concentration of Mg in the haemodialysis solution in mmoles/l.

Answer: From computer fitting of the calibration line Mg = 0.770 mmoles/l

Self-test 6.5

Zinc (Zn) is added to insulin to retard its rate of absorption into the bloodstream. The total concentration of Zn in Zn insulin suspension is determined by atomic absorption spectrophotometry. From the following data, calculate the total concentration of Zn in a Zn insulin suspension in percentage of w/v:

- Concentration of Zn in the standard solution used to prepare the calibration line = 50.5 mg/100 ml.
- Dilution 1:5 ml of standard solution was diluted to 500 ml with 0.01 M HCl (diluted standard solution).
- The calibration line was prepared as follows: 10, 20, 30, 40 and 50 ml amounts of diluted standard solution were diluted to 100 ml with 0.01 M HCl.
- The following absorption readings were obtained: 0.151, 0.313, 0.454, 0.605 and 0.755. 2 ml of the Zn insulin suspension (100 units/ml) was diluted to 200 ml with 0.01 M HCl, and the following reading was obtained: 0.595.

Answer: 0.019883% w/v

Some examples of limit tests employing AAS
Assay of lead in sugars

AAS is used in BP assays to conduct limit tests for lead and nickel in sugars and polyols. In this case, the concentrations of the metals are very low compared with the concentration of the sugar, and thus it is not even possible to compensate for the interference by the sugar using the method of standard additions. In this case, the lead is extracted from a solution of the sugar by forming an organosoluble complex with ammonium pyrrolidinedithiocarbamate (APDC) and by then extracting the complex into organic solvent. The solution of the metal complex in the organic solvent is then assayed by AAS in comparison with a series of standards added to the sugar solution to form a calibration series based on the method of standard additions.

A limit test for lead in mannitol (the BP limit is set at 0.5 ppm) was carried out as follows:

(i)   A solution containing 100 g of mannitol in 250 ml of water was prepared.
(ii) A standard solution containing 101.4 mg/100 ml of lead was prepared with 0.01 M HNO_3.
(iii) 10 ml of this solution was diluted to 1000 ml (diluted standard solution).
(iv) 4 × 50 ml aliquots of the mannitol solution were mixed, respectively, with:
      (a) 0, (b) 0.5 ml, (c) 1.0 ml and (d) 1.5 ml of diluted standard solution.
(v)   Each sample was then mixed with a solution of APDC, and the samples were extracted with 10 ml 4-methylpentan-2-one. The organic layer was then separated and analysed by AAS.
(vi) The following readings were obtained: (a) 0.057, (b) 0.104, (c) 0.156 and (d) 0.217.

Calculate the lead content in the mannitol in ppm: ppm = μg/g of substance.

Calculation example 6.4

Diluted lead standard solution contains $\dfrac{101.4}{10} = 10.4$ mg/100 ml $= 0.0104$ mg/ml $= 10.4\ \mu$g/ml.

101.4 g of mannitol were dissolved in 250 ml of solution; therefore in each 50 ml aliquot there was 20.28 g.

The amount of lead added to the four samples was 0, $0.5 \times 10.4 = 5.2\ \mu$g, $1 \times 10.4 = 10.4\ \mu$g and $1.5 \times 10.4 = 15.6\ \mu$g.

The equation for the line obtained by plotting amount of lead added against the readings is
$y = 0.010\ x + 0.054$ (r = 0.998).

The negative intercept ($y = 0$) gives the content of lead in the sample.

$x = \dfrac{0.054}{0.01} = 5.4\ \mu$g.

5.4 μg of lead is present in a solution containing 20.28 g of mannitol.

Lead content in the mannitol $= \dfrac{5.4}{20.28} = 0.266\ \mu$g/g $= 0.266$ ppm.

Self-test 6.6

The procedure used to determine lead in mannitol was also used to determine nickel in a sample of mannitol. Calculate the content of nickel in a sample of mannitol from the following data:

- 100.5 g of mannitol was dissolved in 250 ml of water.
- A standard solution containing nickel at 10.6 ppm (10.6 μg/ml) was used to prepare a calibration series by adding 0.5 ml, 1.0 ml and 1.5 ml of the standard to 50 ml aliquots of the mannitol solution.
- The following readings were obtained: 0.378, 0.543, 0.718, 0.891. Calculate the content of nickel in ppm in the sample of mannitol.

Answer: 0.58 ppm

Trace metals in a silicone foam cavity wound dressing

This expandable wound dressing is prepared by mixing a silicone elastomer with an organotin catalyst to form an expandable dressing immediately prior to application. Most of the tin is not extractable from the dressing matrix, but a limit test for extractable tin is carried out as follows:

(i) 5 g of dressing cut into pieces is shaken with 50 ml of 0.9% w/v sodium chloride for 4 h.

(ii) The solution is filtered and the tin is determined by AAS using a nitrous oxide/acetylene flame and measuring the absorption at 235.5 nm. The limit set for the tin is 6 ppm (6 μg/g).

(iii) The same solution is used to determine whether the sample passes 5 ppm limits for cadmium, copper, lead and zinc but using an air/acetylene flame and using the lamps appropriate for the detection of these elements.

Applications of AAS in BP assays

AAS is used in a number of limit tests for metallic impurities, e.g. magnesium and strontium in calcium acetate, palladium in carbenicillin sodium and lead in bismuth subgallate. It is also used to assay metals in a number of other preparations: zinc in zinc insulin suspension and tetracosactrin zinc injection; copper and iron in ascorbic acid; zinc in acetylcysteine; lead in bismuth subcarbonate; silver in cisplatinum; lead in oxprenolol; aluminium in albumin solution and calcium, magnesium, mercury and zinc in water used for diluting haemodialysis solutions.

Inductively coupled plasma emission spectroscopy

If high enough temperatures can be reached, any element can be excited to a level where it will produce emission of radiation. Such high temperatures can be achieved by using plasma emission. A schematic diagram of an inductively coupled plasma (ICP) 'torch' is shown in Figure 6.6.

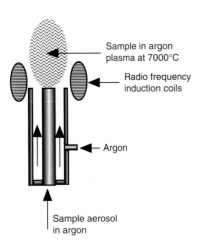

Sample in argon plasma at 7000°C

Radio frequency induction coils

Argon

Sample aerosol in argon

Fig. 6.6
Schematic diagram of an ICP torch.

High temperatures are achieved by heating argon with high-intensity radio-frequency radiation. At such high temperatures all elements will emit radiation as they are excited and then return to the ground state. In order to derive spectral information from the process, an efficient monochromator and computer processing of the data are required in order to unscramble the large number of lines that are derived from a particular sample. ICP has been used to determine a complex of the metal ion dysprosium, which is used as a magnetic resonance imaging contrast agent, in serum.[1]

ICP has potential as a tool for providing rapid analysis of active ingredients because of its high sensitivity and specificity. Recently an ICP method was developed for the analysis of the calcium salt of an investigational drug.[2] The short analysis time required to carry out ICP analysis, in comparison with an HPLC method, was advantageous during formulation development, where it is necessary to have a method which can assess a process quickly.

References

1. Lai J-J, Jamieson GC. *J Pharm Biomed Anal*. 1993;11:1129-1134.
2. Whang L, Marley M, Jahansouz H, Bahnck C. *J Pharm Biomed Anal*. 2003;33:955-961.

Further reading

Beckett AH, Stenlake J, eds. *Practical Pharmaceutical Chemistry*. Vol. 2. London: Athlone Press; 1988.

Dean JR, Ando DJ, eds. *Atomic Absorption and Plasma Spectroscopy*. 2nd ed. Chichester: J. Wiley and Sons; 1997.

Evans EH, Day JA, Palmer C, Smith CMM. Advances in atomic spectrometry and related techniques. *J Anal At Spectrom*. 2010;25:760-784.

Evans EH, Day JA, Palmer CD, Smith CMM. Advances in atomic spectrometry and related techniques. *J Anal At Spectrom*. 2011;26:1115-1141.

Jenniss SW, Katz SA, Lynch RW, eds. *Applications of Atomic Spectrometry to Regulatory Compliance Monitoring*. 2nd ed. Chichester: A Wiley-VCH Publication; 1997.

Contains information on AAS and ICP.

www.spectroscopynow.com

Molecular emission spectroscopy

7

Fluorescence spectrophotometry

KEYPOINTS

Principles
- Certain molecules, particularly those with a chromophore and a rigid structure, can be excited by UV/visible radiation, and will then emit the radiation absorbed at a longer wavelength. The radiation emitted can then be measured

Applications
- Determination of fluorescent drugs in low-dose formulations in the presence of non-fluorescent excipients
- In carrying out limit tests where the impurity is fluorescent or can be simply rendered fluorescent
- Useful for studying the binding of drugs to components in complex formulations
- Widely used in bioanalysis for measuring small amounts of drugs and for studying drug-protein binding

Strengths
- A selective detection method and can be used to quantify a strongly fluorescent compound in the presence of a larger amount of non-fluorescent material
- Can be used to monitor changes in complex molecules such as proteins, which are being used increasingly as drugs

Limitations
- The technique applies only to a limited number of molecules
- Fluorescence is subject to interference by UV-absorbing species and heavy ions in solution and is affected by temperature

Introduction

Figure 7.1 illustrates the behaviour of an excited electron in a fluorescent molecule. In a non-fluorescent molecule, when an electron is excited to the electronic excited state, it returns back to the ground state by losing the energy it has acquired through conversion of the excess electronic energy into vibrational energy. If a molecule has a rigid structure, the loss of electronic energy through its conversion into vibrational energy is relatively slow, and there is a chance for the electronic energy to be emitted as ultraviolet (UV) or visible radiation. The energy emitted is of lower energy than the energy absorbed because, as indicated in Figure 7.1, the excited electron moves to the lowest energy vibrational state in the excited state before returning to the ground state. Thus fluorescence emission is typically shifted by 50–150 nm toward a longer wavelength in comparison with the wavelength of the radiation used to produce excitation. The fluorescence spectrum of a molecule is, ideally, a mirror image of the longest wavelength band in the absorption spectrum of the molecule, but often the spectrum is distorted due to partial overlap between the absorption and the emission spectra. Vibrational fine structure of the fluorescence band may be observed if the molecule does not interact with the solvent strongly (cf. UV spectra) and can be observed in the fluorescence spectra of polycyclic aromatic hydrocarbons such as anthracene. The shape of the fluorescence spectrum is independent of the wavelength used for excitation, since the transition producing the fluorescence spectrum is always from the first excited state to the ground state. In a molecule containing a number of UV absorption bands, the longest wavelength maximum is the one associated most strongly with the production of fluorescence. In addition, the wavelength usually used to produce excitation is close to the λ max of the longest wavelength absorption band in the spectrum of the analyte.

Instrumentation

Figure 7.2 shows a schematic diagram of a fluorescence spectrophotometer. Since emission is being observed, the light being emitted is observed at right angles to the light being used to excite the sample.

The instrument has two monochromators: one to select the wavelength to be used for excitation of the sample, the other to scan the wavelength range of the light emitted by the sample.

Fig. 7.1

Energy changes upon absorption of UV/visible radiation resulting in fluorescence.

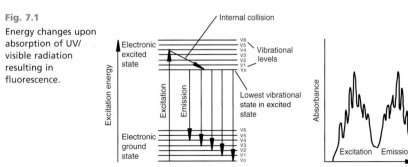

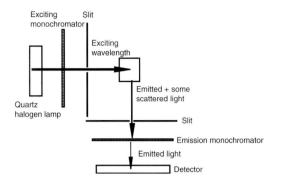

Fig. 7.2
Schematic diagram of monochromator fluorescence spectrophotometer.

The lamp used, which is a quartz halogen lamp or xenon, produces radiation of high intensity to take advantage of the fact that the strength of the fluorescence is related to the number of photons absorbed multiplied by the fluorescence quantum yield (ϕ). For strongly fluorescent compounds, ϕ is close to 1; for non-fluorescent compounds, $\phi = 0$. The wavelength which gives maximum excitation is not necessarily exactly the same as the longest wavelength absorbance maximum in the compound, since the intensity of light emitted by the quartz halogen lamp varies markedly with wavelength, unlike the deuterium and tungsten lamps used in UV/visible spectrophotometers. The lamp gives radiation of maximum intensity between 300 and 400 nm. (see Animation 7.1)

Although the radiation emitted is observed at right angles to the exciting radiation, some of the exciting radiation can be detected by the emission detector because it is scattered by solvent molecules (Rayleigh scatter) or by colloidal particles in solution (Tyndall scatter). The presence of this scatter makes the use of the second monochromator necessary and also means that, for fluorescence measurements to be made without interference, the fluorescence band has to be shifted by at least 20 nm beyond the excitation band. Another, weaker, type of scatter which may be observed is Raman scatter. In Raman scatter, which is solvent dependent, the wavelength of the incident radiation is shifted to a longer wavelength by about 30 nm when methanol is used as a solvent and about 10 nm when chloroform is used as a solvent. Raman scatter is discussed in more detail later in this chapter.

Molecules which exhibit fluorescence

It is not entirely possible to predict how strongly fluorescent a molecule will be. For example, adrenaline and noradrenaline differ in their structures by only a single methyl group, but noradrenaline exhibits fluorescence nearly 20 times more intensely than adrenaline. Generally, fluorescence is associated with an extended chromophore/auxochrome system and a rigid structure. Quinine (Fig. 7.3) is an example of a strongly fluorescent molecule, as might be expected from its extended chromophore and rigid structure. The chromophore in ethinylestradiol is just an aromatic ring, but the presence of a phenolic hydroxyl group in combination with a rigid ring structure in the rest of the molecule renders it fluorescent (Fig. 7.3).

Fig. 7.3
Examples of
fluorescent
molecules.

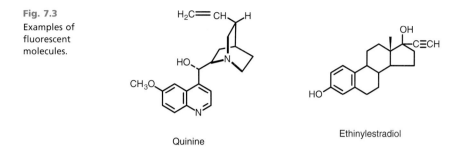

Quinine

Ethinylestradiol

Figure 7.4 shows the fluorescence spectrum of ethinylestradiol. When the fluorescence spectrum of the molecule is scanned with a wavelength of 285 nm being used for excitation, two maxima are seen. The maximum at 285 nm is due to scatter of the exciting radiation, and the second, more intense, maximum at 310 nm is due to fluorescence. The separation of the exciting radiation and emitted radiation is not great in this example, but this is partly because excitation is taking place at a relatively short wavelength, where the displacement of wavelength with energy is lower. For example, the difference between 285 and 310 nm is 0.35 eV, whereas with an excitation wavelength at 385 nm, an energy displacement of 0.35 eV would give an emission wavelength at 443 nm.

Like ethinylestradiol, many other phenols exhibit fluorescence, and, as is the case for ethinylestradiol, this fluorescence is pH dependent and does not occur under alkaline conditions, when the phenolic group becomes ionised. Table 7.1 shows some examples of fluorescent drug and vitamin molecules.

Fig. 7.4
Fluorescence spectrum of a
20 μg/ml solution of
ethinylestradiol.

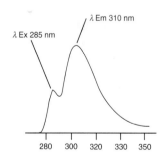

λ Em 310 nm

λ Ex 285 nm

280   300   320   330   350

Table 7.1 Examples of drugs which yield fluorescence spectra			
Compound	**Excitation**	**Emission**	**Limit of detection (μg/ml)**
Pentobarbitone	265	440	0.1
Adrenaline	295	335	0.1
Chlorpromazine	350	480	0.1
Riboflavin	444	520	0.01
Procaine	275	245	0.01
Noradrenaline	285	325	0.006
Quinine	350	450	0.002

Factors interfering with fluorescence intensity

If the concentration of a solution prepared for fluorescence measurement is too high, some of the light emitted by the sample as fluorescence will be reabsorbed by other unexcited molecules in solution. For this reason, fluorescence measurements are best made on solutions with an absorbance of less than 0.02 at their maximum, i.e. solutions of a sample 10–100 times weaker than those which would be used for measurement by UV spectrophotometry.

Heavy atoms in solution quench fluorescence by colliding with excited molecules so that their energy is dissipated; e.g. chloride or bromide ions in solution cause collisional quenching.

Formation of a chemical complex with other molecules in solution can change fluorescence behaviour; e.g. the presence of caffeine in solution reduces the fluorescence of riboflavin. This alteration of fluorescence upon binding is used to advantage when examining binding of fluorescent molecules to proteins or other constituents of cells.

Fluorescence is also temperature dependent, since temperature can promote the loss of excitation by collision and bond vibration. A molecule that is not fluorescent at room temperature may become fluorescent at lower temperatures. In addition, more viscous solvents tend to promote fluorescence.

Applications of fluorescence spectrophotometry in pharmaceutical analysis

Determination of ethinylestradiol in tablets

The British Pharmacopoeia utilises a fluorescence assay to determine ethinylestradiol in tablets. The tablets contain low dosages of the drug, so interference by excipients is likely to cause problems in UV/visible spectrophotometric measurements. The sample is measured using an excitation wavelength of 280 nm and measuring the emission at 320 nm. As was seen when the fluorescence spectrum of ethinylestradiol was discussed earlier, the optimum excitation wavelength for ethinylestradiol is 285 nm and the emission maximum is 310 nm. Thus, this assay as described brings out two important points, which may have been either consciously or empirically adjusted for in the design of the assay:

(i) The use of a slightly shorter excitation wavelength reduces possible interference from Raman scatter, which may overlap with the fluorescence spectrum and is dependent on the wavelength of the exciting radiation, whereas the fluorescence maximum is not.

(ii) The intensity of Rayleigh and Tyndall scatter at shorter wavelengths is greater, and thus the emission is observed at the slightly longer wavelength of 320 nm to reduce interference from this source.

After the fluorescence of the sample extract in methanol has been determined, 1 M sodium hydroxide solution is added to the sample solution and the fluorescence is determined again. The addition of sodium hydroxide removes the fluorescence by ionising the phenol group of the ethinylestradiol, and thus any residual fluorescence which is due to excipients can be subtracted from the reading. In the BP assay, the ethinylestradiol content of the tablet extract is determined by comparison with the fluorescence of a solution containing a known amount of ethinylestradiol standard analysed using the same conditions.

Calculation example 7.1

A methanolic extract from ethinylestradiol tablets is measured using fluorescence spectrophotometry. A standard containing the pure drug is also measured under the same conditions. Calculate the content per tablet of the drug from the following data:

Weight of 20 tablets = 2.5673 g

Weight of tablet powder taken for assay = 0.5257 g

Volume of methanol extract of tablets = 50 ml

Fluorescence reading of methanol extract of tablets = 64.1

Fluorescence reading of sample after addition of 0.1 M NaOH = 3.5

Concentration of standard solution of ethinylestradiol = 4.85 μg/ml

Fluorescence reading of standard solution = 62.3

Fluorescence reading of standard solution after addition of 0.1 M NaOH = 4.1

Corrected reading for tablet extract = 64.1 − 3.5 = 60.6

Corrected reading for standard = 62.3 − 4.1 = 58.2

Amount of ethinylestradiol in tablet extract = 60.2/58.2 × 4.85 = 5.02 μg/ml

Total amount in extract = 50 × 5.02 = 251 μg

Number of tablets in tablet powder analysed = 2.5673/0.5257 = 4.884

Content of ethinylestradiol per tablet = 251/4.885 = 51.4 μg

Determination of the dissolution rate of digoxin tablets

Some compounds which are not naturally fluorescent can be rendered fluorescent by simple chemical reactions. For instance, digoxin can be converted to a fluorescent derivative by dehydration with HCl, followed by oxidation with H_2O_2. The drug has a narrow therapeutic index and it is important to ensure that the correct dose of drug is delivered by the dosage form. To ensure effective release of the drug from the tablet matrix, the BP indicates that dissolution testing should be carried out. The drug is given in low dosage (*ca* 100 μg per tablet), making measurement of the concentration released into the dissolution medium difficult. The BP assay for release indicates that 75% of the drug from six tablets should be released into 600 ml of dissolution medium after 2 h. The fluorescence measurements are made on the dissolution medium after derivative formation using an excitation wavelength of 360 nm and an emission wavelength of 490 nm. The drug in solution is quantified in comparison with a solution containing a known concentration of standard treated in the same way as the sample.

Determination of aluminium in water for injection as a fluorescent complex

Fluorescence measurements are useful in limit tests where the trace impurity is fluorescent or can be rendered fluorescent by chemical modification. An example is the determination of aluminium in water for use in haemodialysis solutions by formation of its salt with 8-hydroxyquinolone (Fig. 7.5), followed by quantification of the complex using fluorescence spectrophotometry. The excitation

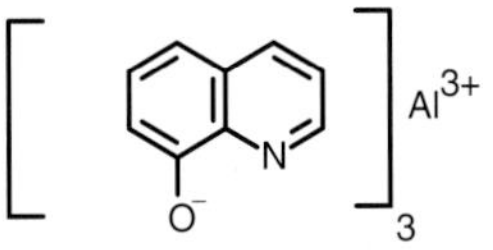

Fig. 7.5
Fluorescent complex of aluminium with hydroxyquinolone.

wavelength is set at 392 nm, and the emission is measured at 518 nm. This type of fluorescent complex can be used to determine low levels of a number of metal ions.

Determination of stability of peptide drugs in solution

The structural complexity of peptide drugs, which are being produced increasingly by biotechnology, means that additional quality control checks are necessary, both for low-level contaminants such as immunogenic proteins and for changes in the tertiary (three-dimensional) structure of the protein in solution, which may affect its activity. During stability studies, peptide drugs are likely to form aggregates, and this eventually results in precipitation. Such changes can alter the efficacy of the drug. In addition, it is important to monitor for the inhibition of such changes where stabilisers and other formulation aids are added to the protein solution. Fluorimetry provides a method of following such changes in solution and was recently used in a study of the stability of recombinant fibroblast growth factor in solution.[1] Fluorescence in this peptide is largely due to the presence of tyrosine residues (excitation 277 nm and emission 305 nm) and a tryptophan residue (excitation 290 nm and emission 350 nm) in its structure. Protein denaturation is accompanied by a gradual fall in the emission peak of the tyrosine residues at 305 nm and a gradual rise in the emission peak of the tryptophan residue at 350 nm. This effect is shown in Figure 7.6 and illustrates the fact that the strength of fluorescence is dependent on the local environment of the chromophore.

Measurement of the effect was found to be capable of quantifying the amount of denatured protein in solution.

Fluorescent derivatives and flow injection analysis

Flow injection analysis (FIA) is discussed in more detail in Chapter 3 (p. 81). Some simple chemical reactions which result in the formation of fluorescent derivatives are shown in Table 7.2. All of these reactions could be adapted to enable analysis by FIA.

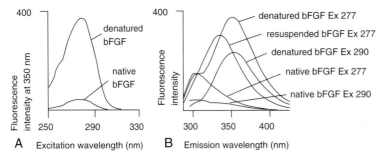

A   Excitation wavelength (nm)   B   Emission wavelength (nm)

Fig. 7.6
The effect of denaturation on the fluorescence spectrum of fibroblast growth factor. (A) Excitation spectra of native and denatured bFGF. (B) Emission spectra of native and denatured bFGF. *(Reproduced with permission from Shahrokh Z, Eberlein G, Wang YJ. J Pharm Biomed Anal. 1994;12:1035-1041.)*

Table 7.2 Examples of chemical conversion of drug molecules into fluorescent derivatives

Compound	Reagent	Excitation (nm)	Emission (nm)
Adrenaline	$K_3Fe(CN)_6$	410	530
Primary amines/amino acids	Fluorescamine	380	480
Chlorphenamine (chlorpheniramine)	H_2O_2	350	436
Fluphenazine	H_2O_2	350	405

Raman spectroscopy

KEYPOINTS

Principles
- The Raman effect is analogous to fluorescence except that it is not wavelength dependent and does not require the molecule to have a chromophore. The energy shift in cm^{-1} due to inelastic scattering of laser radiation is measured, rather than wavelength. The shifts measured correspond to the wavenumbers of the bands present in the middle-infrared (IR) spectrum of the molecule.

Applications
- Has potential for identifying complex samples, e.g. drugs in formulations and in pack.
- Samples such as peptide pharmaceuticals can be analysed for changes in their three-dimensional structure.
- Provides additional fingerprint identity information complementary to middle-IR spectroscopy.

Strengths
- Complementary to middle-IR spectroscopy but requires very little sample preparation, since near-infrared (NIR) radiation with its good penetration properties can be used for the analysis.
- Increasingly a readily available option on middle-IR FT–IR instruments.

Limitations
- Not yet fully established as a quantitative technique.
- The solvent may interfere if samples are run in solution.

Introduction

All molecules can be polarised so that the electrons within them are displaced slightly in the direction of the applied field. This effect is not subject exactly to the laws of quantum mechanics, but the wavenumber of the displacement of radiation by a particular group is the same as the wavenumber of the radiation absorbed by that particular group in middle-IR spectroscopy. In fact, the Raman effect is encountered when making fluorescence measurements in the UV/visible region, although it is usually weak in comparison with Rayleigh and Tyndall scatter. It is analogous to fluorescence except that it is not wavelength dependent and does not require the molecule to have a chromophore, and the energy shift is measured in cm^{-1} rather than in wavelength. Figure 7.7 illustrates the Raman effect; the radiation can be shifted to either slightly higher energy (anti-Stokes shift) or slightly lower energy (Stokes shift). The Stokes shift is usually determined in Raman spectroscopy.

Comparison of the FT-Raman spectrum and FT–IR spectra of dichloroacetophenone (Fig. 7.8) illustrates the fact that the Raman shift for a particular group is similar in energy to the energy of IR absorption for the group in the middle-IR

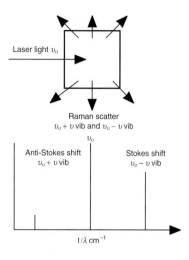

Fig. 7.7
Raman scatter.

region.[2] The two spectra provide complementary information. The general rule is that those bands that absorb weakly in the middle-IR region will absorb strongly in the Raman region and vice versa. For example, in dichloroacetophenone, it can be seen that the aromatic C–H groups which absorb IR radiation weakly give a strong Raman effect, while the C=O group in the structure absorbs IR radiation strongly but gives a weak Raman effect.

Instrumentation

The geometry of a Raman spectrometer (Fig. 7.9) is analogous to that for a fluorescence instrument. Since the Raman effect is weak but proportional to the intensity of energy applied, lasers are used to provide high-intensity radiation in the visible region, generally somewhere between 450 and 800 nm. Lasers provide several emission lines, and, in the case of a fluorescent molecule, a line may be selected that gives Raman scatter where fluorescence does not interfere with the measurement. In recent years, NIR lasers in conjunction with Fourier transform instruments have become available.[2] The use of NIR radiation has two advantages:

(i) Unlike UV/visible radiation, it does not excite fluorescence in molecules, which can result in interference in measurements.
(ii) It has good penetration properties, so a sample in the solid phase can be examined without any sample preparation.

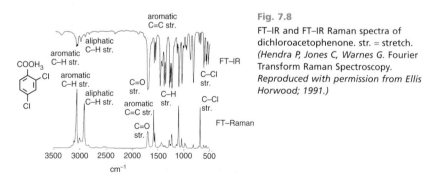

Fig. 7.8
FT–IR and FT–IR Raman spectra of dichloroacetophenone. str. = stretch. *(Hendra P, Jones C, Warnes G. Fourier Transform Raman Spectroscopy. Reproduced with permission from Ellis Horwood; 1991.)*

Fig. 7.9
Schematic diagram of a
Raman spectrometer.

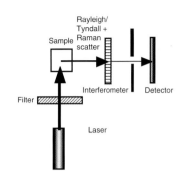

NIR Raman spectroscopy has good potential for the analysis of pharmaceutical formulations and biological materials.

Applications

Rapid fingerprinting of drugs

The Raman spectra of heroin, morphine and codeine (Fig. 7.10) are highly characteristic because of the change in the bands due to the aromatic ring.[2] The FT–IR spectra of these compounds are quite similar. Near-IR Raman spectroscopy can provide a rapid method for characterising drugs with minimal sample preparation and analysis time.

Analysis of drugs in their formulations

Drugs can be characterised directly in formulated materials. For example, diclofenac formulated in sodium alginate was characterised by subtracting the spectrum of the alginate matrix from the spectrum of the formulation containing diclofenac (Fig. 7.11). It is also possible to analyse drugs which are packaged by subtracting the spectrum of the pack. This allows, for instance, a final quality control check on blister-packed tablets.

A quantitative application

FT–Raman is potentially a quantitative technique but does not currently have the sensitivity of NIR when it comes to determination of individual components in complex mixtures. Raman spectroscopy was used to determine glycine and

Fig. 7.10
Raman spectra of heroin (A),
morphine (B) and codeine (C).
*(Hendra P, Jones C, Warnes G.
Fourier Transform Raman
Spectroscopy. Reproduced
with permission from Ellis
Horwood; 1991.)*

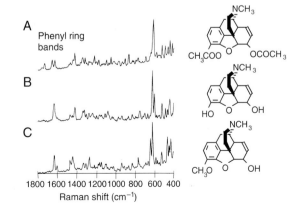

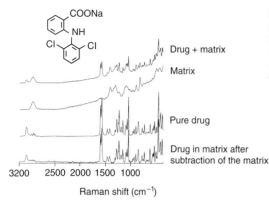

Fig. 7.11

FT–IR Raman spectrum of diclofenac in a sodium alginate matrix. *(Reproduced with permission from Kontoyannis CG. J Pharm Biomed Anal. 1995;13:73-76.)*

calcium carbonate in an antacid tablet.[3] The intensities of the bands at 1088 cm^{-1} for calcium carbonate and 893 cm^{-1} for glycine were used as the basis for quantitation (Fig. 7.12). Precisions of $< \pm 3.5\%$ were achieved for the contents of the ingredients in the tablet.

Control of the polymorphic forms of drugs in tablets

Raman spectroscopy is being increasingly used for the control of polymorphic forms of a drug that may be present in the solid state. A recent study, using NIR Raman spectroscopy, found that it was possible to quantify the polymorphic forms I and II of ranitidine hydrochloride, in the presence of each other, down to a level of 1.8%.[4] The method was more sensitive than X-ray powder diffraction and middle-IR methods. In another study, polymorphic forms of eight different drugs were quantified in tablets using NIR Raman spectroscopy.[5] Figure 7.13 shows the spectra obtained for seven commercial brands of meprobamate tablets. The tablets all contain polymorphic form I of the drug but are distinguishable from each other on the basis of the overall pattern of the spectra that contain contributions from excipients as well as from the active ingredient.

The development of spatially offset Raman spectroscopy (SORS) as a process control tool

Recent advances in Raman spectroscopy have resulted from reconfiguration of the basic instrument geometry. The most powerful method for the collection of

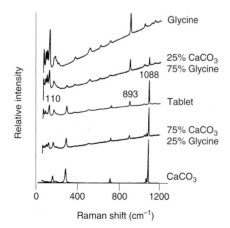

Fig. 7.12

Raman spectra of a tablet containing calcium carbonate and glycine and mixtures containing various proportions of the two components. *(Reproduced with permission from Kontoyannis CG. J Pharm Biomed Anal. 1995;13:73-76.)*

Fig. 7.13

Raman spectra obtained from three polymorphs of meprobamate and seven brands of meprobamate tablets. The bands at 1090.9 cm^{-1} and 1081.3 cm^{-1} are present in all the tablets and are typical of polymorphic form I. *(Reproduced with permission from Auer ME, Griesser UJ, Sawatzki J. J Mol Structure. 2003;661-662, 307-317.)*

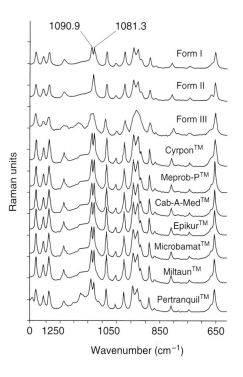

information is where the instrument geometry allows collection of scattered light from deeper layers within the sample.

The use of a probe to obtain SORS spectra can provide a quick check of raw materials feeding into a manufacturing process. Figure 7.14 shows a comparison of sodium citrate which was identity checked through several layers of paper sacking and compares the spectrum obtained by conventional Raman with the spectrum obtained by using SORS. Similarly Figure 7.15 shows the use of SORS to check the identity of ethylene glycol in glass bottles feeding into a process. Finally Figure 7.16 shows an identity check using SORS to fingerprint the polymorphic form of an active pharmaceutical ingredient (API) feeding into a process. Compared with conventional Raman spectroscopy, SORS gives a clear fingerprint for polymorphic form I.

Fig. 7.14

The use of SORS to check the identity of citric acid in paper sacks feeding into a pharmaceutical manufacturing process. *(Reproduced with permission from Bloomfield M, Andrews D, Loeffen P, et al. Pharm Biomed Anal. 2013;76:65-69.)*

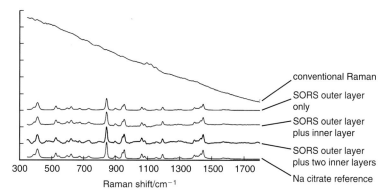

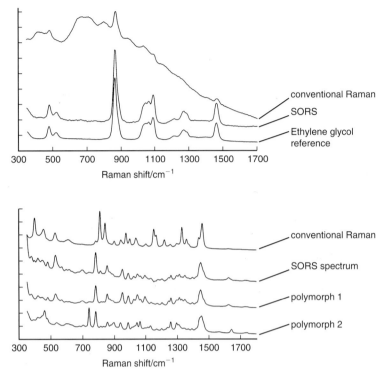

Fig. 7.15
Use of SORS to identity check a solvent feeding into a manufacturing process. *(Reproduced with permission from Bloomfield M, Andrews D, Loeffen P, et al. Pharm Biomed Anal. 2013;76:65-69.)*

conventional Raman

SORS

Ethylene glycol reference

Raman shift/cm^{-1}

Fig. 7.16
Use of SORS to control of the polymorphic form of an API in plastic drums going into a manufacturing process, comparing the conventional Raman spectrum and the SORS spectra against reference spectra. *(Reproduced with permission from Bloomfield M, Andrews D, Loeffen P, et al. Pharm Biomed Anal. 2013;76:65-69.)*

conventional Raman

SORS spectrum

polymorph 1

polymorph 2

Raman shift/cm^{-1}

Further reading

Auer ME, Griesser UJ, Sawatzki J. *J Mol Structure.* 2003;307-317, 661-662.

Bloomfield M, Andrews D, Loeffen P, et al. *Pharm Biomed Anal.* 2013;76:65-69.

Brand L, Johnson ML, eds. *Methods in Enzymology, vol. 278. Fluorescence Spectroscopy.* Elsevier, BV, Amsterdam, 1997.

http://cfs.umbi.umd.edu.

Contains a lot of background material of fluorescence spectroscopy.

Ferraro JR, Nakamoto K, eds. *Introductory Raman Spectroscopy,* Vol. 2. London: Academic Press; 1994.

Gore M, ed. *Spectrophotometry and Spectrofluorimetry: A Practical Approach.* Oxford University Press; 2000.

http://www.ijvs.com/index.html.

Hendra P, Jones C, Warnes G. *Fourier Transform Raman Spectroscopy.* Ellis Horwood; 1991.

Kontoyannis CG. *J Pharm Biomed Anal.* 1995;13:73-76.

Pratiwi D, Fawcett JP, Gordon KC, Rades T. *European J Pharm Biopharm.* 2002;54:337-341.

Shahrokh Z, Eberlein G, Wang YJ. *J Pharm Biomed Anal.* 1994;12:1035-1041.

Lots of material on Raman spectroscopy.

8 Nuclear magnetic resonance spectroscopy

KEYPOINTS

Principles

Radiation in the radiofrequency region is used to excite atoms, like protons or carbon-13 atoms, so that their spins switch from being aligned with to being aligned against an applied magnetic field. The range of frequencies required for excitation and the complex splitting patterns produced are very characteristic of the chemical structure of the molecule.

Applications in pharmaceutical analysis

- A powerful technique for the characterisation of the *exact structure* of raw materials, intermediates and finished products.
- Can determine impurities, including enantiomeric impurities, without separation, down to *ca* the 10% level and 1% level with two-dimensional spectroscopy.
- Can potentially be used for fingerprinting mixtures.
- Has good potential for non-destructive quantitative analysis of drugs in formulations without prior separation.

Strengths

- Provides much more information about molecular structure than any other technique.
- Results are reproducible among the different instruments available in the market.
- A very stable system that does not need any instrument maintenance contract.

Limitations

- A relatively insensitive technique for samples < 1 mg for proton nuclear magnetic resonance (NMR) and < 5 mg for carbon-13 NMR.
- Expensive instrumentation requiring a specialist operator, although automation is increasingly available for routine methods.

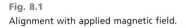

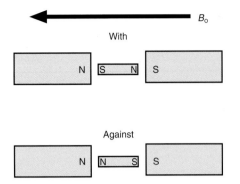

Fig. 8.1
Alignment with applied magnetic field.

Introduction

The spinning nuclei of certain atoms, ^{1}H, ^{13}C, ^{15}N, ^{19}F, ^{29}Si and ^{31}P, gives them the properties of a magnetic vector. When such nuclei are placed in a magnetic field they will tend to align with the field (Fig. 8.1). The energy difference between the spin being aligned with the field and against the field depends on the strength of the magnetic field applied. The greater the field strength, the greater the energy difference ΔE:

$$\Delta E = h\gamma B_o$$

where h is Planck's constant; γ is the magnetogyric ratio of a particular nucleus and B_o is the applied magnetic field.

Figure 8.2 illustrates the absorption of energy to produce alignment against the applied magnetic field. Compared to other spectroscopic techniques, the energy difference between the ground and excited state is not large and thus ΔN, the difference between the number of protons in the low-energy (N_1) and high-energy states (N_2), is very small. This is because the energy difference between the two states is low relative to the thermal energy in the environment. This means that nuclear magnetic resonance (NMR, see Animation 8.1) is a relatively insensitive technique because the net energy absorption by the population of low-energy protons in a sample is low. The wavelength of the radiation used

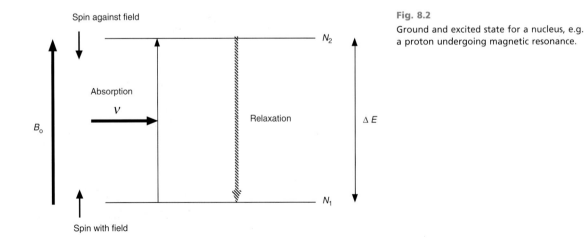

Fig. 8.2
Ground and excited state for a nucleus, e.g. a proton undergoing magnetic resonance.

in NMR is of low energy and is in the radiofrequency region. The units of energy used in NMR are in Hertz, which is a unit of frequency (c/λ, where $c = 3 \times 10^{10}$ cm/s and λ is in cm). The stronger the magnetic field applied, the greater the radiation frequency in Hertz (the shorter the wavelength) required to cause the spin of a nucleus to align against the field (see Animation 8.2 and Animation 8.3). The values for the strength of the applied magnetic field are in the range 14 000–140 000 Gauss (1.4–14 Tesla). A proton in the ground state will absorb radiation having a frequency of *ca* 60 MHz at 1.4 T and *ca* 600 MHz at 14 T. NMR instruments are described in terms of the frequency at which they cause protons to resonate; thus a 600 MHz instrument is one which causes protons to resonate at a frequency of *ca* 600 MHz. At higher magnetic field strength, greater sensitivity is obtained because of the greater difference in the populations of the higher and lower energy states. For a 60 MHz instrument the population difference between the ground and excited state for a proton is *ca* 1 in 100 000, whereas for a 600 MHz instrument the population difference is *ca* 1 in 10 000, i.e. about a 10-fold increase in sensitivity.

Instrumentation

Figure 8.3 gives the basic layout of a continuous wave NMR spectrometer, which has largely been replaced by Fourier transform instruments. However, the principles of operation are broadly similar:

(i) The sample is placed in 3, 5, 10 millimetre glass NMR tubes and is spun in the fixed magnetic field in cases of one-dimensional experiments at *ca* 30 revolutions/s by means of an air turbine, thus ensuring uniformity of the magnetic field across the sample in a horizontal direction. The sample is analysed in solution in a deuterated solvent to ensure there is no interference with the signal from protons in the relatively much larger amount of solvent.

Fig. 8.3
Schematic diagram of a continuous wave nuclear magnetic resonance spectrometer. (see also Animation 8.4)

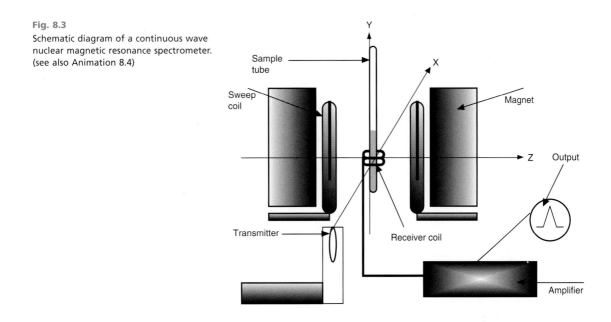

(ii) The reference point in parts per million (ppm) is determined by the resonance of the residual protons of the solvent which are used to lock the protons in a spectrum, e.g. the residual proton in deuterated chloroform is at 7.25 ppm.

(iii) In order to obtain a proton spectrum, the radiofrequency radiation is swept across a range of *ca* 10 ppm, e.g. 1000 Hz when the magnetic field is recorded on a 100 MHz instrument or 6000 Hz when the spectrum is recorded on a 600 MHz instrument. The receiver coil measures the absorption of radiation as the frequency is swept over the range being examined.

(iv) As well as determining the frequency at which protons in the molecule absorb, that is recorded as chemical shifts in ppm, the area of each signal proportional to the number of protons absorbing radiation is documented in integrals.

(v) Modern instruments, rather than being based on a continuous wave, are based on a pulsed wave. In brief, the short powerful pulse used in this type of spectroscopy behaves as a spread of frequencies covering the Hz range of interest, e.g. the range in which protons resonate. Most of the principles of the continuous wave instrument still hold but, rather than the absorption of radiation by the sample being observed, emission is observed as the excited protons relax back to their ground state following the short high-energy pulse of radiation. Thus spectra are accumulated using a high-intensity pulse followed by a time delay of a few seconds while the relaxation data of different protons in the molecule are collected. This type of procedure enables a spectrum to be acquired every few seconds, as opposed to a few minutes required to collect the data using a frequency sweep on a continuous wave instrument. The data from a number of pulses are accumulated using a computer, undergo mathematical manipulation known as Fourier transformation and are combined to produce a spectrum in which the signal-to-noise characteristics are much improved compared to a spectrum obtained on a single-scan continuous wave instrument.

Proton (^{1}H) NMR
Chemical shifts

Proton (^{1}H) NMR is the most commonly used form of NMR because of its sensitivity and the large amount of structural information it yields. The chemical shift is the position on the δ (delta) scale (in ppm) where the peak occurs (Fig. 8.4).

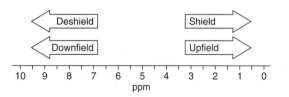

Fig. 8.4
The δ scale (in ppm) of a ^{1}H spectrum.

There are three major factors that influence chemical shifts:

1. Inductive effects by electronegative groups
2. Deshielding due to reduced electron density (due to the presence of electronegative atoms)
3. Anisotropy (due to magnetic fields generated by π bonds).

The exact absorption or resonance frequency of a proton depends on its environment. For example, a proton attached to carbon atom is affected predominantly by the groups which are separated from the carbon atom to which it is attached by one bond or, to a lesser extent, two bonds. As discussed earlier, the chemical shift of a proton is determined in relation to the residual protons of the deuterated solvent. Shift values for individual protons in a molecule are expressed in ppm, and the frequency value of 1 ppm in Hertz depends on the strength of the applied magnetic field, which determines the energy required to excite a proton. For example, at field strength of 100 MHz a shift of 1 ppm has a frequency value of 100 Hz. Proton shifts in organic compounds range from slightly below 0 to 14 ppm, i.e. from a δ value of slightly less than 0 to a δ value of 14. The frequency difference between the shifts of the protons in Hz proportionally increases with the field strengths of the magnetic field corresponding to Larmor proton frequencies of ω_o = 60, 100, 300 and 600 MHz, as exemplified in Figure 8.5.

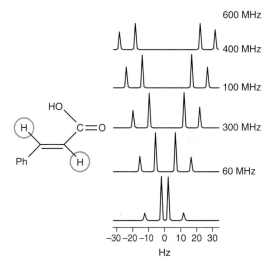

Fig. 8.5

The spectra are shown at different values of the strength of the magnetic field corresponding to Larmor proton frequencies of ω_o = 60, 100, 300, 400 and 600 MHz.

The chemical shift is determined by the extent to which a proton is deshielded by the groups to which it is attached. The more a proton is shielded by the electron density around it, the lower its δ value. If a proton is attached to a system that withdraws electrons from its chemical environment, such as an electronegative group, or to a group which affects its environment by creating a field opposing the applied magnetic field, such as occurs in the case of protons attached to an aromatic ring, its δ value will increase, i.e. it will resonate at lower field (lower frequency) while aliphatic protons will resonate at higher field (higher frequency). It is often convenient to describe the relative positions of the resonances in an NMR spectrum. For example, a peak at a chemical shift of 10 ppm is said to be *downfield* or *deshielded* with respect to a peak at 5 ppm, while the peak at 5 ppm is *upfield* or *shielded* with respect to the peak at 10 ppm (Fig. 8.4). Tables 8.1 and 8.3 show δ values in ppm for protons attached to some common organic groups.

Note:

(i) Alkyl protons such as those in CH_3 and CH_2 groups not attached to adjacent electronegative groups resonate between δ 0.2 and 2.0 ppm.

(ii) Protons on CH_3, CH_2 and CH groups attached to electronegative atoms or groups such as O, N, F, Cl, CN, C=C and C=O resonate between δ 2 and 5 ppm. Electronegative groups attached to the **C-H** system decrease the electron density around the protons, and there is less shielding (i.e. deshielding) so the chemical shift increases (Table 8.2). These effects are cumulative, so the presence of more electronegative groups produces more deshielding and, therefore, larger chemical shifts, as in the case of CH_4, CH_3Cl, CH_2Cl_2, and $CHCl_3$, which exhibit resonances at δ 0.23, 3.05, 5.30 and 7.27, respectively. Protons on an unsubstituted benzene resonate at $\delta = 7.27$, the presence of an electron withdrawing and donating substituent either shields or deshields the protons of a phenyl system, specifically those on the *ortho* and *para* position, as shown in Table 8.3. The proton at the *meta* position is the less affected.

(iii) Protons attached directly to C=C resonate between δ 4 and 7 while protons attached to aromatic rings resonate between δ 6 and 9. Electrons in π systems interact with the applied field, which induces a magnetic field that causes anisotropy (Fig. 8.6). The word '**anisotropic**' means 'non-uniform'. Depending on the position of the proton on the π system, it can be either shielded (smaller δ, +) or deshielded (larger δ, −), which implies that the energy required for, and the frequency of the absorption will change.

Table 8.1 Approximate chemical shift values for non-aromatic protons attached to carbon

Group	δ ppm	Group	δ ppm	Group	δ ppm
CH_3-C	0.9	R-CH_2-C	1.4	CH-C	1.5
CH_3-C-O	1.3	R-CH_2-C-N	1.4	CH-C-O	2.0
CH_3-C=C	1.6	R-CH_2-C-O	1.9	CH-CO-N	2.4
CH_3-CO	2.0	R-CH_2-CO-N	2.2	CH-CO	2.7
CH_3-CO-N	2.0	R-CH_2-C=C	2.3	CH-N	2.8
CH_3-N	2.4	R-CH_2-CO	2.4	CH-Ar	3.3
CH_3-Ar	2.3	R-CH_2-N	2.5	CH-O	3.9
CH_3-O	3.3	R-CH_2-Ar	2.9	CH-N-CO	4.0
CH_3N^+ $(R)_3$	3.3	R-CH_2-O	3.6	CH-Cl	4.2
CH_3-O-CO	3.7	R-CH_2-O-CO	4.1	R-CH=C	4.5–6.0

Table 8.2 ^{1}H shifts of CH_3 moiety in relation to the electronegative substituent

X	Compound, CH_3X						
	F	O	Cl	Br	I	H	Si
Electronegativity of X	4.00	3.50	3.10	2.80	2.50	2.10	1.80
Chemical shift, δ/ppm	4.26	3.40	3.05	2.68	2.16	0.20	0

Table 8.3 Chemical shift values for protons attached to an aromatic ring. The effects of the substituents are either added to or subtracted from the chemical shift for benzene at $\delta = 7.27$

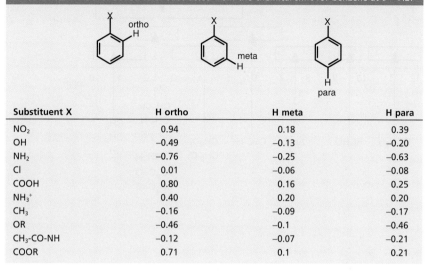

Substituent X	H ortho	H meta	H para
NO_2	0.94	0.18	0.39
OH	−0.49	−0.13	−0.20
NH_2	−0.76	−0.25	−0.63
Cl	0.01	−0.06	−0.08
COOH	0.80	0.16	0.25
NH_3^+	0.40	0.20	0.20
CH_3	−0.16	−0.09	−0.17
OR	−0.46	−0.1	−0.46
CH_3-CO-NH	−0.12	−0.07	−0.21
COOR	0.71	0.1	0.21

Fig. 8.6

Effect of anisotropy on the proton chemical shift.

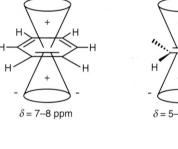

$\delta = 7$–8 ppm

$\delta = 5$–7 ppm

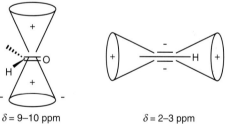

$\delta = 9$–10 ppm

$\delta = 2$–3 ppm

(iv) Protons that are involved in hydrogen bonding (like those of -O*H*s or -N*H*s) are typically observed over a large range of chemical shift values (Fig. 8.7). The more hydrogen bonding there is, the more a proton is deshielded. Hydrogen bonding is susceptible to factors such as solvation, acidity, concentration and temperature and can often be difficult to predict. These H atoms are described to be *exchangeable* and can be observed by using aprotic solvents (e.g. $CDCl_3$, DMSO, pyridine). Their presence can be confirmed by deuterium substitution experiments in D_2O or MeOD.

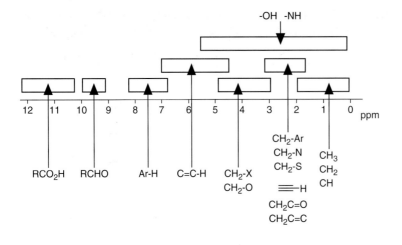

Fig. 8.7
Schematic of the chemical shifts of
various functional moieties.

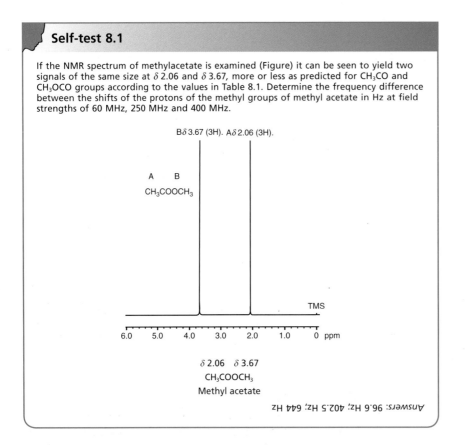

Self-test 8.1

If the NMR spectrum of methylacetate is examined (Figure) it can be seen to yield two
signals of the same size at δ 2.06 and δ 3.67, more or less as predicted for CH_3CO and
CH_3OCO groups according to the values in Table 8.1. Determine the frequency difference
between the shifts of the protons of the methyl groups of methyl acetate in Hz at field
strengths of 60 MHz, 250 MHz and 400 MHz.

Bδ 3.67 (3H). Aδ 2.06 (3H).

A   B
CH_3COOCH_3

TMS

6.0   5.0   4.0   3.0   2.0   1.0   0 ppm

δ 2.06 δ 3.67
CH_3COOCH_3
Methyl acetate

Answers: 96.6 Hz; 402.5 Hz; 644 Hz

Self-test 8.2

Predict the approximate shifts in ppm of the CH₃ and CH₂ groups in the following molecules and the number of protons producing the signal at each shift:

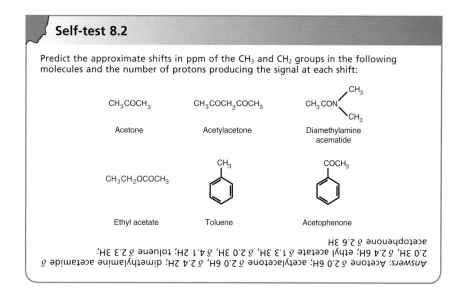

CH₃COCH₃

Acetone

CH₃COCH₂COCH₃

Acetylacetone

CH₃CON(CH₃)₂

Diamethylamine acematide

CH₃CH₂OCOCH₃

Ethyl acetate

Toluene

Acetophenone

Answers: Acetone δ 2.0 6H; acetylacetone δ 2.0 6H, δ 2.4 2H; dimethylamine acetamide δ 2.0 3H, δ 2.4 6H; ethyl acetate δ 1.3 3H, δ 2.0 3H, δ 4.1 2H; toluene δ 2.3 3H; acetophenone δ 2.6 3H.

Self-test 8.3

Determine the shifts of the protons in the following molecules:

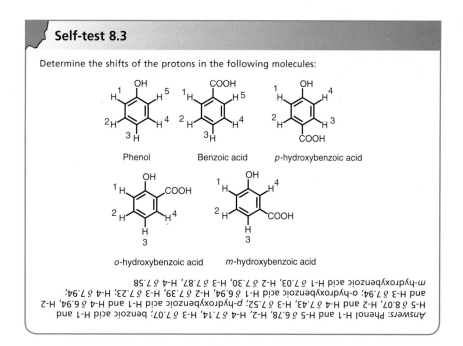

Phenol

Benzoic acid

p-hydroxybenzoic acid

o-hydroxybenzoic acid

m-hydroxybenzoic acid

Answers: Phenol H-1 and H-5 δ 6.78, H-2, H-4 δ 7.14, H-3 δ 7.07; benzoic acid H-1 and H-5 δ 8.07, H-2 and H-4 δ 7.43, H-3 δ 7.52; *p*-hydroxybenzoic acid H-1 and H-4 δ 6.94, H-2 and H-3 δ 7.94; *o*-hydroxybenzoic acid H-1 δ 6.94, H-2 δ 7.39, H-3 δ 7.23; H-4 δ 7.94; *m*-hydroxybenzoic acid H-1 δ 7.03, H-2 δ 7.30, H-3 δ 7.87, H-4 δ 7.58

Integration and equivalence

The integration is the area under the peak of a resonating signal which is proportional to the number of protons absorbing radiation at a particular frequency. Three protons will give an area three times that of a signal due for one proton in the same molecule. As shown in the ¹H NMR spectrum of phenethyl propionate (Fig. 8.8), the chemically equivalent protons of the phenyl protons resonate as a broad singlet integrating for five protons while the methylene and methyl units integrate as two and three protons, respectively. The integration also provides

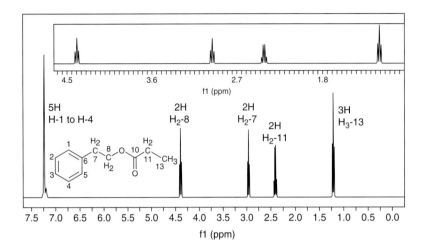

Fig. 8.8
¹H NMR spectrum of phenethyl propionate.

information on the relative amounts of individual compounds in mixtures or for the levels of impurities in a bulk sample.

An integral of two or more protons (or indeed with two or more carbons) resonating at similar chemical shifts would indicate magnetic and/or chemical equivalence as observed for a methyl (CH_3) unit where all three protons are equivalent (Fig. 8.9A). Methylene (CH_2) protons resonating at two chemical shifts would imply chemical and magnetic non-equivalence as exhibited by methylene units vicinal to a chiral centre. In the examples below (Fig. 8.9A–D), the different types

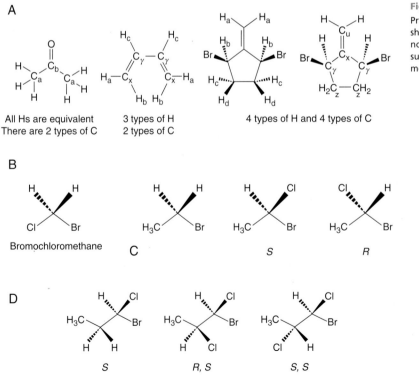

Fig. 8.9
Proton and carbon nomenclature showing equivalence and non-equivalence according to substitution patterns within molecules.

of atoms are given a subscript; atoms which are equivalent will have the same subscript.

Equivalence defines the three types of protons:

1. **Homotopic:** Replacement of the groups gives the same product. For example, it doesn't matter which of the H atoms in bromomethane is replaced with chlorine, and we always get bromochloromethane (Fig. 8.9B). Hence, these three H are said to be **homotopic**.
2. **Enantiotopic:** Replacement of the groups gives enantiomers. Consider the **H** atoms in the methylene group in bromoethane. If we replace one of those **H** with a Cl, we create a chiral centre. Therefore, depending on which of the two **H** is replaced, we get one enantiomer or the other (Fig. 8.9C). Hence these two **H** are said to be **enantiotopic**.
3. **Diastereotopic:** Replacement of the groups gives diastereomers. Consider the **H** atoms in the methylene group in 1-bromo-1-chloropropane. There is already a chirality centre at C1. If we replace one of those **H** with a Cl, we create a *new* chiral centre (Fig. 8.9D). Therefore, depending on which of the two H is replaced, we get one diastereomer or the other. Hence these two H are said to be diastereotopic.

Calculation example 8.1

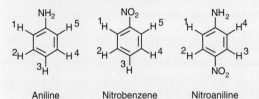

Aniline   Nitrobenzene   Nitroaniline

Aniline: In aniline, the 1 and 5 and 2 and 4 protons are equivalent:
H-1 and H-5 shift = 7.27 − 0.76 = 6.51 ppm
H-2 and H-4 shift = 7.27 − 0.25 = 7.02 ppm
H-3 shift = 7.27 − 0.63 = 6.64 ppm.

Thus the spectrum of aniline would contain:
2H 6.51 ppm; 2H 7.02 ppm and 1H 6.64 ppm.

Nitrobenzene: In nitrobenzene, the 1 and 5 and 2 and 4 protons are equivalent:
H-1 and H-5 shift = 7.27 + 0.94 = 8.21 ppm
H-2 and H-4 shift = 7.27 + 0.18 = 7.45 ppm
H-3 shift = 7.27 + 0.39 = 7.66 ppm.

Thus the spectrum of nitrobenzene would contain:
2H 8.21 ppm; 2H 7.45 ppm and 1H 7.66 ppm.

Nitroaniline: In nitroaniline, the 1 and 4 and 2 and 3 protons are equivalent:
H-1 and H-4 shift = 7.27 − 0.76 + 0.18 = 6.69 ppm
H-2 and H-3 shift = 7.27 − 0.25 + 0.94 = 7.96 ppm.

Thus the spectrum of nitroaniline would contain:
2H 6.69 ppm and 2H 7.96 ppm.

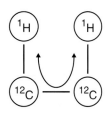

$L = n + 1$
L = number of lines in a coupling pattern
n = number of neighbouring protons

A proton with zero neighbours,
$n = 0$, appears as a single line,
A proton with one neighbour,
$n = 1$ as two lines of equal intensity,
A proton with two neighbours,
$n = 2$, as three lines of intensities 1:2:1, etc.

Fig. 8.10
Coupling of adjacent protons: $L = n + 1$, where
L = no. of lines in a coupling pattern and
n = numbering of neighbouring protons. A
proton with zero neighbours, $n = 0$, appears
as a single line. A proton with one neighbour,
$n = 1$, as two lines of equal intensity. A proton
with two neighbours, $n = 2$, as three lines of
intensities 1:2:1, etc.

Multiplicity and spin–spin coupling

In some of the molecules considered above we have neglected an additional shift effect, which is caused by the spin of the protons on the atoms next to a particular proton (Fig. 8.10). Each proton signal is split into two or more lines by the presence of neighbouring proton(s) following the n+1 rule, where n is the number of neighbouring protons. The proximity of 'n' equivalent H on neighbouring carbon atoms causes the signals to be split into 'n+1' lines. This is known as the multiplicity or splitting or coupling pattern of each signal. A more complex pattern will arise if the neighbours' coupling constants are not equivalent.

The relative intensities of the lines in a coupling pattern are given by a binomial expansion or more conveniently by the Pascal's triangle. To derive Pascal's triangle, start at the apex, and generate each lower row by adding the two numbers above and to either side in the row above together as shown in Figure 8.11.

In examining the proton NMR spectrum of ethyl acetate (Fig. 8.12), it can be seen that its spectrum is more complicated than that of methyl acetate and that the signal due to the CH_3 group B in the alcohol part of the ester is now three lines instead of one, the middle line of the three corresponding to the chemical shift estimated from Table 8.1. The protons of the adjacent CH_2 group C can align their spins in three different ways relative to the CH_3, as seen in Figure 8.13. For alignment 1, there are two equivalent alignments where the effects of the adjacent protons cancel each other out and do not perturb the signal of the methyl group from its predicted shift (*ca* 1.30 ppm). This produces a triplet where the central line is twice the height/area of the two lines produced by alignments 2 and 3. The CH_2 group itself is also split by the effect of the adjacent methyl group. In this case, statistical analysis of the possible combination of the spins of the adjacent

```
              1                      n = 0
            1   1                    n = 1
          1   2   1                  n = 2
        1   3   3   1                n = 3
      1   4   6   4   1              n = 4
    1   5  10  10   5   1            n = 5
```

Fig. 8.11
Pascal's triangle indicating the pattern of lines produced by a particular number of adjacent protons having the same coupling constants to a particular signal.

Fig. 8.12

270 MHz ^{1}H nuclear magnetic resonance spectrum of ethyl acetate.

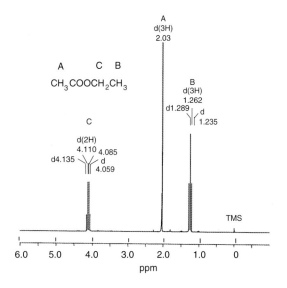

methyl protons indicates that the signal of the CH$_2$ protons should be a quartet, with the lines in the quartet being in the ratio 1:3:3:1; the mid-point between the two central lines gives the predicted chemical shift of 4.1 ppm. The methyl group A appears, as it does in methyl acetate, as a singlet since it is isolated from any adjacent protons. The effect of adjacent protons on the signal for a given group is known as coupling and coupling constants are given in Hz; the range of coupling constants between adjacent protons is 0–20 Hz. The coupling constant, J, is a measure of the interaction between a pair of protons. In a vicinal system of the general type $\mathbf{H_a}$–C–C–$\mathbf{H_b}$, then J_{ab} is the coupling of $\mathbf{H_a}$ with $\mathbf{H_b}$, which must be equal to the coupling of $\mathbf{H_b}$ with $\mathbf{H_a}$, J_{ba}, therefore $J_{ab} = J_{ba}$. Coupling resonances show a roof effect by which the relative binomial intensities of the peaks tend to lean toward the coupling partner.

When two protons are close in chemical shift, coupling can cause their signals to overlap. The coupling constant is independent of the applied magnetic field, and thus the size of coupling constants in ppm will decrease with increasing field strength although their values in Hz remain the same. The higher the field strength, the less likely it is that signals from individual protons will overlap. The spectrum of ethyl acetate in Figure 8.12 was obtained on a 270 MHz (1 ppm = 270 Hz) instrument. The shifts in ppm obtained for the three lines in the CH$_3$ group signal are 1.235, 1.262 and 1.289. Therefore these lines are evenly spaced 0.027 ppm apart, which is equivalent to 270×0.027 Hz = 7.29 Hz. Figure 8.14 shows the spectrum of ethyl acetate obtained on a 60 MHz (1 ppm = 60 Hz)

Fig. 8.13

Possible spin alignments of two protons.

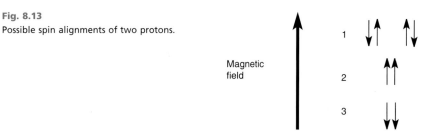

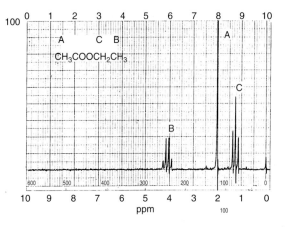

Fig. 8.14
60 MHz ^{1}H nuclear magnetic resonance spectrum of ethyl acetate. *(Reproduced with permission of Aldrich Chemical Co.)*

instrument; in this case the space between the lines is large (*ca* 0.12 ppm) relative to the ppm scale but will result to a similar coupling constant of *ca* 7 Hz, as to that observed using the 270 MHz instrument.

Self-test 8.4

What would be the multiplicity of the following of the marked protons in the following structures? Remember: Number of lines in coupling pattern, L = n + 1:

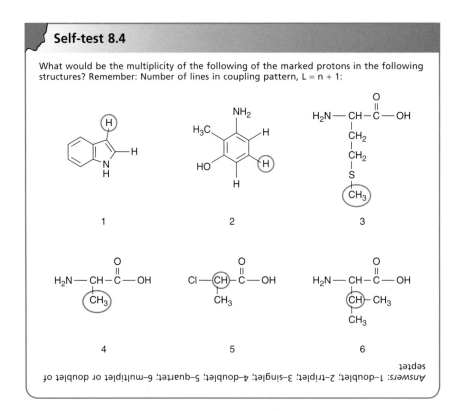

1

2

3

4

5

6

Answers: 1–doublet; 2–triplet; 3–singlet; 4–doublet; 5–quartet; 6–multiplet or doublet of septet

---

Scalar *J* coupling information does reveal the configuration and conformation of a compound. In an aliphatic ring system, the magnitude of the *J* coupling is dictated by the torsion angle between the two coupling nuclei according to the Karplus equation (see Animation 8.5) or so-called gauche effect as shown in Figure 8.15.

Fig. 8.15
The Karplus relation.

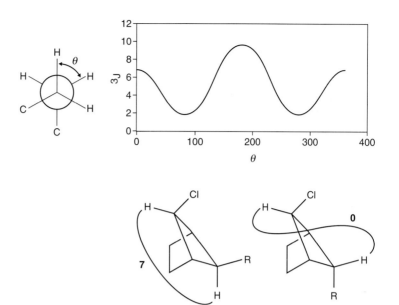

Fig. 8.16
Long range '*ω*' coupling.

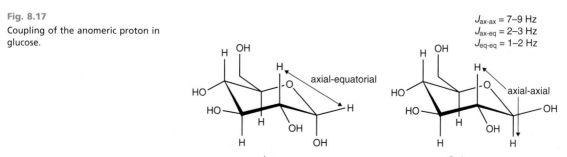

Notes:

(i) Long-range ^4J coupling is not often observed, but one type of system does reveal a dramatic dependence on geometry, often called '*ω*' coupling because of the relationship between the two protons. ^4J for allylic coupling, **H–C=C–C–H** varies from –3 to +2 Hz, depending again on the angle between the two H–C bonds (Fig. 8.16).

(ii) Coupling constants also reveal a dependence on the configuration of the proton on an aliphatic system as in differentiating α and β sugars. An equatorially oriented anomeric proton (H-1) of an α-sugar couples with H-2 at the axial position, which will give a relatively small coupling constant of $J_{ax-eq} = 2$–3 Hz, while in a β-sugar the anomeric proton is axial and couples with an axially oriented H-2, resulting in a large $J_{ax-ax} = 7$–9 Hz (Fig 8.17).

(iii) In an olefinic system, *cis* and *trans* configuration can be determined through their coupling constants of 6 to 11 Hz and 12 to 18 Hz, respectively.

(iv) Coupling constants also reveal the substitution pattern in an aromatic system. Vicinal *ortho* protons give a coupling constant of 6 to 9 Hz, while

Fig. 8.17
Coupling of the anomeric proton in glucose.

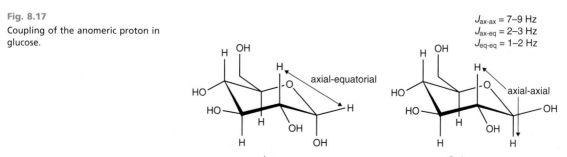

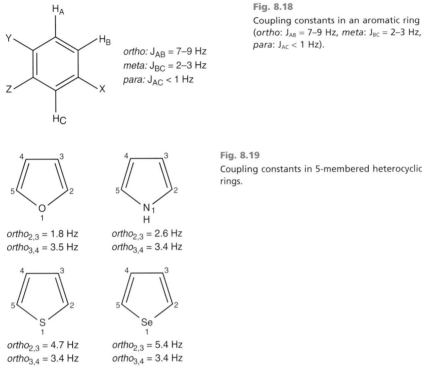

Fig. 8.18
Coupling constants in an aromatic ring
(*ortho*: J_{AB} = 7–9 Hz, *meta*: J_{BC} = 2–3 Hz,
para: J_{AC} < 1 Hz).

ortho: J_{AB} = 7–9 Hz
meta: J_{BC} = 2–3 Hz
para: J_{AC} < 1 Hz

Fig. 8.19
Coupling constants in 5-membered heterocyclic
rings.

ortho$_{2,3}$ = 1.8 Hz
ortho$_{3,4}$ = 3.5 Hz

ortho$_{2,3}$ = 2.6 Hz
ortho$_{3,4}$ = 3.4 Hz

ortho$_{2,3}$ = 4.7 Hz
ortho$_{3,4}$ = 3.4 Hz

ortho$_{2,3}$ = 5.4 Hz
ortho$_{3,4}$ = 3.4 Hz

protons *meta* to each other couple at 2 to 3 Hz and *para*-coupled protons
at less than 1 Hz (Fig. 8.18).

(v) In heterocyclic aromatic systems, there is a marked decrease in *ortho*
coupling constants across the adjacent bond, in line with the effects of
electronegative substituents (Fig. 8.19).

(vi) There is a marked decrease in coupling constants of *ortho* protons passing
from a 6-membered to 5-membered ring system. The magnitude of the
coupling constants of the vicinal protons decreases as they get closer to
the proximity of the electronegative heteroatom (Fig. 8.20).

Splitting diagrams and spin systems

As the number of adjacent protons in a molecule increases, the splitting pattern
of the protons increases in complexity, as shown in compound 6 in Self-test 8.4.
Figure 8.21 shows the proton NMR spectrum of propyl acetate. In this case the
CH_3 group B is present as a triplet as in ethyl acetate, but the CH_2 group C now

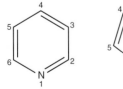

Fig. 8.20
Coupling constants in 6-membered heterocyclic
rings.

ortho$_{2,3}$ = 4.0–5.7 Hz
ortho$_{3,4}$ = 6.8–9.1 Hz

ortho$_{2,3}$ = 2.6 Hz
ortho$_{3,4}$ = 3.4 Hz

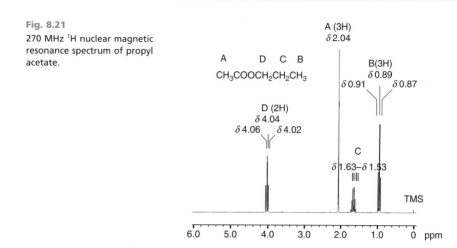

Fig. 8.21
270 MHz ^{1}H nuclear magnetic resonance spectrum of propyl acetate.

has six lines due to the presence of five adjacent protons – three on group B and two on group D. The ratio of the lines in this case is $1:5:10:10:5:1$.

If the protons of groups B and D in propyl acetate did not have similar coupling constants with the protons on group C, a more complicated pattern of lines would result, as indicated in Figure 8.22. In the case shown in Figure 8.23A, the protons can be viewed as being split into four lines by an adjacent methyl group and each of the four lines are further split into three lines by a CH_2 group, giving a total of 12 lines (a quartet of triplets). The appropriate coupling constants of these 'multiplet of multiplets' direct the splitting pattern where the multiplicity of H_A in an $A_nM_pX_m$ spin system is $(p+1)(m+1)$ as demonstrated in Figure 8.24. Their relative intensities still follow the rule of binomial coefficients.

If the differences in coupling constants of adjacent protons are small, not widely different, the patterns tend to merge into those that would be expected if all the adjacent protons coupled identically. This is the case with propyl acetate, where coupling to five adjacent protons on two carbons produces six lines. In reality, coupling patterns are often more complex than the simple n+1 rule since the neighbouring protons are often not equivalent to each other (i.e. there are different types of neighbours). Different types of neighbours interact with

Fig. 8.22
Coupling of CH_2 with adjacent and CH_2 and CH_2 groups where the coupling constants to the adjacent groups are unequal.

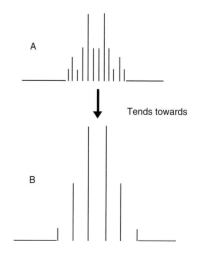

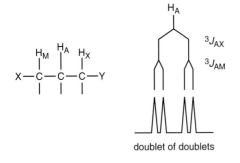

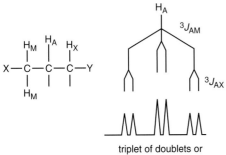

Fig. 8.23
Multiplet of multiplets.

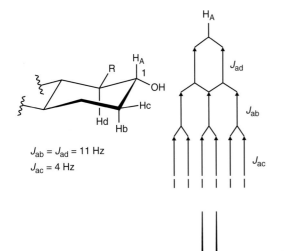

Fig. 8.24
A splitting diagram.

Fig. 8.25
Characteristic splitting patterns for
a tri-substituted phenyl system.

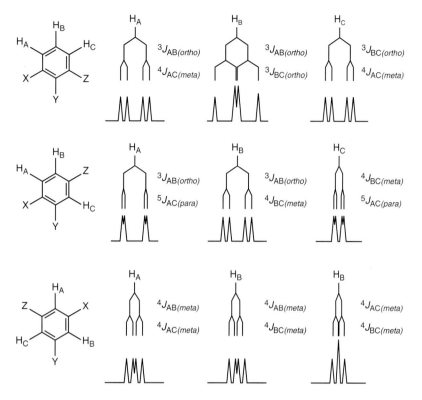

different coupling constants. In these cases the 'n+1' rule has to be refined so that each type of neighbour causes n+1 lines. For a proton with two types of neighbours, the number of lines are L = (n1 + 1)(n2 + 1). This can be properly illustrated by splitting pattern diagrams. A splitting diagram is a simple procedure of analysing a first-order spectrum where line spacing is measured and identical splitting can be identified, as demonstrated in Figure 8.24. In tri-substituted phenyl systems, as shown in Figure 8.25, the positions of the functional groups can be indicated by characteristic splitting patterns. The splitting pattern thus provides the information on the spin system.

A spin system is a group of coupled protons and cannot go beyond a molecule. However, a molecule can have more than one spin system, where groups of protons are separated by a heteroatom or atoms which are not substituted with a proton. For example, isopropyl propionate has two spin systems (Fig 8.26).

Fig. 8.26
Spin systems found in isopropyl propionate.

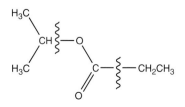

Self-test 8.5

Identify the number of spin systems in each of the molecules below:

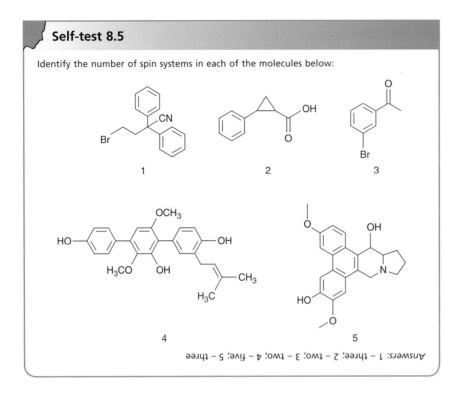

Answers: 1 – three; 2 – two; 3 – two; 4 – five; 5 – three

In naming spin systems, consecutive letters (ABC) are used when the ratio ($\Delta v/J$) of the separation of chemical shifts (Hz) and the coupling constant (J) between them is ≈ 3.0. A break in the alphabet (AMX) is used when the ratio is > 3.0, where A has the smaller and C or X has the considerably larger chemical shift. Subscripts are applied for magnetically equivalent protons, and chemical equivalence is represented by primes.

Notes:

(i) AB spin systems involve two protons coupling only with each other. In some cases the coupling arises from three intervening bonds or vicinal protons; hence the term $^3J_{\text{H-H}}$ coupling for an alkene system. An AB spin is also applied to non-equivalent geminal (CH_2) protons. The spin system is referred to as AB if the chemical shifts are quite close together and AX if they are far apart. As the chemical shifts of two non-equivalent protons move closer together and thus approach the coupling constants line perturbation occurs, where the outside lines become smaller. As can be seen in Figure 8.27, the line intensities of olefin protons in cinnamic acid change according to the strength of the magnetic field applied, because at higher field strengths the differences in the chemical shifts of the protons in Hz become large relative to the coupling constants.

(ii) An AA'BB' spin system consists of four protons consisting of two equivalent pairs due to structure symmetry (Fig. 8.28). The signals are exemplified by pairs of 'pseudo' *ortho* doublets, each integrating for two protons. These doublets exhibit shoulder peaks, indicating that the protons are magnetically non-equivalent due to the further *meta* and *para*

Fig. 8.27
AB and AX spin systems.

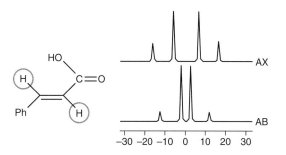

coupling. The simple explanation is that the pairs A and A′ and B and B′ are not always equivalent, since at a given instant they may be affected differently by the protons they are interacting with. Such spectra are known as second-order spectra and can only be analysed accurately by using quantum mechanical calculations.

(iii) An ABC or ABX or AMX spin system refers to three different protons coupling to one another and follows the 2nI+1 rule. Each proton is described as a doublet of doublets, since the two coupling constants are numerically different. In the example shown in Figure 8.29A, H_c has a chemical shift at a considerably lower field than protons H_b and H_c, and it thus appears as a doublet of doublets with minimal line perturbation. It couples with H_b most strongly where the dihedral angle is 180° and less strongly to H_a where the dihedral angle is 60°. Protons H_a and H_b are close in chemical shift and, in addition to coupling to H_c, they also couple to each other strongly via geminal coupling. The close chemical shifts of these protons in combination with strong geminal coupling produce a strong line perturbation. In the second example shown in Figure 8.29B, the ABX system is simpler. A and B are close in chemical shift, but only weakly coupled via *meta* coupling and line perturbation, depends on the ratio of chemical shift difference to strength of coupling is minimal. H_b is further split by strong ortho-coupling to H_c, which has a chemical shift well upfield due to shielding by the ortho hydroxyl group. The weak *para* coupling between H_c and H_a is not observed.

Fig. 8.28
Examples of AA′BB′ spin systems.

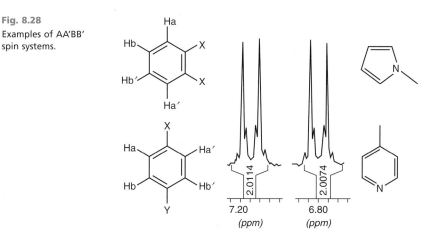

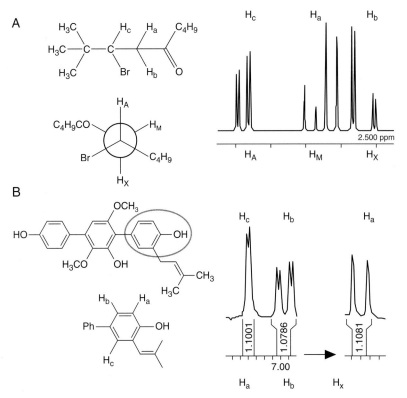

Fig. 8.29
Examples of ABX and AMX spin
systems.

(iv) Four different protons all coupling to one another is described as an
   ABCD spin system, where all protons are non-equivalent. In the NMR
   spectrum of indole protons (Fig. 8.30) H_a and H_d are doublets due to *ortho*
   coupling to H_b and H_c, respectively, while H_b and H_c are triplets coupling
   to each other and protons H_a and H_d, respectively. The coupling constants
   between all the protons are very similar and there is an absence of
   long-range coupling.

   As indicated, splitting patterns can be complex, but the NMR spectra of many
drug molecules do not reach this level of complexity. Some classes of molecules,
such as the steroids or prostaglandins, provide examples of spectra where complex
splitting patterns occur, but the majority of drug molecules contain one or two

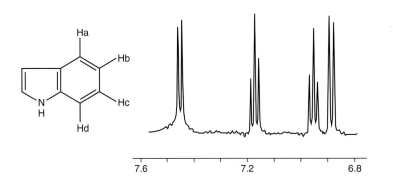

Fig. 8.30
Example of an ABCD spin system.

aromatic rings with varying types of relatively simple side chains. In the case of complex molecules such as steroids, two-dimensional NMR techniques involving proton–proton and proton–carbon correlations have simplified spectral interpretation. The most complex applications of NMR are found in the structure elucidation of natural products.

Application of NMR to structure confirmation in some drug molecules

Proton NMR spectrum of paracetamol

The NMR spectrum of paracetamol run in CD_3OD is shown in Figure 8.31. The spectrum shows a signal for an isolated CH_3 group at δ 2.07 ppm due to CH_3CONH. The broad signal at δ 4.88 is due to the proton in CD_3OH, which forms as a result of exchange of deuterium with the NH and OH protons of paracetamol; this is why the protons attached to these groups are not seen in the spectrum. The other signals in the spectrum are two doublets with mean shifts of δ 6.72 ppm and δ 7.30, which, from the information given in Table 8.3, can be said to be assigned to the equivalent protons 2 and 3 and 1 and 4, respectively. Proton 1 is coupled to proton 2 and proton 4 is coupled to proton 3, thus causing the signals to appear as doublets.

Proton NMR spectrum of aspirin

Figure 8.32 shows the proton NMR spectrum for aspirin run in CD_3OD. The methyl group is isolated and appears at δ 2.28, which could be predicted from Table 8.1. There is a broad peak at δ 4.91 due to CD_3OH formed by exchange with the –COOH group on aspirin. The aromatic region is more complex than that observed for paracetamol because the four aromatic protons are non-equivalent. The four proton signals have mean shifts of 7.13 ppm, 7.34 ppm, 7.60 ppm and 8.02 ppm, and from Table 8.3 it is possible to assign these signals to protons 4, 2, 3 and 1, respectively. H-1 is a doublet due to coupling to H-2; H-2 appears as a triplet due to overlap of two doublets caused by coupling to H-1 and H-3. Similarly, H-3 is a triplet due to coupling equally with H-2 and H-4, and H-4 is a doublet due to coupling with H-3. It is actually possible with a closer

Fig. 8.31
270 MHz ^1H nuclear magnetic resonance spectrum of paracetamol.

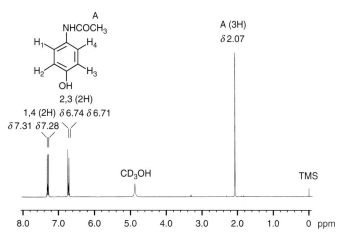
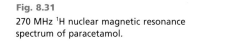

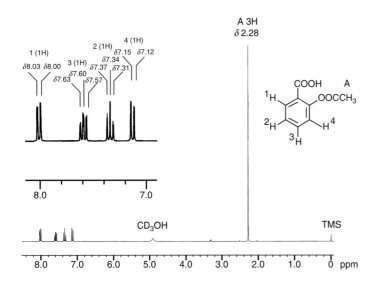

Fig. 8.32
270 MHz ¹H nuclear magnetic resonance
spectrum of aspirin.

view to see additional splitting of all of the aromatic proton signals, and this is due to long-range coupling between the protons *meta* to each other, i.e. H-1 and H-3 and H-2 and H-4, which can occur in aromatic systems and can be up to 3 Hz. *Para* coupling can also occur but it is only *ca* 1 Hz.

Proton NMR spectrum of salbutamol: a more complex example

Figure 8.33 shows the NMR spectrum of salbutamol obtained in CD₃OD and in this case the spectrum is somewhat more complex. The signal at δ 1.40 arises from the t-butyl group A, in which the CH₃ groups are all equivalent and have no adjacent protons to which they could couple. The signal at δ 4.65 is due to the CH₂ group D, which is also not coupled to any other protons. The protons on the aromatic ring are also readily assigned: the doublet at δ 6.80 is due to H-3, which is coupled to H-2. H-2 appears at δ 7.22 and is split into a doublet via coupling to H-3 and each peak in the doublet is split again through meta-coupling

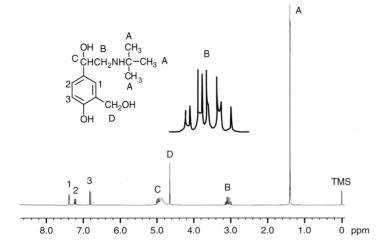

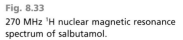

Fig. 8.33
270 MHz ¹H nuclear magnetic resonance
spectrum of salbutamol.

Fig. 8.34
Line intensities in AB systems.

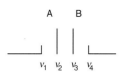

to H-1, which appears at δ 7.37 and is split into a closely spaced doublet through meta-coupling to H-2. A signal centred at δ 4.97, appearing on the shoulder of a broad peak due to CD_3OH, is due to proton C. This proton is attached to a chiral centre and is coupled to the two adjacent protons B1 and B2, which are non-equivalent since they are immediately next to a chiral centre. Thus proton C has two different coupling constants to protons B1 and B2, and appears as a doublet of doublets. The most complex signal in the spectrum is due to protons B1 and B2, and this requires a more detailed explanation. These protons are AB type signals because the protons are close in chemical shift (less than 30 Hz apart), and they give lines which are of unequal sizes, as shown in Figure 8.34.

The place to start with the analysis of the signal for the B protons in salbutamol is with signal C, which gives the couplings of the B1 and B2 protons with the proton on position C. From analysis of this signal the two couplings are 4 and 10 Hz. The total width of the B signal is 44 Hz; thus its width in the absence of coupling to the C proton would be 37 Hz (see Fig. 8.23 for clarification). To make the full analysis, one has to try some values for the AB coupling that make approximate sense in relation to the final signal. If the coupling of the B protons to each other is 12 Hz, then the pattern when plotted on graph paper (Fig. 8.35) gives more or less the pattern seen for the B protons in salbutamol (leaving 13 Hz from the total signal width for separation of the inner lines). Two other points should be noted: the ratio of the outer to the inner lines is *ca* 1:3, as predicted

Fig. 8.35
A typical AB system split by a third (X) proton with coupling constants observed for the B1 and B2 protons in salbutamol.

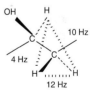

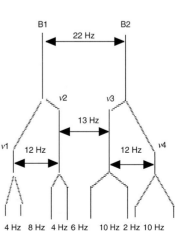

from the equation shown in Figure 8.29, and the original separation of the B1 and B2 signals is given by the following equation:

$$\delta_{B1} - \delta_{B2} = \sqrt{(v_4 - v_1)(v_3 - v_2)}$$

If the differences between the frequencies are substituted in the equation, this gives a difference in frequency of B1 and B2 of 22 Hz, i.e. the geminal coupling (coupling of protons on the same carbon) of the two signals gives shifts of 7.5 Hz in one direction and 4.5 Hz in the other direction instead of the usual even splitting.

Self-test 8.6

Using the values given in Tables 8.1 and 8.3, predict the approximate NMR spectra of the following drug molecules with respect to chemical shift, the number of protons in each signal and the multiplicity of their proton signals:

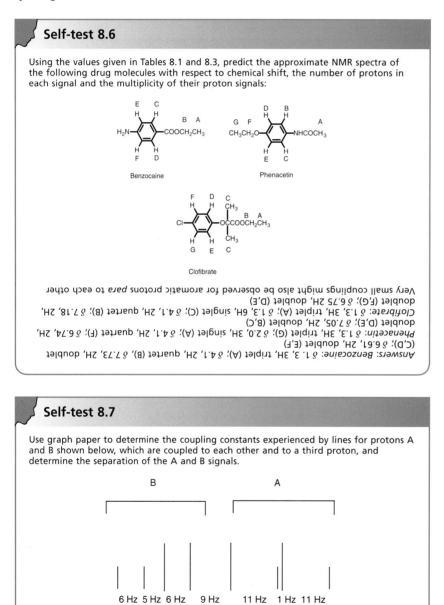

Benzocaine

Phenacetin

Clofibrate

Answers: Benzocaine: δ 1. 3, 3H, triplet (A); δ 4.1, 2H, quartet (B); δ 7.73, 2H, doublet (C,D); δ 6.61, 2H, doublet (E,F).
Phenacetin: δ 1.3, 3H, triplet (G); δ 2.0, 3H, singlet (A); δ 4.1, 2H, quartet (F); δ 6.74, 2H, doublet (D,E); δ 7.05, 2H, doublet (B,C).
Clofibrate: δ 1.3, 3H, triplet (A); δ 1.3, 6H, singlet (C); δ 4.1, 2H, quartet (B); δ 7.18, 2H, doublet (F,G); δ 6.75 2H, doublet (D,E).
Very small couplings might also be observed for aromatic protons para to each other

---

Self-test 8.7

Use graph paper to determine the coupling constants experienced by lines for protons A and B shown below, which are coupled to each other and to a third proton, and determine the separation of the A and B signals.

B

A

6 Hz 5 Hz 6 Hz   9 Hz   11 Hz 1 Hz 11 Hz

Answer: on page 203

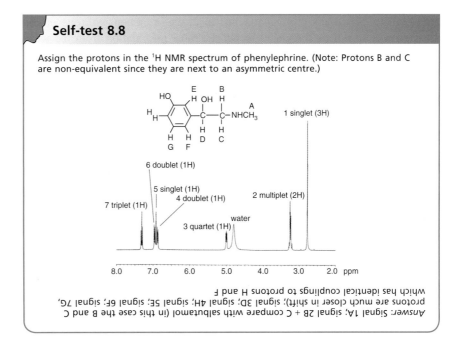

Self-test 8.8

Assign the protons in the ¹H NMR spectrum of phenylephrine. (Note: Protons B and C are non-equivalent since they are next to an asymmetric centre.)

Carbon NMR
Chemical shifts

Nuclei other than ¹H give nuclear magnetic resonance spectra. One of the most useful is ¹³C, but, since the natural abundance of ¹³C is only 1.1% of that of ¹²C, the ¹³C resonance is relatively weak. ¹³C resonance occurs at a frequency *ca* 25.1 MHz when proton resonance is occurring at *ca* 100 MHz (i.e. at 2.33 Tesla). Thus it is at lower energy than proton resonance and the spread of resonances for ¹³C is over *ca* 180 ppm; thus there is less likelihood of overlapping lines in ¹³C NMR. Table 8.4 shows the chemical shifts of some ¹³C signals. It is possible to calculate these quite precisely, and the table is only an approximate guide. A ¹³C

Table 8.4 Typical chemical shifts of ¹³C atoms

Group	δ ppm	Group	δ ppm	Group	δ ppm
H_3C^{13}-C	5–20	$C\text{-}H_2C^{13}$-N	35–65	$(C)_3C^{13}$-C-N	50–70
H_3C^{13}-C=C	15–30	$C\text{-}H_2C^{13}$-O	55–75	$(C)_3C^{13}$-C-O	70–90
H_3C^{13}-Ar	ca 20	$(C)_2HC^{13}$-C	25–55		
H_3C^{13}-COO	ca 20	$(C)_2HC^{13}$-CO	40–70	$ArC^{13}H$	115–135
H_3C^{13}-CO	22–32	$(C)_2HC^{13}$-Ar	ca 40	ArC^{13}-C	137–147
H_3C^{13}-N	25–40	$(C)(O)HC^{13}$-Ar	70–80	ArC^{13}-Cl	135
H_3C^{13}-O	45–55	$(C)_2HC^{13}$-N	45–75	$ArC^{13}CO$	137
$C\text{-}H_2C^{13}$-C	16–46	$(C)_2HC^{13}$-O	65–85	ArC^{13}-N	145–155
$C\text{-}H_2C^{13}$-CO	30–50	$(C)_3C^{13}$-C	35–55	ArC^{13}-O	150–160
$C\text{-}H_2C^{13}$-Ar	ca 30	$(C)_3C^{13}$-C-CO	45–65	C^{13}=O	170–200
$O\text{-}H_2C^{13}$-Ar	60–70	$(C)_3C^{13}$-C-Ar	45–65		

atom will couple to any protons attached to it, e.g. a carbon with one proton attached will appear as a doublet; to get the most information from the weak carbon spectrum, it is better if this coupling is removed. In the salbutamol example the coupling is removed using the *J* mod technique.

An example of a ^{13}C spectrum

Figure 8.36 shows the *J* mod spectrum of salbutamol sulphate. As can be seen, the *J* mod ^{13}C spectrum of salbutamol is much simpler than its proton spectrum. The carbons can be assigned as follows: A δ 26; C δ 58.8; E δ 61; D δ 70.4; 3 δ 116; 2 + 6 δ 127.1; 5 δ 129.5; 1 δ 133 and 4 δ 156 (carbons 3 and 5 are shifted upfield through being ortho to an OH group). The signal due to carbon B is missing, and this illustrates one of the problems of ^{13}C NMR, which is that the relaxation times of the carbon atoms tend to vary more widely than those for protons in ^{1}H NMR and thus their signals may be missed or not fully accumulated. This is particularly true for quaternary carbons, and it can be seen in Figure 8.36 that the quaternary carbons 1, 4 and 5 give weaker signals than the other carbons which have protons attached. In the case of quaternary carbon B, its signal has been completely missed. Thus the signals in ^{13}C are non-quantitative when compared to ^{1}H NMR signals. A *J* mod spectrum is one of the modern equivalents of the ^{13}C spectrum; it allows the number of protons attached to the carbon atoms to be known while at the same time removing the signal broadening due to the coupling between ^{13}C and its attached protons.

Self-test 8.9

Assign the signals in the *J* mod C-13 spectrum of procaine shown below (C and CH$_2$ up, CH$_3$ and CH down) obtained on a 400 MHz instrument.

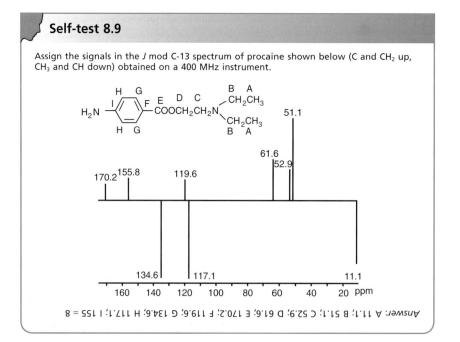

Answer: A 11.1; B 51.1; C 52.9; D 61.6; E 170.2; F 119.6; G 134.6; H 117.1; I 155 = 8

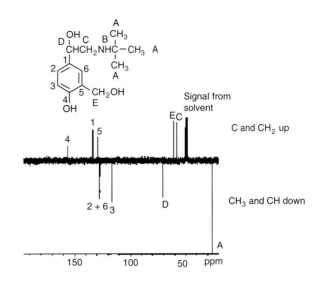

Fig. 8.36

J mod C nuclear magnetic resonance spectrum of salbutamol sulphate.

Two-dimensional NMR spectra
Simple examples

Computer control of NMR instruments has led to great advances in both data acquisition and processing and has given rise to advanced NMR structural elucidation techniques. In two-dimensional experiments, *both* the *x* and the *y* axes have chemical shift scales, and the two-dimensional spectra are plotted as a grid like a map. Information is obtained from the spectra by looking at the peaks in the grid and matching them to the *x* and *y* axes. The most common two-dimensional experiments used in structure elucidation are:

- *J* correlated through bonds-based experiments:COSY – Proton-Proton Correlation Spectroscopy
- TOCSY – Total Correlation – Homonuclear Hartmann Hahn (HOHAHA)
- HMBC – Long-range Correlation Spectroscopy
- HMQC – CH Direct Correlation Spectroscopy.

Nuclear Overhauser through space-based experiments for stereochemistry analysis:

- NOESY – Nuclear Overhauser Effect Spectroscopy
- ROESY – Rotating Frame Overhauser Effect Spectroscopy.

Three-dimensional experiments use a combination:

- NOESY – TOCSY
- NOESY – NOESY.

Proton–proton correlation or COSY is among the first two-dimensional experiments carried out in the early stages of elucidating a structure. This technique enables correlations to be observed between coupling protons. It is used to define the presence of the various spin systems in a structure. Taking the simple example of the aromatic proton region of aspirin, as shown in the COSY spectrum (Fig. 8.37); the diagonal gives the correlation of the signals with themselves, i.e. A with A, B with B, etc. On either side of the diagonal, identical information is

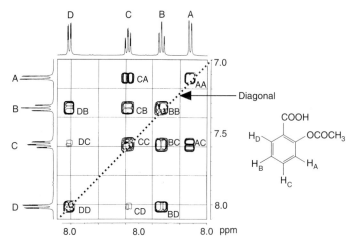

Fig. 8.37
The proton–proton correlation spectrum of the aromatic region of aspirin.

presented; thus only one side of the diagonal is required for spectral interpretation. From the information given in Figure 8.37, it can be seen that A is coupled to C; B is coupled to C and D and C is weakly coupled to D via long-range meta-coupling. COSY has simplified interpretation of complex NMR spectra.

In sorting out the various resonances for the different overlapping spin systems in a molecule, TOCSY or Total Correlation Spectroscopy provides the best solution. This can be well illustrated by analysing the NMR spectra of lactose (Fig. 8.38). Lactose consists of two monosaccharides, β-glucose and galactose with impurities in the form of the free sugars. The anomeric protons are distinctly separated. However, resonances for H-3 to H-6 in both monomers are overlapping between 3.2 and 4.6 ppm. With the aid of a TOCSY spectrum, cross peaks are sorted out and aligned to unambiguously assign the peaks that belong to each of the monomers. A similar technique is employed in identifying the amino acids in a peptide structure.

There are a number of techniques stemming from the basic two-dimensional technique, which allows correlation between carbon atoms and the protons attached to them (CH direct or HMQC spectroscopy) and correlations of carbon atoms with protons one (^2J) and two bonds (^3J), or sometimes three bonds (^4J) away from them by heteronuclear multiple bond correlation spectroscopy (HMBC). Long-range CH correlations especially with quaternary carbons confirm their positions in the molecule. HMBC is used to connect the different spin systems or substructures to elucidate the entire molecular structure as demonstrated for ethyl butenoate in Figure 8.39.

A more complex example

The anti-haemorrhagic drug tranexamic acid when drawn in a two-dimensional representation may look as if all four protons on position 2 and all four protons on position 3 are equivalent. However, when the structure is drawn as indicated on the left in Figure 8.40, it is apparent that, because the molecule is forced for steric reasons to remain with the carboxylic acid and methylamine groups more or less in the plane of the paper, the axial (a) protons, which are held above and below the plane of the paper, and the equatorial (e) protons, which are held more

Fig. 8.38
COSY and TOCSY spectra of lactose.

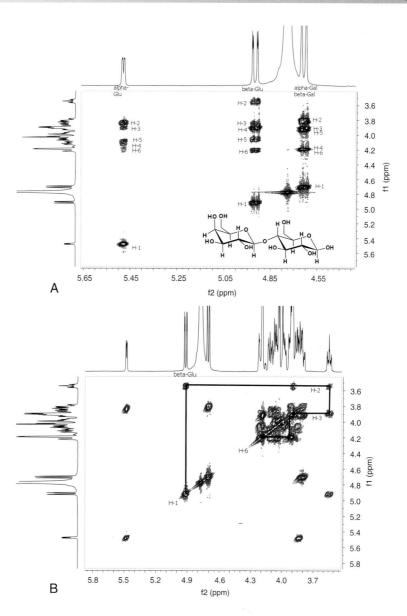

or less in the plane of the paper, are no longer in an equivalent environment. This introduces a number of additional couplings between the protons in the molecule, leading to an increased complexity of its spectrum. Assignment of the protons in this spectrum is simplified by two-dimensional NMR and, as for the aspirin example, the correlations can be derived from the signals either side of the diagonal. The place to start in this type of assignment is usually with the simplest signal, which in this case is due to the 4′ protons, which only couple to the 4 protons. The 4 protons themselves present the most complex signal since they are separately coupled to the 4′, 3a and 3e protons, producing $3 \times 3 \times 3 = 27$ lines, which are not all seen because of the overlap of the signals. Two additional factors that are applicable to the interpretation of more complex molecules

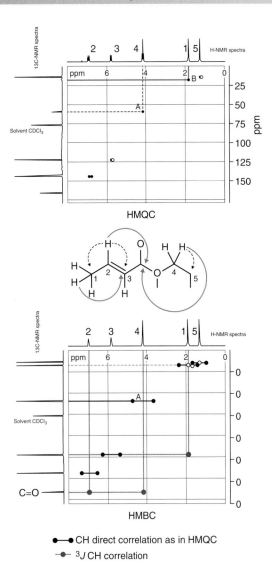

Fig. 8.39
HMQC and HMBC spectra for
ethyl butenoate.

●——● CH direct correlation as in HMQC
—●— ^3J CH correlation

emerge from examination of the signals due to axial and equatorial protons in Figure 8.40:

(i)   The signals due to 2a and 3a experience three couplings due to coupling to the equatorial protons attached to the same carbon (geminal coupling) and due to coupling (9–13 Hz) to two adjacent axial protons, resulting overall in broad signals. The signals due to 2e and 3e protons are narrower since they only experience one large germinal coupling to the axial proton attached to the same carbon. The axial/equatorial and equatorial/equatorial couplings (e.g. 2e/3a and 2e/3e) are small (2–5 Hz), resulting in narrower signals overall.

(ii)   Axial protons (2a and 3a) are usually upfield from equatorial protons (2e and 3e) since they are shielded by being close in space to other axial protons.

Fig. 8.40

The proton–proton correlation spectrum of tranexamic acid.

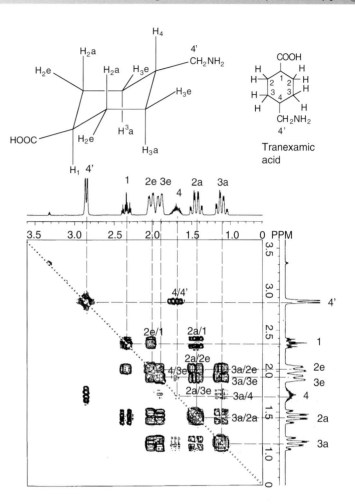

Application of NMR to quantitative analysis

NMR can be used as a rapid and specific quantitative technique. For example, a drug can be rapidly quantified by measuring suitable protons (often isolated methyl protons) against the intense singlet for the methyl groups in t-butanol. The amount of drug present can be calculated using the following formula for the methyl groups in t-butanol used as an internal standard (int. std.):

$$\text{Amount of drug} = \frac{\text{Area signal for drug protons}}{\text{Area signal for int. std. protons}} \times \text{mass of int. std. added}$$

$$\times \frac{\text{MW drug}}{\text{MW int. std.}} \times \frac{\text{No. protons from int. std.}}{\text{No. protons from drug}}$$

An advantage of this method of quantitation is that a pure external standard for the drug is not required since the response is purely proportional to the number of protons present, and this can be measured against a pure internal standard. Thus the purity of a substance can be determined without a pure standard for it being available. Figure 8.41 shows the spectrum of an extract from tablet powder containing aspirin, paracetamol and codeine with 8 mg of t-butanol added as an

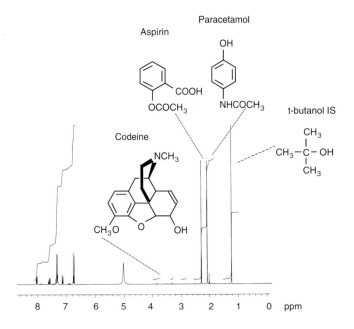

Fig. 8.41
NMR spectrum obtained from a tablet containing aspirin, paracetamol and codeine with 8 mg of t-butanol added as an internal standard.

internal standard. In the analysis, deuterated methanol containing 8 mg/ml of t-butanol was added to the sample of tablet powder, and the sample was shaken for 5 min, filtered and transferred to an NMR tube. The t-butanol protons gave a signal at $\delta\,1.31$; the CH_3CO group in aspirin gave a signal at $\delta\,2.35$; the CH_3CON group in paracetamol gave a signal at $\delta\,2.09$ and the CH_3O group in codeine gave a signal at $\delta\,3.92$. The low amount of codeine present would be likely to make its quantitation inaccurate in the example shown, which was only scanned for a few minutes. Since its signal is close to the baseline, a longer scan would improve the signal : noise ratio, giving better quantitative accuracy.

The data obtained from the analysis is as follows:

- Stated content/tablet = aspirin 250 mg, paracetamol 250 mg, codeine phosphate 6.8 mg
- Weight of 1 tablet = 0.6425 g
- Weight of tablet powder taken for analysis = 0.1228 g
- Weight of t-butanol internal standard added = 8.0 mg
- Area of internal standard peak = 7.2
- Area of aspirin CH_3 peak = 5.65
- Area of paracetamol CH_3 peak = 6.73
- Area of codeine phosphate CH_3 peak = 0.115
- Molecular weight t-butanol = 74.1
- Molecular weight aspirin = 180.2
- Molecular weight paracetamol = 151.2
- Molecular weight codeine phosphate = 397.4
- Number of protons in t-butyl group = 9
- Number of protons in methyl groups of aspirin, paracetamol and codeine = 3.

Calculation of the paracetamol in the tablets is shown in Example 8.2.

Other specialised applications of NMR

There are a number of other specialised applications of NMR, which are valuable in pharmaceutical development. Chiral NMR employs chiral shift reagents, e.g. europium tris(d,d-dicamphoylmethanate), which can be used to separate signals from enantiomers in a mixture and thus quantify them. Solid state NMR can be used to examine crystalline structures and characterise polymorphs and crystal hydrates. Biological NMR uses wide-bore sample tubes and can be used to examine drugs and their metabolites directly in biological fluids such as urine or cerebrospinal fluid. High-pressure liquid chromatography (HPLC) NMR has been investigated so that impurities or drug metabolites can be chromatographically separated by HPLC and identified by using an NMR spectrometer as a detector. However, LC-NMR has never really found its wide application due to the expense of using deuterated solvents in a coupled system. Diffusion spectroscopy (DOSY) is a pulse-field gradient spin-echo experiment which was first established 10 years ago. The resonance for each component decays at different diffusion rates by varying the gradient strength. The method practically allows non-destructive separation of the different components in an extract without using chromatography. It has become the cost-effective alternative of LC-NMR. Signals for an individual component in a mixture can be pseudo-isolated according to its diffusion coefficient (Figs 8.36 and 8.37) because, using a complex mathematical transformation, the signals of a particular component can be linked to its diffusion coefficient. Figure 8.42 illustrates the separation of the ^{1}H spectra of paracetamol and para-aminophenol in a mixture. The Y axis exhibits the diffusion coefficient of each component and the signals belonging to the two components in this simple mixture are linked to a diffusion coefficient and can be summed to give a concentration of each of the drug in the sample mixture. Para-aminophenol is a smaller molecule than paracetamol and thus has a higher diffusion coefficient.

Fig. 8.42
400 MHz DOSY spectrum of a paracetamol with a para-aminophenol impurity.

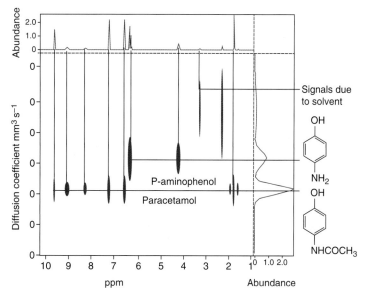

The best results can be attained by calibrating the exponential decay of each of the major components in the mixture through an array experiment. The calibration should be done on isolated well-resolved peaks. However, the method can only resolve a limited number of up to five components. Resolution for data sets from mixtures of more than five components can be analysed by employing a single channel method which only utilises a limited or smaller sweep width. DOSY can also find its application as a quality control tool in the analysis of phytopharmaceuticals. With the emergence of high-resolution NMR, it is possible to employ this spectroscopic method for dereplication studies on crude extracts. At an early stage, it becomes possible to determine the expected type of chemistry of different metabolites in an active extract as shown in Figure 8.43. In dereplication studies, there is a need to do rapid but sensitive spectral acquisitions where more precise data can be obtained at a shorter period of time without using up the sample.

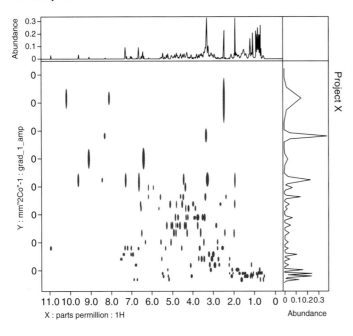

Fig. 8.43
400 MHz DOSY spectrum of a biologically active plant fraction.

Calculation example 8.2

Weight of aspirin and paracetamol expected in the tablet powder $= 250 \times \dfrac{0.1228}{0.6425} = 47.97$ mg

Weight of codeine expected in the tablet powder $= 6.8 \times \dfrac{0.1228}{0.6425} = 1.300$ mg

Calculation for aspirin
Substituting into the formula given above:

$$\text{mg or aspirin present in extract} = \frac{5.65}{7.2} \times 8 \times \frac{180.2}{74.1} \times \frac{9}{3} = 45.80 \text{ mg}$$

$$\text{Percentage of stated content} = \frac{45.8}{47.97} \times 100 = 95.48\%$$

Self-test 8.10

From the above data calculate the percentage of stated content for paracetamol and codeine phosphate.

Answers: paracetamol 95.42%, codeine phosphate 158.5%

NMR in drug metabolism and related areas

NMR has been developed recently, in conjunction with chemometrics, as a tool for the diagnosis of disease and also for the assessment of drug toxicity – metabonomics. It has also found wide application in magnetic resonance imaging, a technique that may be used for imaging soft tissues using the NMR signal produced by the protons within the tissues.

Self-test 8.7 – Answer

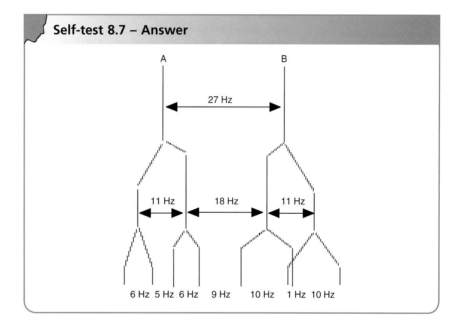

Further reading

Berger S, Braun S. *200 and More NMR Experiments: A Practical Course.* 3rd ed. Weinheim: Wiley VCH; 2004.

Breitmaier E. *Structure Elucidation by NMR in Organic Chemistry: A Practical Guide.* 3rd ed. Hoboken, NJ: Wiley-Blackwell; 2002.

Claridge TDW. *High-Resolution NMR Techniques in Organic Chemistry: 27 (Tetrahedron Organic Chemistry).* 2nd ed. London: Elsevier Science; 2008.

Friebolin H, ed. *Basic One- and Two-Dimensional NMR Techniques.* 5th ed. Weinheim: Wiley VCH; 2010.

Keeler J. *Understanding NMR Spectroscopy.* Hoboken, NJ: Wiley-Blackwell; 2010.

Simpson JH. *Organic Structure Determination Using 2-D NMR Spectroscopy: A Problem-Based Approach (Advanced Organic Chemistry).* 1st ed. London: Academic Press; 2008.

Williams DH, Fleming I. *Spectroscopic Methods in Organic Chemistry.* 6th ed. New York: McGraw-Hill Higher Education; 2007.

www.metabometrix.com

Contains information on the uses of NMR in disease diagnosis.

www.spectroscopynow.com

www.varianinc.com

Websites contain background information of NMR and links to tutorials.

Mass spectrometry

9

KEYPOINTS

Principles
- Charged molecules or molecular fragments are generated in a high-vacuum region, or immediately prior to a sample entering a high-vacuum region, using a variety of methods for ion production. The ions are generated in the gas phase so that they can then be manipulated by the application of either electric or magnetic fields to enable the determination of their molecular weights.

Applications
- Mass spectrometry provides a highly specific method for determining or confirming the identity or structure of drugs and raw materials used in their manufacture.
- Mass spectrometry in conjunction with either gas chromatography (GC–MS) or liquid chromatography (LC–MS) provides a method for characterising impurities in drugs and formulation excipients.

(Continued)

KEYPOINTS *(Continued)*

- GC–MS and LC–MS provide highly sensitive and specific methods for determining drugs and their metabolites in biological fluids and tissues.
- Mass spectrometry has become an important tool in proteomics, which is currently a major tool in drug discovery.

Strengths
- The best method for getting rapid identification of trace impurities, which should ideally be carried out using chromatographic separation in conjunction with high-resolution mass spectrometry so that elemental compositions can be determined
- The method of choice for monitoring drugs and their metabolites in biological fluids because of its high sensitivity and selectivity.
- With the advent of electrospray mass spectrometry and the re-emergence of time of flight mass spectrometry, the technique will be of major use in the quality control of therapeutic antibodies and peptides.

Limitations
- Mass spectrometry is not currently used in routine quality control (QC) but is placed in a research and development (R&D) environment, where it is used to solve specific problems arising from routine processes or in process development.
- The instrumentation is expensive and requires support by highly trained personnel and regular maintenance. However, these limitations are gradually being removed, with open access instruments becoming more common.

Introduction

A mass spectrometer works by generating charged molecules or molecular fragments either in a high vacuum or immediately prior to the sample entering the high-vacuum region. The ionised molecules have to be generated in the gas phase. In classical mass spectrometry there was only one method of producing the charged molecules but now there are quite a number of alternatives. Once the molecules are charged and in the gas phase, they can be manipulated by the application of either electric or magnetic fields to enable the determination of their molecular weight and the molecular weight of any fragments which are produced by the molecule breaking up. Thus mass spectrometry can be divided into two sections: ion generation and ion separation.

Ion generation

The two most popular methods for ion generation are electrospray ionisation (ESI) and electron impact ionisation (EI). Also popular in certain areas of application is matrix assisted laser desorption ionisation (MALDI).

Electrospray ionisation (ESI) (see Animation 9.1)

ESI began to be popularised around 20 years ago and has revolutionised the applicability of MS as an analytical tool. Thus ESI is now the most widely applied method of ionisation because of its ready compatibility with high-pressure liquid chromatography (HPLC). The ionisation takes place under atmospheric pressure. The basis of the technique is shown in Figure 9.1.

The eluent from an HPLC system (see Animation 9.2) passes through a quartz or metal needle to which a high electrical potential, e.g. 4.5 kV, is applied. If a positive potential is applied, then the negative ions in the eluent are stripped away by being attracted to the needle, thus leaving positively charged solvent droplets

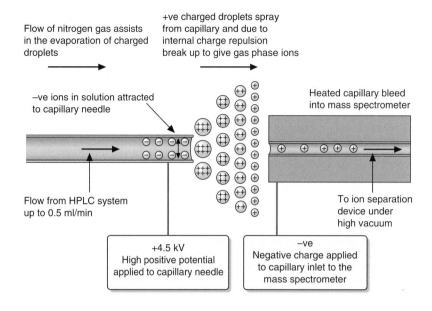

Fig. 9.1
The electrospray
ionisation (ESI) process.

which spray out of the capillary. Under the influence of a coaxial flow of nitrogen gas, the droplets evaporate and, as they do so, break up due to internal charge–charge repulsion. In the end gas phase ions are produced which are attracted into the mass spectrometer by an opposite charge applied to a heated capillary which allows a slow bleed from the atmosphere into the mass spectrometer, which has to operate under high vacuum. In order to maintain high vacuum in the instrument two pumping stages are used, an intermediate stage immediately after the heated capillary and a high-vacuum stage in the ion separation stage.

Figure 9.2 shows an electrospray spectrum of the basic drug acebutolol. The positive charge on the molecule is generated by its basic centre being protonated. This occurs even in a weakly acidic HPLC mobile phase. The main ion seen at m/z 337.2 (m/z stands for mass over charge ratio) is due to the molecular weight of the drug plus a proton. ESI is known as a soft ionisation technique, and in

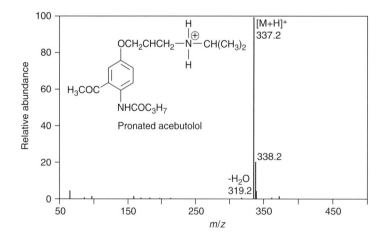

Fig. 9.2
A positive electrospray ionisation (ESI)
spectrum of acebutolol.

Figure 9.2 it can be seen that there is little fragmentation of the molecule. A very minor fragment can be observed at *m/z* 319.2, which is due to the loss of water (18 amu). Two additional features of the spectrum should be noted:

1. The ion separation used in this case was based on a quadrupole (discussed later) which measures masses to approximately one decimal place and the mass measured for protonated acebutolol ($C_{18}H_{29}N_2O_4$) is greater than the mass of 337 amu, which would be obtained by adding up all the atoms making it up according to their nominal masses, i.e. C=12, H=1, N=14 and O=16. The greatest deviation from nominal mass is for hydrogen (Table 9.1), which has an exact mass of 1.00783. Hydrogen is very abundant in drug molecules, and the presence of 29 hydrogen atoms in protonated acebutolol increases its mass by $29 \times 0.00783 = 0.23$ above its nominal mass of 337 and thus the quadrupole measures it at approximately 337.2 amu.

2. There is an additional peak which is abundant in the mass spectrum at *m/z* 338.2. This is due to protonated acebutolol where one of the 18 carbon atoms making up the molecule is due to a ^{13}C atom. There is a 1.1% probability that a ^{13}C atom will occur, and where there are 18 C atoms there is a $1.1 \times 18 = 19.8\%$ probability that one of them will be a ^{13}C atom. Thus the ion at *m/z* 338.2 is approximately 20% of the intensity of the ion at *m/z* 337.2. The abundances of the isotopes for H, N and O are much lower and do not contribute very much in this case. The halogen atoms chlorine and bromine have abundant isotopes, and their isotope peaks can be useful in structure elucidation. The exact masses and isotope abundances of atoms commonly found in drug molecules are summarised in Table 9.1.

ESI can also produce negative ions if the polarity on the spray needle is reversed so that it attracts positive ions, thus producing a negatively charged spray. Figure 9.3 shows the ESI mass spectrum of ketoprofen, which forms a negatively charged anion at *m/z* 253.1 (see Animation 9.3). In addition, the spectrum is dominated by an adduct ion formed between ketoprofen and formate, which was used as an additive in the HPLC mobile phase. Adduct formation can occur both

Table 9.1 Elements commonly found in drug molecules with their exact masses, isotopes and isotope abundances

Element	Main isotope	Mass	Relative abundance	Other isotopes	Mass	Relative abundance
Hydrogen	^1H	1.00783	100%	^2H	2.01410	0.0115%
Carbon	^{12}C	12.00000	100%	^{13}C	13.00335	1.1%
Nitrogen	^{14}N	14.00307	100%	^{15}N	15.00011	0.37%
Oxygen	^{16}O	15.99491	100%	^{18}O	17.99916	0.21%
Fluorine	^{19}F	18.99840	100%			
Phosphorus	^{31}P	31.97376	100%			
Sulphur	^{32}S	31.97207	100%	^{33}S	33.97146	0.76%
				^{34}S	33.96787	4.52%
Chlorine	^{35}Cl	34.96885	100%	^{36}Cl	36.96590	31.96%
Bromine	^{79}Br	78.91834	100%	^{81}Br	80.91629	97.28%
Iodine	^{127}I	126.90447	100%			

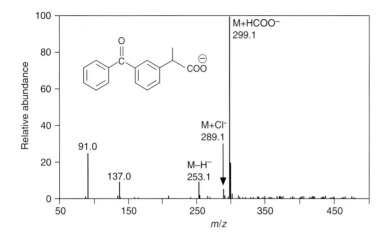

Fig. 9.3
A negative ion electrospray ionisation (ESI) spectrum of ketoprofen.

in positive and negative ion mode but is usually more pronounced in negative ion mode. It can occur even with trace levels of contaminants in the mobile phase, and it can be seen that the spectrum of ketoprofen also contains an ion at *m/z* 289.1, which is due to adduct formation with traces of Cl⁻ in the mobile phase. It can also be observed that there are more background ions present in the spectrum of ketoprofen and the ions at *m/z* 91.0 and 137.0 are due to clusters of 2 and 3 formic acid molecules. Table 9.2 lists common adduct ions which are observed in ESI spectra.

Self-test 9.1

Ampicillin forms many adducts. The drug was introduced into the mass spectrometer in a mobile phase containing methanol. Identify the adducts of ampicillin:

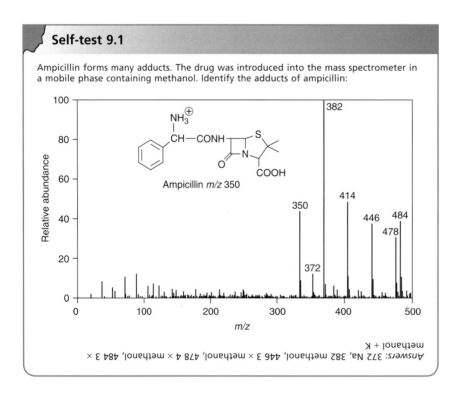

Answers: 372 Na, 382 methanol, 446 3 × methanol, 478 4 × methanol, 484 3 × methanol + K

Table 9.2 Some of the commonly observed additions to molecular ions observed under electrospray ionisation (ESI) conditions

	Adduct	Comment
Addition +ve ion amu		
18	NH_4^+	More likely to occur with ammonium in the mobile phase
22	Na^+	Forms readily with traces of Na^+ in mobile phase
32	CH_3OH	With methanol in mobile phase
39	K^+	Less common than Na, adduct forms with traces of K^+ in the mobile phase
41	CH_3CN	Formed with acetonitrile in mobile phase
54	CH_3OH/Na^+	Formed with methanol in mobile phase + traces of Na^+
63	CH_3CN/Na^+	Formed with acetonitrile in mobile phase + traces of Na^+
Addition −ve ion amu		
35	Cl^-	Formed with traces of Cl^- in mobile phase
45	$HCOO^-$	With formate in mobile phase
60	CH_3COO^-	With acetate in mobile phase

Atmospheric pressure chemical ionisation (APCI)

Atmospheric pressure chemical ionisation (APCI) is closely related to ESI, and instruments carrying out ESI can be readily switched to operate in APCI mode. In APCI mode the eluent from the HPLC does not pass through a charged needle before entering the mass spectrometer source but via a heated tube so that it forms an aerosol. Upon exiting the heated tube an electric discharge is passed through the aerosol, generating reactive species such as H_3O^+ and N_2^+, which promote the ionisation of the analytes. The technique has never achieved the level of popularity of ESI since most drug molecules can be ionised under ESI conditions; however, APCI can be employed for the analysis of drug molecules of low polarity that do not ionise efficiently under ESI conditions.

Electron impact ionisation (EI) (see Animation 9.4)

EI is not compatible with the use of HPLC as a method for introducing the sample into the mass spectrometer. Before ESI was developed several interfaces were developed which were compatible with EI type ionisation, such as particle beam, thermospray and FRIT-EI interfaces, but these have been almost completely superseded by the ESI interface. However, EI is still used in conjunction with sample introduction either via a direct heated probe or via gas chromatography (GC):

(i)   The sample is introduced into the instrument source by heating it on the end of a probe until it evaporates, assisted by the high vacuum within the instrument or via a capillary GC column.

(ii) Once in the vapour phase, the analyte is bombarded with the electrons produced by a rhenium or tungsten filament, which are accelerated toward a positive target with an energy of 70 eV (Fig. 9.4). The analyte is introduced between the filament and the target, and the electrons cause ionisation as follows:

$$M + e \rightarrow M^{+\cdot} + 2\,e$$

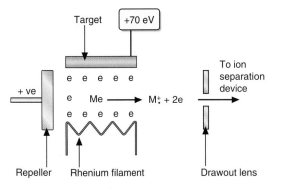

Fig. 9.4
Ion generation in an electron impact source.

(iii) Since the electrons used are of much higher energy than the strength of the bonds within the analyte (4–7 eV), extensive fragmentation of the analyte usually occurs.

(iv) The molecule and its fragments are pushed out of the source by a repeller plate which has the same charge as the ions generated.

Figure 9.5 shows the EI spectrum of ketoprofen. Ions generated under EI conditions are always positive, and thus the ion at *m/z* 254 is exactly the molecular weight of ketoprofen minus the very small mass of an electron. If there is an electronegative atom in the molecule, such as oxygen or nitrogen, usually the positive charge is located there. Unlike the ESI spectrum of ketoprofen shown in Figure 9.3 the EI spectrum of ketoprofen contains many fragment ions because of the high energy nature of the ionisation process. This is an advantage when it comes to structural confirmation since the spectrum provides a unique fingerprint of the molecule which can be matched against a library spectrum and also can be interpreted. Identifying all of the fragment ions in an EI spectrum is often not easy, and ketoprofen provides a less common example where many of the fragment ions can be explained (Fig. 9.6).

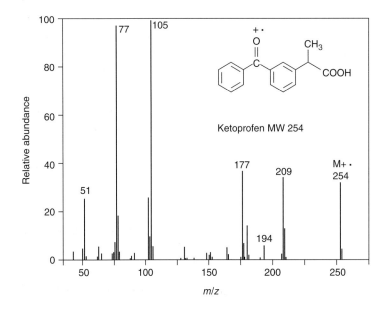

Fig. 9.5
An electron impact spectrum of ketoprofen.

Fig. 9.6
Structure of the ions generated in the electron
impact ionisation (EI) mass spectrum of ketoprofen.

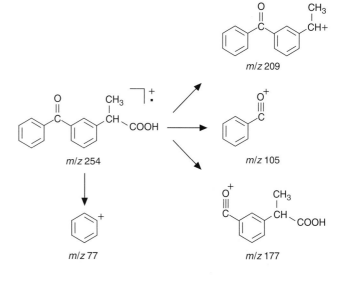

Figure 9.7 shows a generalised scheme for decomposition of a molecule under EI conditions. The principles of the scheme are as follows:

(i) $M^{+\cdot}$ represents the molecular ion which bears one positive charge since it has lost one electron, and the unpaired electron which results from the loss of one electron is represented by a dot. Such an ion is known as a radical cation.

(ii) $M^{+\cdot}$ may lose a radical, which, in a straightforward fragmentation not involving rearrangement, can be produced by the breaking of any single bond in the molecule. The radical removes the unpaired electron from the molecule, leaving behind a cation A^{+}.

(iii) This cation can lose any number of neutral fragments (N), such as H_2O or CO_2, but *no further radicals*.

(iv) The same process can occur in a different order with a neutral fragment (H_2O, CO_2, etc.) being lost to produce B^{+}, and since this ion still has an unpaired electron it can lose a radical to produce C^{+}; this ion can thereafter only lose neutral fragments.

To summarise, the following rules apply to mass spectrometric fragmentation:

(i)   The molecular ion can lose only *one* radical but any number of neutral fragments.

(ii) Once a radical has been lost only neutral fragments can be lost thereafter.

Fig. 9.7
Electron impact ionisation (EI) fragmentation pathways.

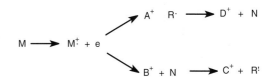

Table 9.3 Common losses from a molecular ion

Loss amu	Radicals/neutral fragments lost	Interpretation
1	H·	Often a major ion in amines, alcohols and aldehydes
2	H_2	
15	CH_3·	Most readily lost from a quaternary carbon
17	OH· or NH_3	
18	H_2O	Readily lost from secondary or tertiary alcohols
19/20	F·/HF	Fluorides
28	CO	Ketone or acid
29	C_2H_5·	
30	CH_2O	Aromatic methyl ether
31	CH_3O·	Methyl ester/methoxime
31	CH_3NH_2	Secondary amine
32	CH_3OH	Methyl ester
33	$H_2O + CH_3$·	
35/36	Cl·/HCl	Chloride
42	$CH_2= C=O$	Acetate
43	C_3H_7·	Readily lost if isopropyl group present
43	CH_3CO·	Methyl ketone
43	$CO + CH_3$·	
44	CO_2	Ester
45	CO_2H·	Carboxylic acid
46	C_2H_5OH	Ethyl ester
46	$CO + H_2O$	
57	C_4H_9·	
59	CH_3CONH_2	Acetamide
60	CH_3COOH	Acetate
73	$(CH_3)_3Si$·	Trimethylsilyl ether
90	$(CH_3)_3SiOH$	Trimethylsilyl ether

Table 9.3 shows typical fragments which are lost under EI conditions to give the complex fingerprint pattern of a particular molecule. Further examples of EI spectra will be discussed later in the chapter.

Matrix assisted laser desorption ionisation (MALDI)

MALDI uses a nitrogen laser to promote ionisation of molecules prior to ion separation in a mass spectrometer. It is usually combined with time of flight (TOF) separation of the ions generated. In order for the sample to be ionised it has to be dissolved in a matrix that absorbs UV radiation at around the wavelength (337 nm) produced by the laser. A simple example of a matrix is dihydroxybenzoic acid, and there are a number of similar aromatic compounds which are used to promote ionisation of different classes of molecules. The sample solution is mixed with matrix solution on a metal plate and allowed to dry prior to being introduced into the instrument. The laser is then directed at the target plate to promote ionisation (Fig. 9.8).

The technique like ESI is a soft ionisation technique, and the ions generated are most commonly due to protonated, or in negative ion deprotonated, molecular ions without extensive fragmentation occurring. It has been widely applied in the characterisation of proteins since it allows ionisation of these high-molecular-weight compounds as singly charged ions, and, in combination with TOF

Fig. 9.8

Matrix assisted laser desorption ionisation (MALDI) carried out on a sample crystallised with a UV absorbing matrix.

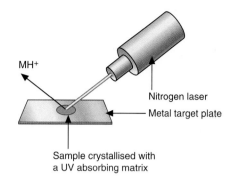

MH+

Nitrogen laser

Metal target plate

Sample crystallised with a UV absorbing matrix

separation, measurement of high-molecular-weight species can be carried out. It is also a useful technique for the determination of very polar compounds such as DNA oligomers (DNA fragments 10–20 base pairs long) which contain a phosphate backbone and do not readily ionise in ESI mode because of the strong association of these molecules with sodium ions.

MALDI is also useful for the ionisation of other polar biomolecules, and Figure 9.9 shows the ions generated from coenzyme A and two acyl CoAs using MALDITOF in negative ion mode. Another use of MALDI in pharmaceutical development is in the characterisation of pharmaceutical polymers. These usually comprise a mixture of chain lengths, and MALDIMS can provide a molecular size distribution for these materials providing one method for setting a quality standard for such materials. The disadvantage of MALDIMS is that it is not readily quantitative and cannot be linked directly with HPLC. However, another area where MALDI has proved useful has been in tissue imaging where a tissue section is coated with matrix and the MALDIMS instrument is used to scan across the tissue in *ca* 0.1 mm steps to image the tissue in terms of the molecules making it up which could lead, for instance, to a better understanding of a disease process or find the site of accumulation of a drug within the tissue.

Figure 9.10 shows a MALDIMS image of an experimental antipsychotic drug in rat brain. One of the major sites of accumulation is in the cerebellum.

Fig. 9.9

Matrix assisted laser desorption ionisation mass spectrometry (MALDIMS) in negative ion mode of a sample containing standards for coenzyme A (CoA), acetyl CoA and propionyl CoA.

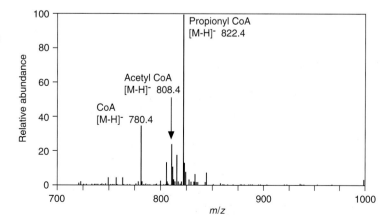

Propionyl CoA
[M-H]⁻ 822.4

Acetyl CoA
[M-H]⁻ 808.4

CoA
[M-H]⁻ 780.4

Relative abundance

m/z

Cerebellum

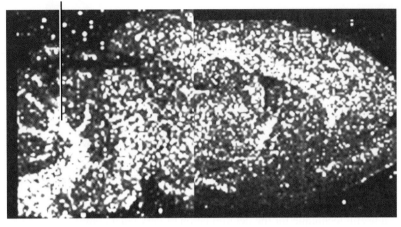

Fig. 9.10
Matrix assisted laser desorption ionisation mass spectrometry (MALDIMS) image of a sagittal section of rat brain following dosing with an experimental antipsychotic drug. Accumulation can be seen in specific regions, e.g. the cerebellum.

Other ionisation methods

Older methods of ionisation such as fast atom bombardment ionisation, thermospray ionisation and particle beam ionisation have been replaced by ESI. A group of techniques that will become increasingly important in the future are surface ionisation techniques, which are useful in forensic investigations for traces of drugs and potentially useful in the characterisation of pharmaceutical polymers and in the type of imaging work described above. Secondary ionisation mass spectrometry (SIMS) has been used for many years to explore the surfaces of materials, and it used high energy heavy ions such as positively charged argon, xenon or cesium to generate ions from surfaces and measure them by mass spectrometry. Two recent techniques which have great potential in this area are desorption electrospray ionisation (DESI) and DART®.

Ion separation techniques
Magnetic sector mass spectrometry

The original mass spectrometric technique was based on separation of charged ions generated in an ion source using a curved magnet. Magnetic sector instruments are still used, but the range of ion separation methods now available means that they only represent a small fraction of the instruments currently used. A schematic view of a magnetic mass spectrometer is shown in Figure 9.11.

Magnetic sector instruments

In a magnetic sector instrument the ions generated are pushed out of the source by a repeller potential of the same charge as the ion itself (most often positive). They are then accelerated in an electric field of *ca* 3–8 kV and travel through an electrostatic field region so that they are forced to fall into a narrow range of kinetic energies prior to entering the field of a circular magnet. They then adopt a flight path through the magnetic field depending on their charge to mass (m/z) ratio; the large ions are deflected less by the magnetic field:

$$m/z = \frac{H^2 r^2}{2V}$$

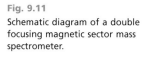

Fig. 9.11
Schematic diagram of a double focusing magnetic sector mass spectrometer.

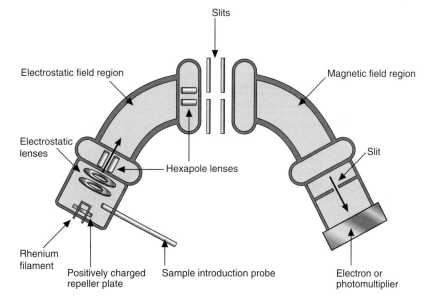

where H is the magnetic field strength, r is the radius of the circular path in which the ion travels, and V is the accelerating voltage.

At particular values for H and V, only ions of a particular mass adopt a flight path that enables them to pass through the collector slit and be detected. If the magnetic field strength is varied, ions across a wide mass range can be detected by the analyser; a typical sweep time for the magnetic field across a mass range of 1000 is 5–10 s, but faster speeds are required if high-resolution chromatography is being used in conjunction with mass spectrometry. The accelerating voltage can also be varied while the magnetic field is held constant, in order to produce separation of ions on the basis of their kinetic energies. Magnetic instruments are capable of making high-resolution mass spectrometry measurements where masses of ions can be measured to four or five decimal places, thus enabling the determination of the elemental composition of molecules.

Quadrupole instruments (see Animation 9.5)

A cheaper and more sensitive mass spectrometer than a magnetic sector instrument is based on the quadrupole analyser (Fig. 9.12), which uses two electric fields applied at right angles to each other, rather than a magnetic field, to separate ions according to their m/z ratios. One of the fields used is DC, and the other oscillates at radio frequency.

The effect of applying the two orthogonal electrostatic fields at right angles is to create a resonance frequency for each m/z value; ions which resonate at the frequency of the quadrupole are able to pass through it and be detected. Thus ions across the mass range of the mass spectrum are selected as the resonance frequency of the quadrupole is varied. A quadrupole instrument is more sensitive than a magnetic sector instrument since it is able to collect ions with a wider range of kinetic energies. The disadvantage of a simple quadrupole mass spectrometer is that it cannot resolve ions to an extent > 0.1 amu, whereas a magnetic sector instrument can resolve ions to a level of 0.0001 amu or more. However,

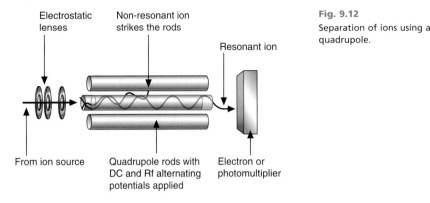

Electrostatic lenses

Non-resonant ion strikes the rods

Resonant ion

From ion source

Quadrupole rods with DC and Rf alternating potentials applied

Electron or photomultiplier

Fig. 9.12
Separation of ions using a quadrupole.

the quadrupole remains the most widely used ion separation device since it is incorporated into triple quadrupole mass spectrometers which are the industry standard for the measurement of drugs in biological fluids.

Time of flight (TOF) ion separation (see Animation 9.6)

The patent for separating ions by TOF was registered in 1952, but the first commercial instruments using the technology did not become available until around 1990. The basis of the separation is that smaller ions move more quickly than larger ions and thus reach the detector first. The technique relies on gating the signal from the ion source, so that one packet of ions is allowed time to reach the detector before the next set is ejected from the ion source, so that there is no overlap between ion packets. The ions leaving the ion source have different kinetic energies, and this compromises the mass resolution; indeed early instruments gave very wide peaks for a single mass. The problem of mass resolution was resolved by using a device called a reflectron, which opposes the direction that the ions are moving by sending them back in the opposite direction. The faster moving ions penetrate deeper into the reflectron, and thus a lag effect is produced for faster moving ions so that they are focused with the slower moving ions which do not penetrate as far into the reflectron. Pushing the ions back in the opposite direction also effectively increases the length of the flight tube, thus increasing instrument resolution. Resolution can be further improved by using a W-configuration where the ions move back and forth twice passing into two relectrons (see Animation 9.7).

TOF separation is often used with MALDI as described above, but it is also used in conjunction with ESI, in this case a hybrid instrument is produced where the ions can be initially filtered through a quadrupole prior to entering the TOF separation stage. Figure 9.13 shows the TOF separation process in combination with electrospray and a quadrupole ion filter. This type of combination is used to produce ion fragmentation in ESI mode and will be discussed further below. This type of configuration is found in instruments such as the QTOF. TOF instruments are capable of making high-resolution mass measurements to four decimal places.

Fig. 9.13
Schematic diagram of a quadrupole time of flight (QTOF) mass spectrometer.

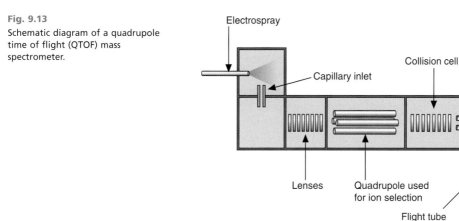

Ion trap separation (see Animation 9.8)

Ion trap technology first became commercialised in the late 1980s. Figure 9.14 shows one version of an ion trap. Ions are injected into the trap and are then trapped in an rf field, which is applied to a circular electrode. The trap is filled with helium which quenches the kinetic energy of the ions. The ions can then be ejected from the trap in order of mass by applying a DC electric field to an endcap electrode. If it is of interest to fragment a particular ion, the trap can be set to empty itself of all the ions apart from the ion of interest. The rf voltage can then be altered so that the ion becomes excited and collides with helium atoms in the trap, thus producing fragments. The fragments derived from the selected ion can then be ejected from the trap and detected. This will be illustrated with an example later in the chapter.

Fig. 9.14
Schematic diagram of an ion trap.

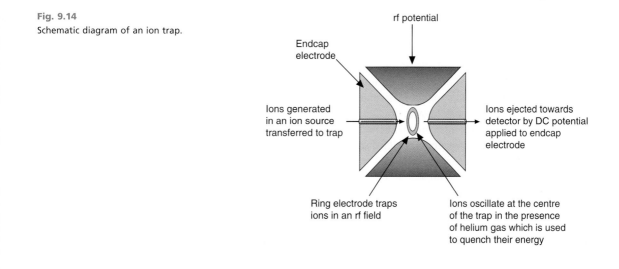

Fourier transform mass spectrometry

Fourier transform mass spectrometers produce very accurate mass measurements. The original cyclotron resonance instruments have been used for many years and are very expensive instruments. These instruments trap ions in a magnetic field in order to measure their masses. However, in 2005 the Orbitrap Fourier transform mass spectrometer was launched and is in the same price range as TOF instruments, making the technique much more routine. The Orbitrap uses an electrostatic field to trap ions so that they orbit around a central spindle electrode (Fig. 9.15). The ion oscillations are detected as an image current which can be converted into highly accurate mass and the Orbitrap can measure masses to five decimal places.

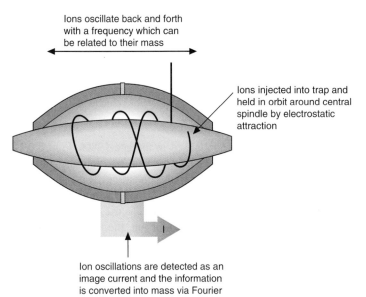

Ions oscillate back and forth with a frequency which can be related to their mass

Ions injected into trap and held in orbit around central spindle by electrostatic attraction

Ion oscillations are detected as an image current and the information is converted into mass via Fourier transformation

Fig. 9.15
The Orbitrap high-resolution ion trap.

Calibration of the mass axes of mass spectrometers

Like all instruments, mass spectrometers have to be calibrated, and a test of fundamental importance in mass spectrometry is to calibrate the mass axis of the mass spectrometer with a suitable tuning compound or tuning mixture. Tuning to exact known masses tells the instrument the exact magnetic field or electric field strength which corresponds to that mass and enables it to plot a calibration curve of mass against magnetic field strength.

The calibration of the instrument drifts with time, and calibration has to be carried out regularly. In systems which use EI, the most popular tuning compounds are perfluorokerosene (PFK) and perfluorotributylamine (PFTBA). The use of fluorinated tuning compounds has the advantage that on the carbon-12 scale of atomic weight fluorine is very close to its nominal mass of 19 whereas the mass hydrogen is considerably greater than its nominal mass of 1 (see Table 9.1). For example, in the electron impact mode PFTBA produces a number of abundant ions below a mass of m/z 219 and weaker ions above this value. Tuning should be carried out on a minimum of three ions covering the mass range of interest. Typically the ions at *m/z* 69, 219 and 502 generated by PFTBA are used to calibrate the mass axis in EI mode, as these ions are also used to determine resolution between masses. In Figure 9.16 the ions have been set with a mass width of 0.6 amu at half height, which is *ca* 1.2 amu at base. The peak for the ion at *m/z* 69 extends between *m/z* 68.4 and 69.6, and thus there will be some slight overlap with the ions at *m/z* 68 and *m/z* 70. However, there is no interference at *m/z* 69.

There is usually a tradeoff between resolution and sensitivity, and if the mass window is narrowed to reduce peak width, sensitivity will be lost. Ions in mass spectra are usually displayed as centroided data, as can be seen in Figure 9.16. The ions in the calibrant at 69, 219 and 502 can be viewed in profile, or just the midpoint of the ion peaks is plotted in the centroid view. In the case of quadrupole mass spectrometers and other low-resolution instruments, such as ion traps, the ions used in tuning are assigned masses to the nearest whole number. When high-resolution calibration is being carried out, masses of four or five decimal places are assigned to calibration ions – thus, for instance, the CF_3^+ ion at *m/z* 69 would be assigned its exact mass of *m/z* 68.9952.

Fig. 9.16

Calibration ions generated from perfluorotributylamine (PFTBA) in electron impact ionisation (EI) mode.

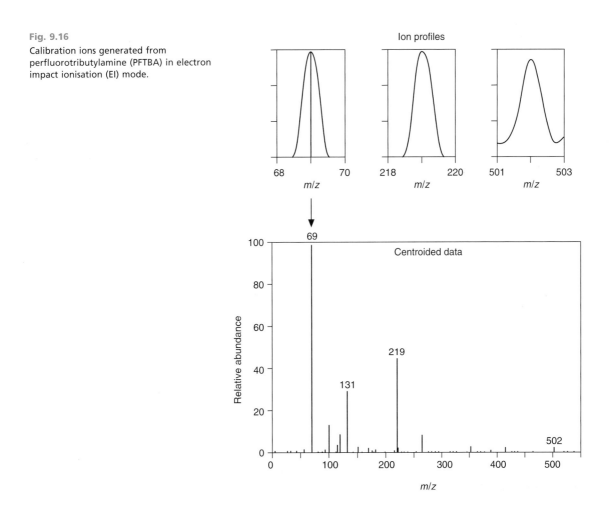

In ESI mode commonly used calibrants are proteins such as horse myoglobin, small peptides and Ultramark™, which can be used to calibrate in ESI mode both in positive and negative ion mode.

A more detailed consideration of mass spectra
Mass spectra obtained under electron impact (EI) ionisation conditions

EI ionisation, as described earlier, produces extensive fragmentation of the bonds within the analyte. It is still very commonly used in standard chemical analyses but is not as readily applicable where molecules are very involatile or unstable. Many of the rules for fragmentation under EI conditions were summarised by McLafferty (see further reading), and to a large extent these rules apply to the type of fragmentation produced when ions obtained under ESI conditions are fragmented. However, in general, apart from one or two obvious fragmentations, it may be difficult to fully interpret mass spectrum, and an important aspect of mass spectrometry is library matching where the fragmentation pattern of an unknown is compared to a library spectrum.

Molecular fragmentation patterns
Homolytic α-cleavage (see Animation 9.9)

Under EI conditions the analyte develops a positive charge through the loss of one electron. If there is an electronegative atom in the structure of the molecule, such as nitrogen or oxygen, this positive charge will be on the electronegative atom(s). If an electronegative atom is absent, the charge is more difficult to locate with certainty.

Figure 9.17 shows the EI spectrum of lidocaine (lignocaine) where the fragmentation is dominated by a type of fragmentation known as homolytic α-cleavage producing a fragment at *m/z* 86. This type of fragmentation is promoted by the presence of a heteroatom such as oxygen, nitrogen or sulphur, and in molecules containing a heteroatom it often gives rise to the most abundant ion in the mass spectrum (the base peak), as can be seen in Figure 9.17 where the molecular ion is barely observed. The single-headed curly arrows in Figure 9.17

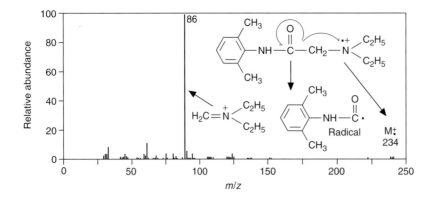

Fig. 9.17
Electron impact ionisation (EI) spectrum of lidocaine (lignocaine) illustrating homolytic α-cleavage.

represent single electrons moving, any bond is composed of two electrons so if the two electrons move out of the bond, the bond breaks. It should also be noted that a radical is generated in the fragmentation of lidocaine, but this is not observed since the mass spectrometer can only separate charged fragments.

Heterolytic cleavage (see Animation 9.10)

Heterolytic cleavage occurs less often as a predominant fragmentation mechanism in drug molecules since they usually contain a lot of heteroatoms to direct the cleavage. In the spectrum of ibuprofen (Fig. 9.18), the two principal ions at m/z 163 and 161 arise from heterolytic cleavage which is denoted by curly arrows with double heads indicating the movement of two electrons in one direction, which leaves a positive charge on the atom that the arrow has moved away from. In ibuprofen the heterolytic cleavage is directed by the fact that the positively charged ions generated can be drawn in the form shown in Figure 9.19, where the positive charge is delocalised into the benzene ring. This type of ion is known as a tropylium ion and is frequently the base peak in compounds with a benzyl group, i.e. CH_2 or CH next to a benzene ring.

The spectrum of ibuprofen also shows a prominent ion at m/z 119, which arises as shown in Figure 9.20 via the loss of CO_2 from the tropylium ion with m/z 163 (Fig. 9.19). This is an example of the loss of a neutral fragment and a molecule can lose several neutral fragments. Other commonly lost neutral fragments include H_2O, CO, H_2CCO and HCOOH. Table 9.3 summarises come common

Fig. 9.18
Electron impact ionisation (EI) spectrum of ibuprofen showing heterolytic cleavage at two positions directed by the presence of the benzene ring.

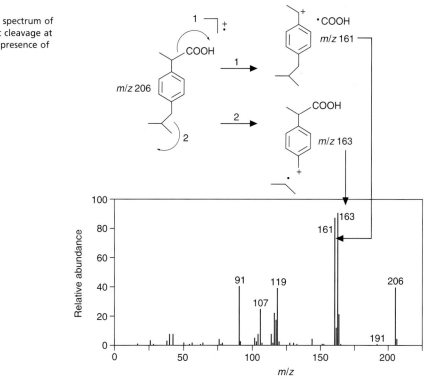

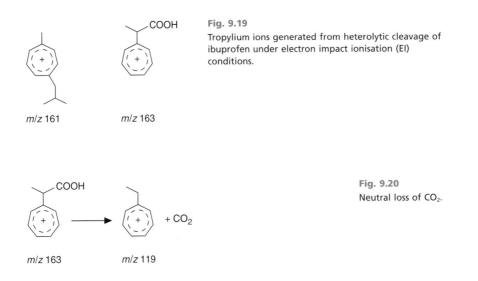

Fig. 9.19
Tropylium ions generated from heterolytic cleavage of
ibuprofen under electron impact ionisation (EI)
conditions.

m/z 161   *m/z* 163

Fig. 9.20
Neutral loss of CO_2.

m/z 163   *m/z* 119

losses from molecules due to heterolytic cleavage or loss of a neutral fragment. Neutral fragment loss generally involves a proton transfer, and in the fragmentation of drug molecules this is very common and can lead to some quite complicated spectra. The EI MS of propranolol (Fig. 9.21), as well as the expected α-homolytic cleavage, which gives rise to an ion at *m/z* 72, has a base peak with *m/z* 115, which is due to a neutral loss involving a proton transfer (Fig. 9.22). In addition, the ions at *m/z* 241 and 215 result from neutral losses of H_2O and isopropane, respectively. The ion at *m/z* 186 is another example of a neutral loss with proton transfer to the neutral fragment. The ion at *m/z* 127 is the result of heterolytic cleavage. The larger the number of heteroatoms in a molecule, the more complex the fragmentation pattern is likely to be.

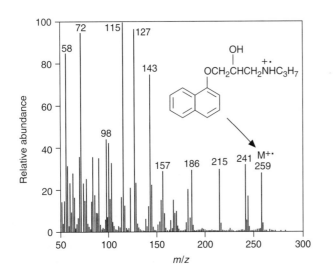

Fig. 9.21
Electron impact
ionization mass
spectrometry (EI MS)
of propranolol

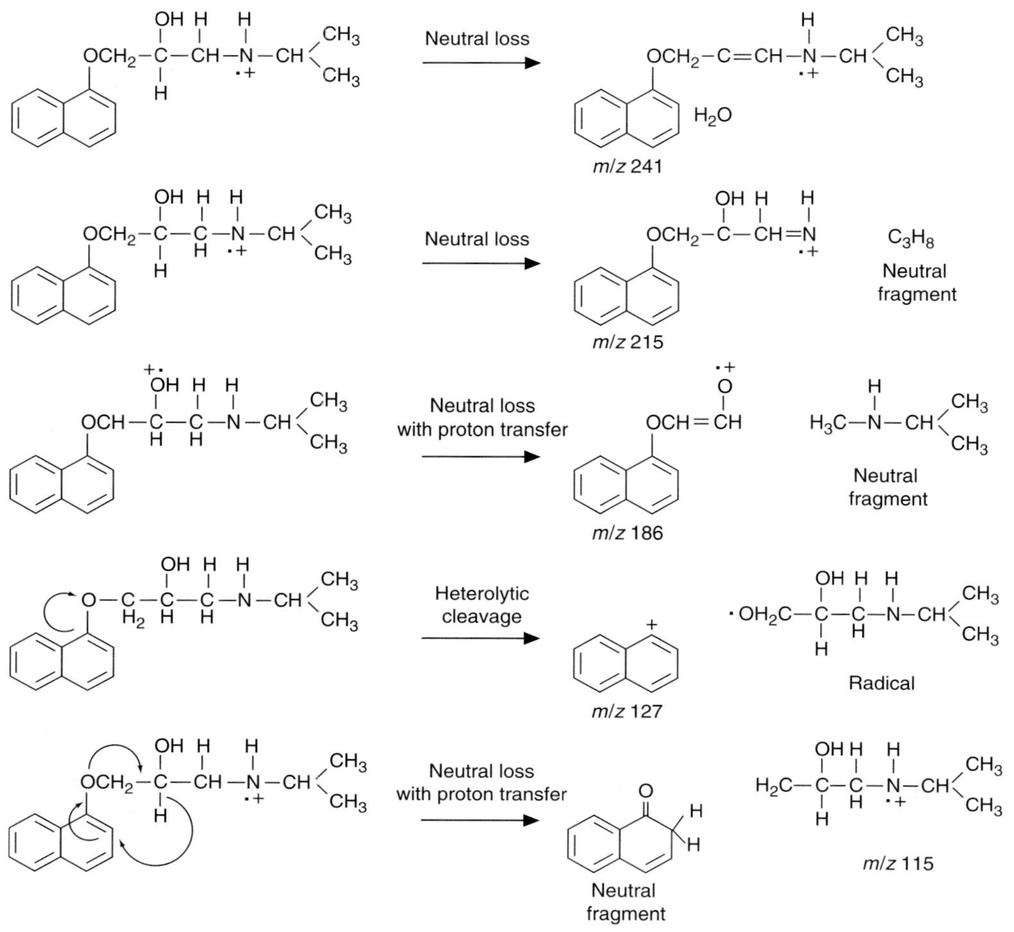

Fig. 9.22
Structures of some the fragments of propranolol where neutral losses produce a number of fragments.

Fragmentation of aliphatic rings involving hydrogen transfer (see Animation 9.11)

When a ring fragments in mass spectrometry at least two bonds have to be broken before a fragment can be lost. The mass spectrum of ketobemidone is shown in Figure 9.23. Ketobemidone contains a heterocyclic ring and one of the bonds at one carbon removed from the nitrogen undergoes α-homolytic cleavage. There is then a rearrangement within the ring involving a single hydrogen transfer with simultaneous breaking of the bond attaching the nitrogen-containing fragment to the rest of the ring (Fig. 9.24). The resulting fragment ion at *m/z* 70 produces the base peak much as α-homolytic cleavage produces a base peak in an open chain structure.

The ring fragmentation shown above is found in the mass spectra of some drugs which have nitrogen-containing rings. However, in many cases where it is possible to form an α-homolytic cleavage fragment, this predominates.

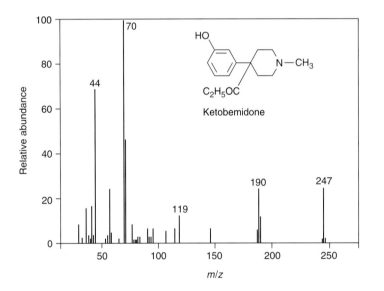

Ketobemidone

Fig. 9.23
Electron impact ionisation (EI) mass spectrum of ketobemidone.

Another form of directed ring fragmentation is promoted by functional groups attached to a ring. For instance, the extra cyclic amine in the structure of the anti-amoebic alkaloid conessine gives rise to the dominant ion in its mass spectrum at *m/z* 84 (Fig. 9.25). This can be explained by the mechanism shown in Figure 9.26, which involves a proton transfer.

Retro Diels–Alder fragmentation (see Animation 9.12)

Retro Diels–Alder fragmentation is another type of fragmentation, which occurs in compounds with ring systems. It is very common in large natural product structures which have many rings but occurs less often in drug molecules. The EI mass spectrum of the analgesic tilidate is shown in Figure 9.27. The base peak at *m/z* 97 results from retero Diels–Alder fragmentation. Figure 9.28 shows the

Fig. 9.24

Fragmentation of ketobemidone under electron impact ionisation (EI) conditions.

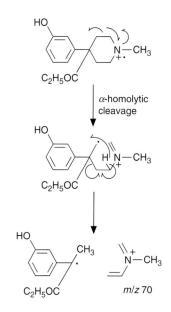

α-homolytic cleavage

m/z 70

mechanism of formation of the retero Diels–Alder fragment. The fragmentation is most likely to occur in a ring containing a single double bond.

McLafferty rearrangement (see Animation 9.13)

The McLafferty rearrangement, although much loved by organic chemists, is relatively uncommon in drug molecules; it is most often encountered in fatty acid esters. Figure 9.29 shows the mass spectrum of the pharmaceutical excipient hydroxy ethyl stearate. The ion at *m/z* 104 is due to the McLafferty rearrangement shown in Figure 9.30. This rearrangement can occur in any carbonyl-containing compound, e.g. amides, ketones and acids.

Fig. 9.25

Electron impact ionisation (EI) mass spectrum of conessine.

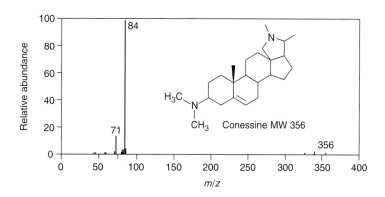

Conessine MW 356

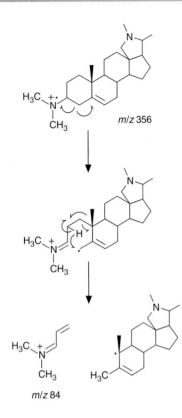

Fig. 9.26
Directed fragmentation of conessine.

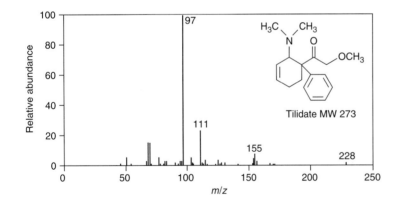

Fig. 9.27
Electron impact ionisation (EI) mass
spectrum of tilidate.

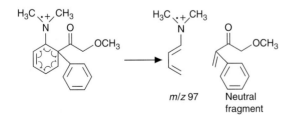

Fig. 9.28
Retro Diels–Alder fragmentation of tilidate.

Fig. 9.29
Electron impact ionisation
(EI) mass spectrum of
hydroxyethyl stearate.

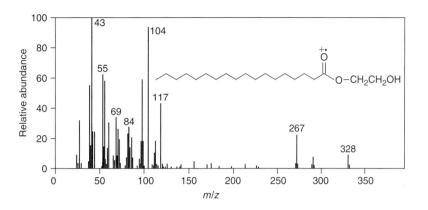

Fig. 9.30
McLafferty rearrangement in the fragmentation of
hydroxyethylstearate.

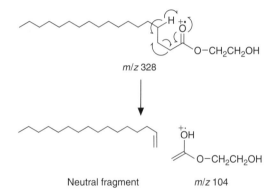

Neutral fragment   *m/z* 104

Self-test 9.2

Draw the mechanism which gives rise to the base peak at *m/z* 58 in the EI spectrum of
ephedrine.

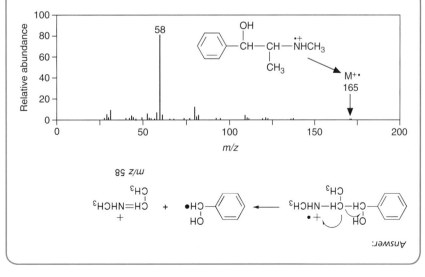

Answer:

Self-test 9.3

Predict the base peaks in the mass spectra of the drugs shown below (N=14, O=16, C=12, H=1).

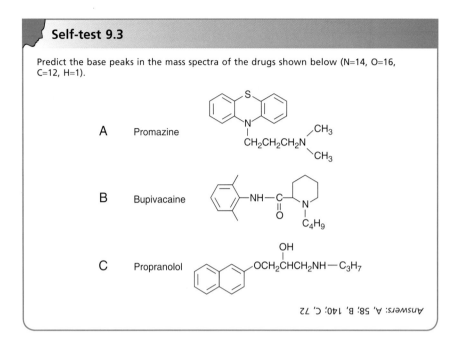

A   Promazine

B   Bupivacaine

C   Propranolol

Answers: A, 58; B, 140; C, 72

EI mass spectra where the molecular ion is abundant

The most important ion in the mass spectrum is the molecular ion, since the molecular weight of a compound is a very specific property. There are many mass spectra of drugs where the molecular ion is abundant. Figure 9.31 shows the mass

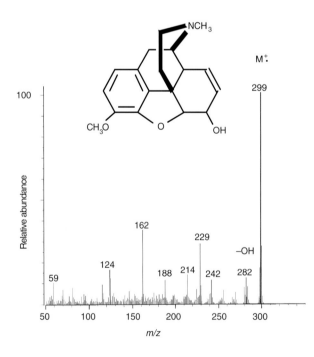

Fig. 9.31
Electron impact ionisation (EI) mass spectrum of codeine.

spectrum of codeine, where the molecular ion at *m/z* 299 is the base peak. The extended ring structure of the molecule means that, apart from the abundant molecular ion, the fragmentation of codeine is not easy to interpret because of the structural rearrangements which occur. The only other ion in the mass spectrum of codeine closely related to the molecular ion is at *m/z* 229, and even formation of this ion involves some rearrangement of the ring structure.

Self-test 9.4

Draw the base peak ions which are formed at 199 and 167 in the EI mass spectra of flurbiprofen and diphenhydramine, respectively.

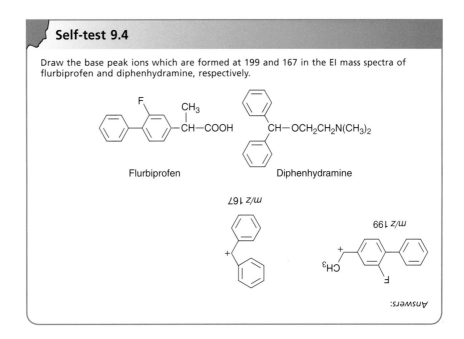

Drugs which yield abundant molecular ions under EI conditions include caffeine, coumatetralyl, cyclazocine, dextromethorphan, dichlorphenamide, diflunisal, dimoxyline, fenclofenac, flurbiprofen, griseofulvin, harmine, hydralazine, hydroflumethiazide, ibogaine, ketotifen, levallorphan, methaqualone, nalorphine. These drugs are characterised by having ring structures without extensive side chains, or, if side chains are present, they do not contain heteroatoms which would direct cleavage to that part of the molecule.

Self-test 9.5

Draw the structure of the fragments in the EI MS of buphenine.

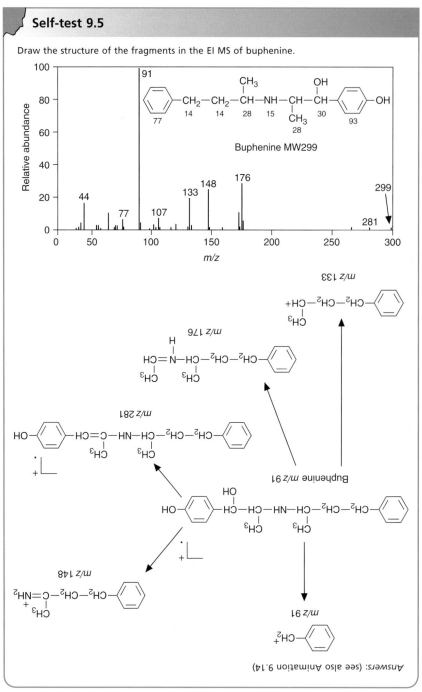

Buphenine MW299

Answers: (see also Animation 9.14)

Gas chromatography–mass spectrometry (GC–MS)

For the chromatographic aspects of GC–MS, refer to Chapter 11. Gas chromatography (GC) was the earliest chromatographic technique to be interfaced to a mass spectrometer. The original type of gas chromatograph had a packed GC column with a gas flow rate passing through it at *ca* 20 ml/min, and the major problem was how to interface the GC without losing the mass spectrometer vacuum. This was solved by use of a jet separator, where the column effluent was passed across a very narrow gap between two jets and the highly diffusible carrier gas was largely removed, whereas the heavier analyte molecules crossed the gap without being vented. The problem of removing the carrier gas no longer exists since GC capillary columns provide a flow rate of 0.5–2 ml/min, which can be directly introduced into the mass spectrometer without its losing vacuum. The ionisation technique most commonly used in conjunction with GC is EI, which has been described in detail above.

It is worth mentioning two other soft ionisation techniques: positive ion chemical ionisation (PICI) and negative ion chemical ionisation (NICI). In PICI a reagent gas is continuously introduced into the ion source, e.g. methane (isobutane and ammonia are also used). The gas interacts with electrons produced by the filament to produce a series of ions – $C_2H_5^+$ and $C_3H_5^+$ – which can either combine directly with the molecular ion or protonate the molecular ion. Thus PICI spectra contain abundant ions related to the molecular ion and very little fragmentation. In NICI the most common form of ionisation mechanism occurring is electron capture ionisation. Again a reagent gas is used and the electrons collide with it so that their energies are reduced to < 10 eV. Molecules with a high affinity for electrons are then able to capture these low-energy thermal electrons generating negatively charged ions with little fragmentation. NICI provides one of the most sensitive methods of analysis with limits of detection in the femtogram range.

Self-test 9.6

Draw the fragment ions at *m/z* 70 in the MS of clozapine and *m/z* 98 in the MS of difenidol.

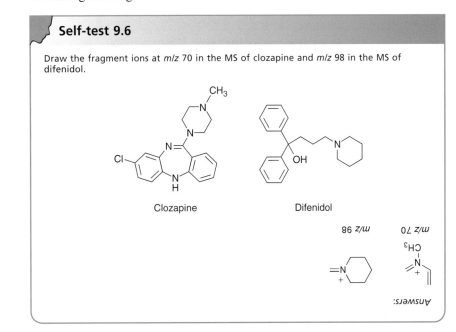

Clozapine   Difenidol

m/z 98   *m/z* 70

Answers:

Self-test 9.7

Draw the structure of the ion at *m/z* 180, which occurs in the EI mass spectrum of ketamine.

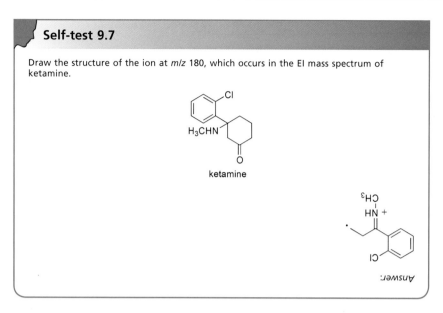

ketamine

Answer:

Self-test 9.8

Indicate how the peak at *m/z* 110 in the spectrum of ticlopidine is formed:

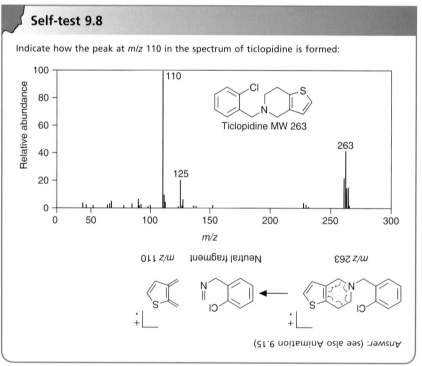

Ticlopidine MW 263

m/z 110   Neutral fragment   *m/z* 263

Answer: (see also Animation 9.15)

Applications of GC–MS with EI
Analysis of an essential oil

Quality control of essential oils is commonly carried out by GC or GC–MS. The use of GC–MS enables identification of adulterants and minor components in an essential oil. Figure 9.32 shows a GC–MS trace obtained for peppermint oil. The

Fig. 9.32

Gas chromatography mass spectrometry (GC–MS) analysis of peppermint oil (DB-1 column 80°C (5 min) and then 7°C/min to 180°C).

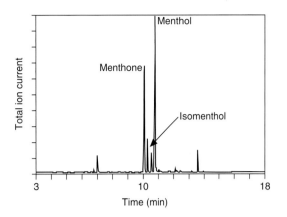

two major components are menthone and menthol. It is possible to identify minor components in the oil according to their mass spectra. For instance, a peak for isomenthol can be identified in the trace above by searching its mass spectrum against the database of spectra in a library. The compound gives a match value of 916 to the library spectrum for isomenthol. It can be seen in Figure 9.33 that,

Fig. 9.33

Electron impact ionisation (EI) spectra of A menthol and B isomenthol.

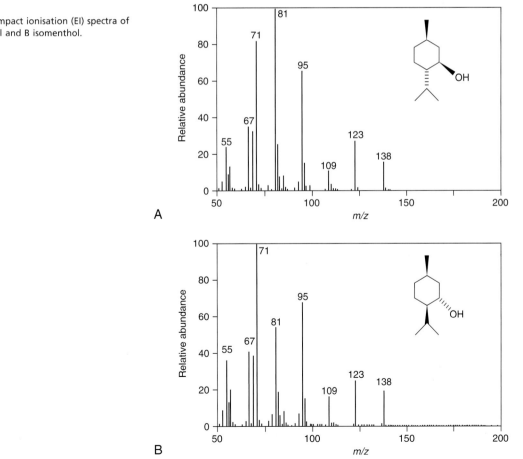

although menthol and isomenthol are isomers and contain more or less the same ions in their mass spectra, there are distinct differences in the intensities of these ions, and this enables the mass spectral library to distinguish between them based on correlating mass/intensity data for the two spectra. As stated earlier the great advantage of EI spectra is that there are libraries of EI spectra containing > 100 000 entries and matches to library spectra are fairly reliable since EI spectra obtained at 70 eV do not vary greatly from instrument to instrument.

GC–MS of process intermediates and degradation products

GC is a technique ideally suited to determining residues of process intermediates, since these are often more volatile than the finished drug and elute from a GC at an earlier time. Figure 9.34 shows a GC–MS trace derived from the injection of a concentrated (4 mg/ml) sample of ketoprofen. The levels of impurities in the sample are really very low, but a number of low-level impurities can be observed. The mass spectra of impurities A and B are shown in Figure 9.35. The EI spectrum of ketoprofen in Figure 9.5 and Figure 9.36 shows an interpretation of the structures of the fragment ions observed in Figure 9.5.

Self-test 9.9

Indicate how the ion at *m/z* 138 arises in the spectrum of pipamperone.

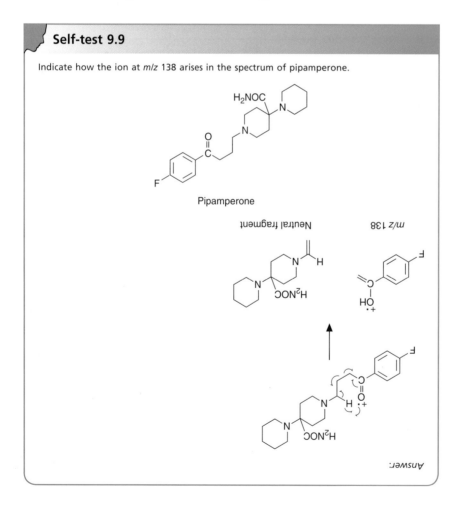

Fig. 9.34

Gas chromatography–mass spectrometry (GC–MS) trace of manufacturing impurities in ketoprofen (2 μl of a 4 mg/ml solution of ketoprofen injected into the GC–MS. 100°C (1 min) and then 15°C/min to 325°C).

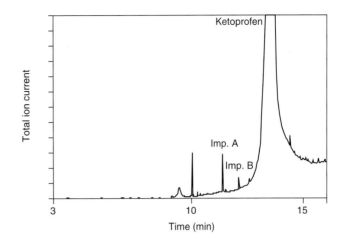

Fig. 9.35

Electron impact ionisation (EI) mass spectra of impurities A and B.

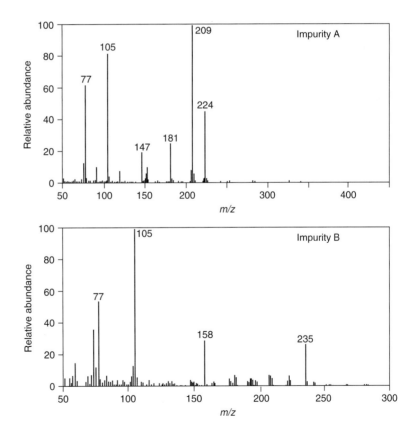

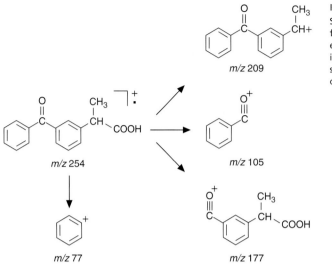

m/z 209

m/z 254

m/z 105

m/z 77

m/z 177

Fig. 9.36
Structures of fragment ions in the electron impact ionisation mass spectrometry (EI MS) of ketoprofen.

Tandem mass spectrometry (see Animation 9.16)

Under ESI conditions there is very little fragmentation induced in a molecule; therefore there is a lack of information about the structure. For example, the ESI MS of acebutolol shown in Figure 9.2 shows little fragmentation, which means only limited information about its structure can be derived. Fragmentation can be induced by applying small accelerating voltage in the source to induce collision with solvent molecules within the source and thus induce fragmentation. In this way EI type spectra are produced. However, this type of fragmentation is not useful where, for instance, trace impurities in a drug substance are being characterised because there is a background due to the HPLC solvent being introduced into the instrument, and this will also produce fragment ions which will contribute to the spectrum of the molecule which is being studied. In order to obtain EI type spectra, a triple quadrupole instrument (Fig. 9.37) can be used, where collision induced dissociation (CID) is used in conjunction with ESI. Typically the molecular ion of the molecule is selected (the precursor ion) by the first

Fig. 9.37
Schematic diagram of a triple quadrupole tandem mass spectrometer with collision induced dissociation (CID) of acebutolol (gas pressure 1 Torr, collision energy 25 V).

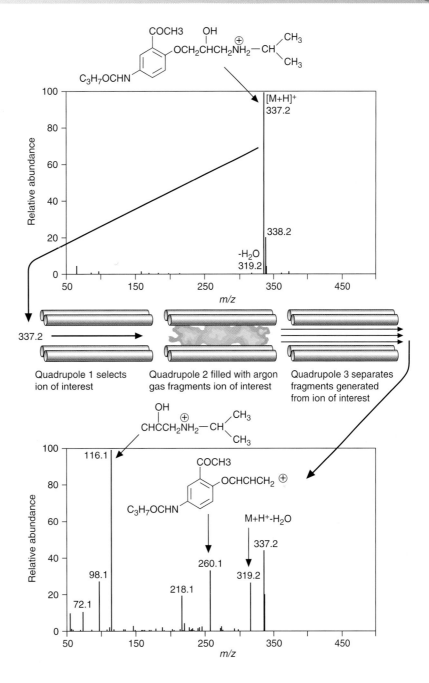

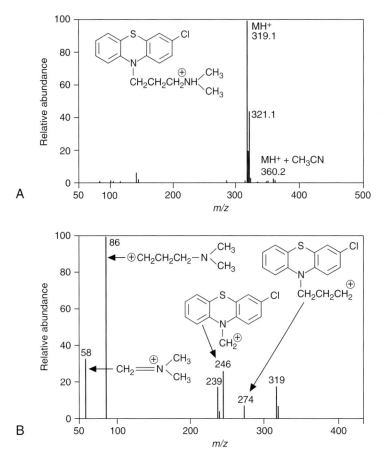

Fig. 9.38
Electrospray ionisation (ESI) spectrum of chlorpromazine A and its product ion spectrum B obtained using tandem mass spectrometry (MS) (gas pressure 1 Torr, collision energy 25 V).

quadrupole, is fragmented and then the fragments (product ions) are separated using a third quadrupole. This process is shown in Figure 9.37 for acebutolol where collision with argon produces a more complex EI type spectrum.

Figure 9.38 shows the ESI spectrum of chlorpromazine and also a tandem MS spectrum for chlorpromazine. In fact the tandem MS is not entirely similar to the EI spectrum of chlorpromazine, which is almost completely composed of an alpha homolytic cleavage fragment at m/z 58.

Self-test 9.10

From the information provided in Figures 9.37 and 9.38 select from the EP listed impurities shown below, the structures which correspond to impurities A and B in ketoprofen.

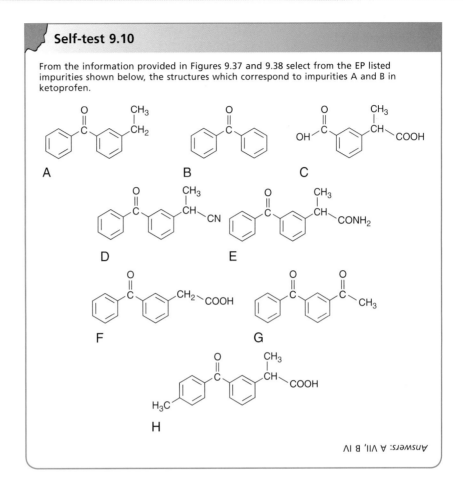

A   B   C

D   E

F   G

H

A feature of CID is that its energy may be controlled; thus if the collision energy used for fragmenting chlorpromazine is increased to 40 V, the ion at *m/z* 86 increases, due to the higher fragmentation energy, and the molecular ion is absent. For this reason it is difficult to form libraries of tandem MS spectra in the way that large databases of EI spectra exist, since the spectrum obtained in tandem MS depends on the gas pressure, type of gas (nitrogen is also used as a collision gas) and fragmentation energy.

Self-test 9.11

Suggest structures for the major ions in the CID spectra of clindamycin and ampicillin obtained at 25 V and 1 Torr gas pressure. The structures do not have to be exact, but it is possible to get close to the structure by breaking the appropriate bond.

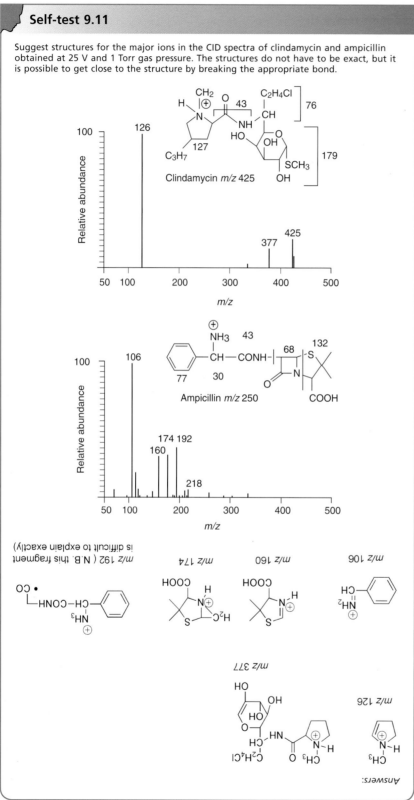

Fig. 9.39
An electrospray ionisation (ESI) spectrum of chlorpromazine obtained on an ion trap instrument A and T B MS^2 spectrum obtained on an ion trap instrument, collision energy 30 V.

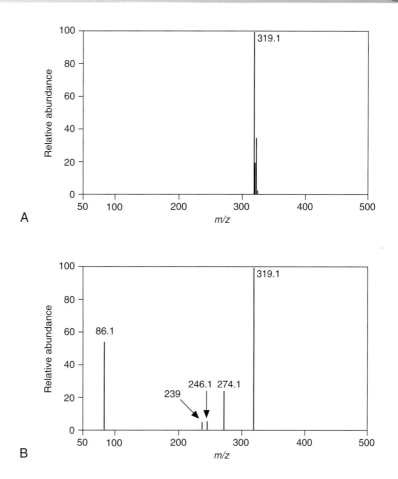

The spectra of chlorpromazine shown in Figure 9.38 was obtained on a triple quadrupole instrument. Figure 9.39 shows the fragmented and unfragmented spectra of chlorpromazine run on an ion trap instrument. On an ion trap instrument spectrum B is called an MS^2 spectrum and is equivalent to the type of spectrum obtained from a triple quadrupole instrument, except that the collision gas is helium. As can be seen by comparison with Figure 9.39 the ions obtained are similar to the tandem spectrum of chlorpromazine, except that there are variations in abundance and the ion at *m/z* 58 is absent. The collisions in an ion trap are of lower energy, since helium is much lighter than argon.

An advantage of ion trap instruments is that repeat fragmentation can be carried out. Figure 9.40 shows the MS^3 spectrum for chlorpromazine. In this example the ion at *m/z* 274 (resulting from the loss of $N(CH_3)_2$) in the MS^2 spectrum is retained in the trap and fragmented again. With each fragmentation the number of ions left in trap is reduced and it can be seen in Figure 9.40 that the background noise for the MS^3 spectrum is greater than in MS^2 spectrum, but in principle this process can be carried out a number of times and instruments are capable of producing up to MS^{12} spectra; however, spectra > MS^4 are uncommon. The selected ion at *m/z* 274 fragments to yield ions at *m/z* 246 and *m/z* 239 due to loss of ethylene and chlorine, respectively, such repeat fragmentation can be useful in structure elucidation of ions of unknown compounds.

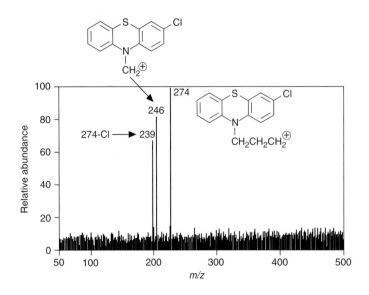

Fig. 9.40
MS³ spectrum of chlorpromazine obtained by selecting the ion at *m/z* 274 in the MS² spectrum for further fragmentation at 30 V.

Fragmentation can also be carried out on negative ions. Figure 9.41 shows the negative ion CID spectrum of ketoprofen. CID was carried out on the formic acid adduct ion (M-HHCOOH⁻) at *m/z* 299 (this can be observed in the ESI MS of ketoprofen shown in Figure 9.3). The CID spectrum just shows a single ion which has the same mass as the base peak in the positive ion CID spectrum, except that in this instance it must carry a negative charge.

Tandem mass spectrometry is useful for characterising unknown compounds, such as drug impurities, and also in the analysis of drugs in biological fluids, where it is a very sensitive method for measuring trace levels of drug to as low as levels around 10^{-12} g/ml. Figure 9.42 shows an HPLC UV chromatogram of a sample of diphenhydramine which was subjected to an accelerated oxidative degradation by treatment with the oxidising agent hydrogen peroxide. As can be seen in Figure 9.42 several minor degradants are produced. The MS and MS² spectra, obtained using an ion trap, of diphenhydramine are shown in Figure 9.43.

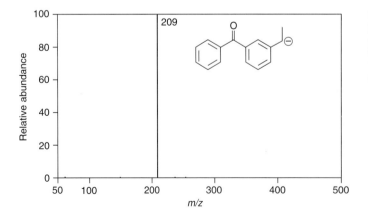

Fig. 9.41
Negative ion electrospray ionisation (ESI)/collision induced dissociation (CID) spectrum of ketoprofen (collision energy 25 V, gas pressure 1 Torr) carried out on formic acid adduct ion at *m/z* 299.

Fig. 9.42

High-pressure liquid chromatography (HPLC) UV trace of a sample of diphenhydramine treated with 10% hydrogen peroxide, which results in the formation of minor degradation products.

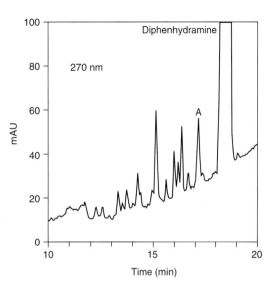

Fig. 9.43

Mass spectrometry (MS) and MS^2 spectra of diphenhydramine at 35 V collision induced dissociation (CID).

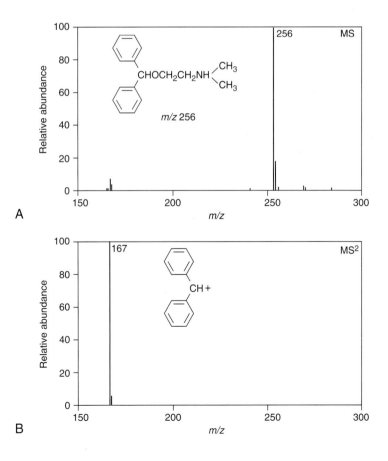

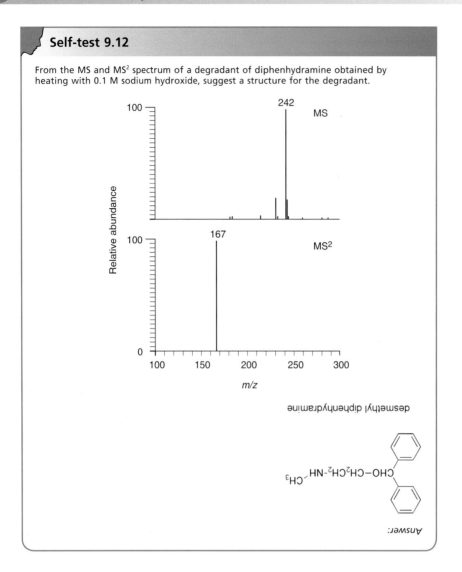

Self-test 9.12

From the MS and MS^2 spectrum of a degradant of diphenhydramine obtained by heating with 0.1 M sodium hydroxide, suggest a structure for the degradant.

Answer:

desmethyl diphenhydramine

The peak for degradant A shown in Figure 9.44 gave an MS spectrum where the molecular ion was 16 amu above the molecular ion of diphenhydramine, indicating addition of an oxygen atom to diphenhydramine. The MS^2 spectrum of degradant A shown in Figure 9.44 indicates that an oxygen had been added somewhere in one of the benzene rings.

High-resolution mass spectrometry

As mentioned earlier in the section on ion separation techniques, a number of ion separation techniques can produce high-resolution measurements where the masses of ions can be measured to four or five decimal places, thus enabling determination of the elemental composition of an ion. Figure 9.45 shows a chromatogram of minor impurities in promethazine. The chromatogram was obtained by using high-resolution Fourier transform mass spectrometry. The elemental

Fig. 9.44
Mass spectrometry (MS) and MS^2 spectra of degradant A obtained with 35 V collision induced dissociation (CID).

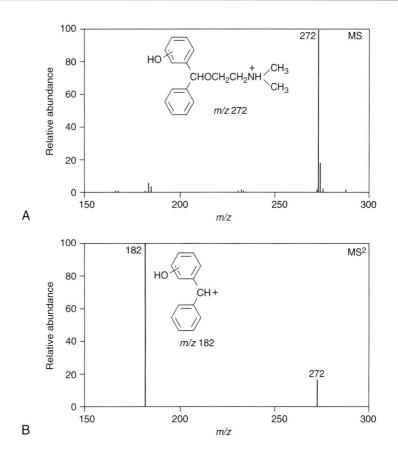

A

B

Fig. 9.45
Total ion chromatogram (TIC) for impurities in promethazine obtained using Fourier transform mass spectrometry (FT-MS) with hydrophilic interaction chromatography on a cyanopropyl column with acetonitrile:water (95:5) containing 3.25 mM ammonium acetate.

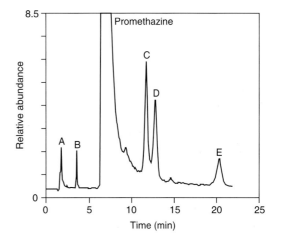

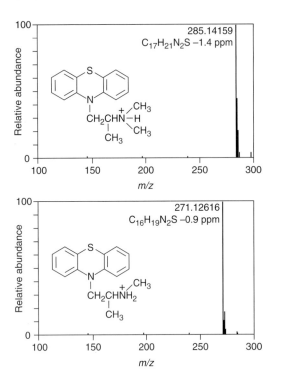

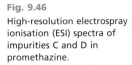

Fig. 9.46
High-resolution electrospray
ionisation (ESI) spectra of
impurities C and D in
promethazine.

composition obtained for the [M+H]⁺ ion promethazine is within −1.4 ppm of an exact mass match and thus accurate to four decimal places (Fig. 9.46).

The close elemental matching allows structures to be proposed for the impurities. Impurities D is one CH_2 less than promethazine and is probably a secondary amine lacking a methyl group. Impurity C is an isomer of impurity D and impurity B is an isomer of promethazine. Figure 9.47 shows the spectra for impurities A and E. Impurity E is produced by the oxidation of the sulphur atom in promethazine, and impurity A contains an oxidised sulphur and lacks the side chain of promethazine; it elutes early under the hydrophilic interaction chromatography conditions used because of its weak basicity (see Chapter 12).

Mass spectrometry of proteins

Since the ESI process can produce multiply charged ions, it can be used to examine large molecules such as proteins. Without being multiply charged, the protein would be outwith the separation range of most instruments, which usually only extends to 4000 amu for singly charged ions. Figure 9.48 shows the ESI spectrum of cytochrome C, a haem-containing protein that is involved in the terminal respiratory chain. The charges on the ions within the spectrum can be obtained from two adjacent ions in the mass spectrum according to the formula:

$$n = \frac{M_A - 1}{M_A - M_B}$$

where n = the charge on M_B, and M_A and M_B are adjacent ions, with M_A the higher in mass.

Fig. 9.47

High-resolution electrospray ionisation (ESI) spectra of impurities E and A in promethazine.

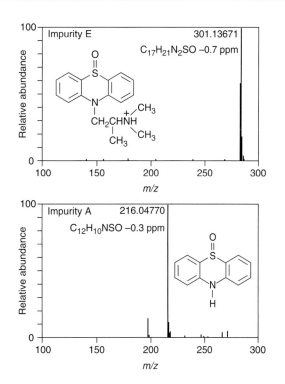

Thus, for example, in the spectrum of cytochrome C, the charge on the ion at m/z 680.8 is calculated as follows:

$$n = \frac{720.8 - 1}{720.8 - 680.8} = \frac{719.8}{40} = 17.99$$

Thus the mass of the sample of cytochrome C is $680.8 \times 18 = 12\,254$ Da.

ES MS provides an excellent means for quality control of recombinant proteins, some of which are now used as drugs, e.g. human insulin, interferons, erythropoietin and tissue plasminogen activating factor.[1] The simplicity of the single ion spectra for each charge number means that small amounts of related

Fig. 9.48

Electrospray ionisation (ESI) spectrum of cytochrome C.

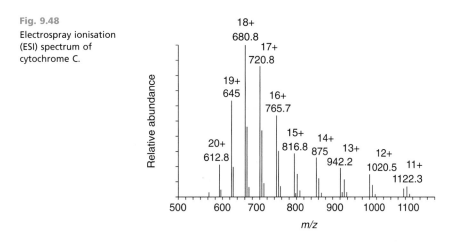

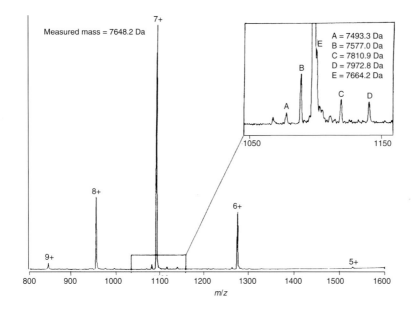

Fig. 9.49
Electrospray ionisation mass spectrometry (ESI MS) of insulin-derived growth factor and minor impurities. *(Reproduced with permission from Elsevier.[1])*

proteins that may contaminate the main protein show up quite clearly. Thus, variations in protein structure, such as degree of glycosylation, or in the terminal amino acids of the protein, can be seen quite clearly.

An example of how ES MS can be used to determine minor impurities in a recombinant protein is shown in Figure 9.49, where some small additional ions in the mass spectrum of recombinant insulin-like growth factor (IGF) can be seen. The major ions in the spectrum are due to IGF itself bearing varying charge, but the minor impurities also give rise to peaks, and these can be interpreted as shown in Table 9.4.

Before the advent of this technique, the determination of protein molecular weight was a laborious process, and control and identification of minor impurities more or less impossible.

Mass spectrometry in drug discovery

- Drug discovery involves a number of phases, including target identification, lead identification, small molecule optimisation and pre-clinical and clinical development.
- Target identification has been speeded up as a result of genomics, but the measurement of gene transcription through detection of RNAs does not

Table 9.4 Minor impurities in insulin-like growth factor (IGF)

Assignment	Molecular weight Da
IGF	7648
IGF-N terminal glycine-proline	7494
IGF-C terminal alanine	7577
IGF oxidised methionine	7664
IGF + hexose	7810
IGF + 2 × hexose	7972

Fig. 9.50

(A) Electrospray ionization mass spectrometry (ESI MS) of leuenkephalin. (B) Collision induced dissociation (CID) spectrum of the ion at *m/z* 556.

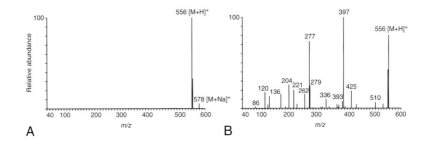

necessarily indicate exactly what the structures of the proteins produced are, since the proteins may be modified after translation by processes such as glycosylation or phosphorylation.

• With advances in mass spectrometry, identification of translated proteins is possible. Such proteins may signal disease processes, in which case their regulation by a potential drug might indicate its efficacy, but equally expression of certain proteins following drug therapy may indicate drug toxicity.

In order to derive more structural information it is necessary to break the protein into small peptide units. This is accomplished most often by treating the protein with trypsin or chymotrypsin, which cleave the protein between specific amino acids. For example, trypsin cleaves proteins at the carboxyl side of either a lysine or an arginine residue. The mixture of peptides produced is separated using capillary liquid chromatography. Figure 9.50A shows the ESI mass spectrum of the opioid peptide leuenkephalin; although it is not a product of cleavage from a larger protein, it illustrates peptide fragmentation. The CID mass spectrum (Fig. 9.50B) reveals the sequence of the amino acids in the peptide, as shown in Figure 9.51. Fragmentation largely occurs between NH and CO (the peptide bond), producing a series of Y ions, derived by sequential losses starting at the N-terminus of the peptide and a series of B ions starting at the C-terminus of the peptide. The spectrum is further complicated by loss of neutral fragments. For example, the ion at *m/z* 397 results from the loss of CO from the ion at *m/z* 425. The spectrum also contains immonium ions that result from the individual amino

Fig. 9.51

The electrospray ionisation collision induced dissociation (ESI CID) spectrum of leuenkephalin illustrating fragmentation of a peptide.

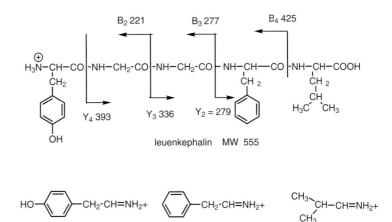

acids in the peptide chain. In the case of leuenkephalin, ions derived from tyrosine, phenylalanine and leucine can be seen (Fig. 9.50). Once the sequences of the mixture of peptides derived from a protein are established, they can be matched against a database in order to try to identify the protein or at least relate it closely to a known protein. The pattern of peptide molecular weights obtained from the tryptic digest can be matched against one of a number of databases by using a linking program such as ProteinProspector (prospector.ucst .edu) or TurboSEQUEST. The one two peptide sequences are often enough to fingerprint a protein, and large databases of protein structures such as SwissProt are available on-line.

Self-test 9.13

Methionine enkephalin differs from leuenkephalin in that it has a methionine at the C-terminus instead of leucine. Explain the ions in the spectrum below at *m/z* 411, 354, 297, 149 and 104.

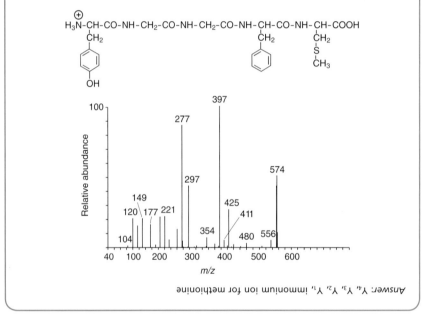

Answer: Y_4, Y_3, Y_2, Y_1, immonium ion for methionine

Reference

1. Poulter LK, Green BN, Kaur S, Burlingame AL. In: Burlingame AL, McCloskey JA, eds. *Biological Mass Spectrometry*. Amsterdam: Elsevier; 1990:119-128.

Further reading

Chapman JR, ed. *Practical Organic Mass Spectrometry: A Guide for Chemical and Biochemical Analysis*. 2nd ed. Chichester: Wiley Interscience; 1995.

Davis R, Frearson M, eds. *Mass Spectrometry*. Chichester: John Wiley and Sons; 1994.

Francese S, Dani FR, Traldi P, et al. MALDI mass spectrometry imaging, from its origins up to today: the state of the art. *Comb Chem High Throughput Screen*. 2009;12:156-174.

Guillarme D, Schappler J, Rudaz S, Veuthey JL. Coupling ultra-high-pressure liquid chromatography with mass spectrometry. *Trac-Trends Anal Chem*. 2010;29:15-27.

Johnstone RAW. *Mass Spectrometry for Chemists and Biochemists*. Cambridge: Cambridge University Press; 1996.

Lee TA. *A Beginner's Guide to Mass Spectral Interpretation*. Chichester: John Wiley and Sons; 1998.

Lee MS. *LC/MS Applications in Drug Development*. New York: Wiley Interscience; 2002.

Leibler DC. *Introduction to Proteomics*. Totowa, New Jersey: Humana Press; 2002.

McLafferty F. *Interpretation of Mass Spectra*. 3rd ed. California: University Science Books; 1980.

Nicoli R, Martel S, Rudaz S, et al. Advances in LC platforms for drug discovery. *Expert Opin Drug Discov.* 2010;5:475-489.

Scigelova M, Makarov A. Advances in bioanalytical LC-MS using the Orbitrap (TM) mass analyzer. *Bioanalysis.* 2009;1:741-754.

van Hove ERA, Smith DF, Heeren RMA. A concise review of mass spectrometry imaging. *J Chromatogr A.* 2010;1217:3946-3954.

Williams DH, Fleming I, eds. *Spectroscopic Methods in Organic Chemistry.* 4th ed. London: McGraw Hill; 1989.

www.jeol.com

The site contains a lot of information on methods of ion generation and separation, with a strong emphasis on high-resolution mass spectrometry.

www.spectroscopynow.com

Comprehensive coverage of mass spectroscopy.

www.agilent.com

Descriptions of different mass spectrometer instruments and their applications.

Chromatographic theory

10

Introduction

Chromatography is the most frequently used analytical technique in pharmaceutical analysis. An understanding of the parameters which govern chromatographic performance has given rise to improvements in chromatography systems, so the ability to achieve high-resolution separations is continually increasing. The system suitability tests which are described at the end of this chapter are now routinely included in chromatographic software packages so that the chromatographic performance of a system can be monitored routinely. The factors determining chromatographic efficiency will be discussed first in relation to high-pressure liquid chromatography (HPLC).

Void volume and capacity factor

Figure 10.1 shows an HPLC column packed with a solid stationary phase with a liquid mobile phase flowing through it.

If a compound does not partition appreciably into the stationary phase, it will travel through the column at the same rate as the solvent. The length of time it takes an unretarded molecule to flow through the column is determined by the void volume of the column (V_o). The porous space within a silica gel packing is usually about $0.7 \times$ the volume of the packing; a typical packing volume in a 0.46×15 cm column is ca 2.5 cm^3. Thus, in theory, it should take solvent or unretarded molecules, flowing at a rate of 1 ml/min, ca 1.8 min to pass through the void volume of such a column (the internal space is likely to be reduced where the silica gel has been surface coated with stationary phase). The length of time it takes a retarded compound to pass through the column depends on its capacity

Fig. 10.1
Schematic diagram of bands for three different compounds travelling through an HPLC column. The compound with the largest capacity factor emerges last.

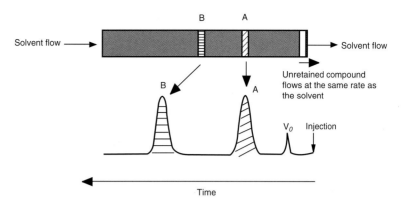

factor (K'), which is a measure of the degree to which it partitions (adsorbs) into the stationary phase from the mobile phase:

$$K' = \frac{V_r - V_o}{V_o} \text{ or } \frac{t_r - t_o}{t_o}$$

where V_o is the void volume of the column; V_r is the retention volume of the analyte; t_o is the time taken for an unretained molecule to pass through the void volume and t_r is the time taken for the analyte to pass through the column. In the example shown in Figure 10.1, compound B has a larger capacity factor than compound A. For example, if a compound had a K' of 4, the V_o of a column was 1 ml and the solvent was flowing through the column at 1 ml/min, the total time taken for the compound to pass through the column would be 5 min, i.e. for the 1 min required to pass through the void space in the column 4 min would be spent in the stationary phase. This is a simplification of the actual process, but it provides a readily understandable model. As can be seen in Figure 10.1 the peaks produced by chromatographic separation actually have width as well as a retention time, and the processes which give rise to this width will be considered later.

Self-test 10.1

Calculate the time taken for the following compounds to emerge from a chromatographic column under the specified conditions.

K' of compound	V_o of column (ml)	Solvent flow rate (ml/min)
6	1	1
10	1	2

Answers: 7 min and 5.5 min

Calculation of column efficiency

The broader a chromatographic peak is relative to its retention time, the less efficient the column it is eluting from. Figure 10.2 shows a chromatographic peak emerging at time t_r after injection; the efficiency of the column is most readily

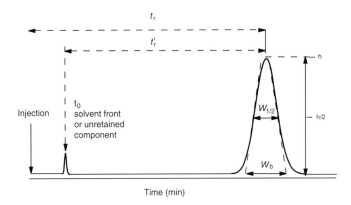

Fig. 10.2
Determination of retention time and peak width at half height.

assessed from the width of the peak at half its height $W_{1/2}$ and its retention time using Equation 1:

$$n = 5.54 \, (t_r/W_{1/2})^2 \qquad \textbf{[Equation 1]}$$

where n is the number of theoretical plates.

Column efficiency is usually expressed in theoretical plates per metre:

$$n \times 100/L$$

where L is the column length in cm.

A stricter measure of column efficiency, especially if the retention time of the analyte is short, is given by Equation 2:

$$N \, eff = 5.54(t'_r/W_{1/2})^2 \qquad \textbf{[Equation 2]}$$

where $N \, eff$ is the number of effective plates and reflects the number of times the analyte partitions between the mobile phase and the stationary phase during its passage through the column and $t'_r = t_r - t_o$.

Another term which is used as a measure is H, the 'height of a theoretical plate':

$$H = L/N \, eff$$

where H is the length of column required for one partition step to occur.

Self-test 10.2

A standard operating procedure states that a column must have an efficiency > 30 000 theoretical plates/m. Which of these 15 cm columns meets the specification?

Retention time of analyte (min)	$W_{1/2}$ (min)
1. 6.4	0.2
2. 5.6	0.2
3. 10.6	0.6

Answer: Column 1

Origins of band broadening in HPLC
Van Deemter equation in liquid chromatography

Chromatographic peaks have width and this means that molecules of a single compound, despite having the same capacity factor, take different lengths of time to travel through the column. The longer an analyte takes to travel through a column, the more the individual molecules making up the sample spread out and the broader the band becomes. The more rapidly a peak broadens the less efficient the column. Detailed mathematical modelling of the processes leading to band broadening is very complex.[1] The treatment below gives a basic introduction to the origins of band broadening. The causes of band broadening can be formalised in the Van Deemter equation (Equation 3) as applied to liquid chromatography:

$$H = \frac{A}{1 + C_m / u^{1/2}} + \frac{B}{u} + C_s u + C_m u^{1/2} \qquad \textbf{[Equation 3]}$$

H is the measure of the efficiency of the column (discussed above); the smaller the term, the more efficient the column.

u is the linear velocity of the mobile phase, simply how many cm/s an unretained molecule travels through the column, and A is the 'eddy' diffusion term; broadening occurs because some molecules take longer erratic paths while some, for instance, those travelling close to the walls of the column, take more direct paths, thus eluting first. As shown in Figure 10.3, for two molecules of the same compound, molecule X elutes before molecule Y. In liquid chromatography the eddy diffusion term also contains a contribution from streaming within the solvent volume itself, i.e. A (see the C_m term) is reduced if the diffusion coefficient of the molecule within the mobile phase is low because molecules take less erratic paths through not being able to diffuse out of the mainstream so easily.

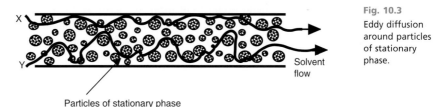

X

Y

Solvent flow

Particles of stationary phase

Fig. 10.3
Eddy diffusion around particles of stationary phase.

B is the rate of diffusion of the molecule in the liquid phase, which contributes to peak broadening through diffusion either with or against the flow of mobile phase; the contribution of this term is very small in liquid chromatography. Its contribution to band broadening decreases as flow rate increases, and it only becomes significant at very low flow rates.

C_s is the resistance to mass transfer of a molecule in the stationary phase and is dependent on its diffusion coefficient in the stationary phase and upon the thickness of the stationary phase coated onto silica gel:

$$C_s = \frac{d^2 \text{ thickness}}{D_s}$$

where d^2 thickness is the square of the stationary-phase film thickness and D_s is the diffusion coefficient of the analyte in the stationary phase.

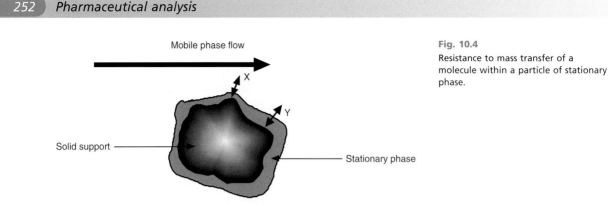

Fig. 10.4
Resistance to mass transfer of a
molecule within a particle of stationary
phase.

Obviously the thinner and more uniform the stationary-phase coating, the smaller the contribution to band broadening from this term. In the example shown in Figure 10.4, molecule Y is retarded more than molecule X. It could be argued that this effect evens out throughout the length of the column, but in practice the number of random partitionings during the time required for elution is not sufficient to eliminate it. As might be expected, C_s makes less contribution as u decreases.

C_m is resistance to mass transfer brought about by the diameter and shape of the particles of the stationary phase and the rate of diffusion of a molecule in the mobile phase.

$$C_m = \frac{d^2 \text{ packing}}{D_m}$$

where d^2 packing is the square of the stationary-phase particle diameter and D_m is the diffusion coefficient of the analyte in the mobile phase.

The smaller and more regular the shape of the particles of the stationary phase, the smaller the contribution to band broadening from this term. In Figure 10.5 molecule X is retarded more than molecule Y in terms of both pathlength (this really belongs to the eddy diffusion term) and contact with stagnant areas of solvent within the pore structure of the stationary phase. With regard to the latter effect, the smaller the rate of diffusion of the molecular species (D_m) in the mobile

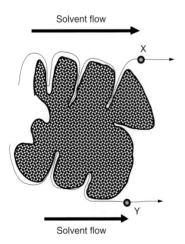

Fig. 10.5
Band broadening due to resistance to diffusion of a molecule
within the mobile phase, contained within the pores of a
stationary phase and due to irregularities in stationary-phase
pore structure.

phase, the greater the retardation will be. There are an insufficient number of random partitionings during elution for these effects to be evened out.

Thus, a low diffusion coefficient for the analyte in the mobile phase increases efficiency with regard to the A term but decreases efficiency with respect to the C_m term. On balance, a higher diffusion coefficient is more favourable. Higher column temperatures reduce mass transfer effects because the rate of diffusion of a molecule in the mobile phase increases.

In practice the contributions of the A, $C_s u$ and $C_m u^{1/2}$ terms to band broadening are similar except at very high flow rates, where the $C_s u$ terms predominate. At very low flow rates, the B term makes more of a contribution. A compromise has to be reached between analysis time and flow rate. Advances in chromatographic techniques are based on the minimisation of the effects of the various terms in the Van Deemter equation, and it has provided the rationale for improvements in the design of stationary phases.

Self-test 10.3

Indicate which of the following parameters can decrease or increase column efficiency in liquid chromatography.

- Very low flow rate
- Large particle size of stationary phase
- Small particle size of stationary phase
- Thick stationary-phase coating
- Thin stationary-phase coating
- Regularly shaped particles of stationary phase
- Irregularly shaped particles of stationary phase
- High temperature
- Low temperature
- Uneven stationary-phase coating
- Even stationary-phase coating
- Uniform stationary-phase particle size
- Non-uniform stationary-phase particle size
- Low diffusion coefficient in the mobile phase
- High diffusion coefficient in the mobile phase
- Low diffusion coefficient in the stationary phase
- High diffusion coefficient in the stationary phase

Answers: Increases column efficiency: small particle size of stationary phase; thin stationary-phase coating; regularly shaped particles of stationary phase; high temperature; even stationary-phase coating; uniform stationary-phase particle size; high diffusion coefficient in the mobile phase; high diffusion coefficient in the stationary phase.

Decreases column efficiency: very low flow rate; large particle size of stationary phase; thick stationary-phase coating; irregularly shaped particles of stationary phase; low temperature; uneven stationary-phase coating; non-uniform stationary-phase particle size; low diffusion coefficient in the mobile phase; low diffusion coefficient in the stationary phase.

Van Deemter equation in gas chromatography

The Van Deemter equation can be applied to gas chromatography with a different emphasis on the relative importance of its terms. In fact, the interactions between an analyte and a stationary phase are much simpler in gas chromatography than those in liquid chromatography since the mobile phase does not modify the stationary phase in any way. The theoretical considerations are different for packed GC columns vs open tubular capillary columns.

In gas chromatography the Van Deemter equation can be written as:

$$H = A + \frac{B}{u} + Cu$$

where H is the measure of column efficiency; A is the eddy diffusion coefficient; B is $2 \times$ the diffusion coefficient of the analyte in the gas phase; C is composed of terms relating to the rate of diffusion of the analyte in the gas and liquid phases (mass transfer, see above) and u is the carrier gas velocity.

For an open tubular capillary column (Fig. 10.6), the eddy diffusion coefficient does not play a part in band broadening, and the C term is largely composed of the transverse diffusion coefficient in the gas phase since the liquid film coating of the capillary column wall is typically 0.1–0.2% of the internal diameter of the column. B/u is most favourable for nitrogen (diffusion coefficients of molecules are lower in nitrogen than in the other commonly used carrier gases hydrogen and helium). However, nitrogen only gives better efficiency where u is small, since the size of the term Cu is governed by the resistance to transverse diffusion, which is greatest for nitrogen, i.e. fast flow rates of nitrogen reduce the interaction of the analyte with the stationary phase. Most often helium is used as a carrier gas in capillary GC since it gives a good efficiency without having to reduce the flow rate, which would give long analysis times. Transverse diffusion effects are reduced by reducing the internal diameter of a capillary column, and thus the smaller the internal diameter of a column, the more efficient it is.

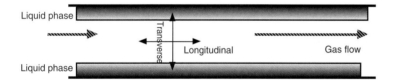

Fig. 10.6
Band broadening factors in open tubular columns.

With a packed GC column the separation efficiency is lower because, although the longitudinal diffusion coefficient is lower, the eddy diffusion coefficient (A) causes band broadening (Fig. 10.3). In addition, mass transfer effects are greater for a packed column because of the irregular structure of the particles of packing and the consequent uneven coating of a relatively thick liquid phase. However, whatever type of GC column is used, the C_m term is not as significant as that in liquid chromatography because of the high diffusion coefficient of molecules in the gas phase.

Parameters used in evaluating column performance

Having optimised the efficiency of a chromatographic separation, the quality of the chromatography can be controlled by applying certain system suitability tests. One of these is the calculation of theoretical plates for a column, and there are two other main parameters for assessing performance: peak symmetry and the resolution between critical pairs of peaks. A third performance test, the peak purity parameter, can be applied where two-dimensional detectors such as diode or coulometric array or mass spectrometry detectors are being used. The reproducibility of peak retention times is also an important parameter for controlling performance.

Resolution

The more efficient a column, the greater degree of resolution it will produce between closely eluting peaks. The resolution between two peaks – A and B (Fig. 10.7) – is expressed in Equation 4:

$$R_s = 2(t_{rB} - t_{rA})/W_{bB} + W_{bA} \qquad \textbf{[Equation 4]}$$

where t_{rB} and t_{rA} are the retention times of peaks A and B and W_{bB} and W_{bA} are the widths of peaks A and B at baseline. An R_s of 1 indicates a separation of 4σ between the apices of two peaks. Complete separation is considered to be $R_s = 1.2$. The retention times of peaks A and B are 26.3 and 27.2 min respectively. The substitution of these values and the values obtained for peak widths at base for A and B into Equation 4 is as follows:

$$R_s = \frac{2(27.2 - 26.3)}{0.56 + 0.56} = 1.6$$

It is obvious without calculation that peaks A and B are well resolved. With incomplete separation, the determination of resolution is more difficult since the end and beginning of the two partially overlapping peaks has to be estimated; if the peak shape is good it is easiest to assume the same symmetry for the leading and tailing edges of the two peaks. If this is carried out for peaks B and C in Figure 10.7, their resolution is found to be 0.85, which is not an entirely satisfactory resolution. More is required of the integrator which is used to measure peak areas when peaks overlap since it must be able to decide where one peak ends and the other begins. Ideally peak overlap should be avoided for quantitative accuracy and precision.

Fig. 10.7
Determination of the degree of resolution between chromatographic peaks.

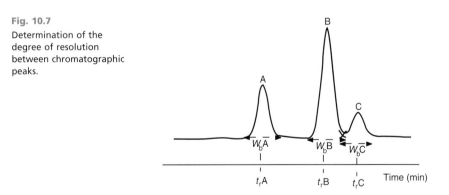

The resolution equation may also be written as follows:

$$R_s = 1.18 \frac{t_{rB} - t_{rA}}{W_{B0.5} + W_{A0.5}}$$

where $W_{B0.5}$ and $W_{A0.5}$ are the widths of peaks A and B at half height. This is the form of the equation that is used by the British and European Pharmacopoeias, whereas the American Pharmacopoeia uses Equation 4. The width of a peak at half height is easier to measure than its width at the base.

Self-test 10.4

The BP assay of betamethasone 17-valerate states that it must be resolved from betamethasone 21-valerate so that the resolution factor is > 1.0. Which of the following ODS columns meet the specification?

Retention time of betamethasone 21-valerate (min)	Retention time of betamethasone 17-valerate (min)	Width at base of betamethasone 21-valerate (min)	Width at base of betamethasone 17-valerate (min)
1. 9.5	8.5	0.4	0.5
2. 9.3	8.6	0.4	0.4

Answer: 1 and 2

The resolution equation may be written in a more complex form for two peaks, A and B, in a chromatogram:

$$R_s = \left(\frac{1}{4}\right) N^{0.5} \left(\frac{\alpha - 1}{\alpha}\right) \left(\frac{K'_B}{1 + K'}\right)$$

N = efficiency

K'_A = capacity factor of peak A

K'_B = capacity factor of peak B   **[Equation 5]**

$$\alpha = \frac{K'_A}{K'_B} = \text{selectivity}$$

$$K' = \frac{K'_A + K'_B}{2}$$

This equation is applicable if the calculated column efficiency is the same for both analytes. If the column efficiency is different for the two analytes then: $\sqrt{N}$ is replaced by $\sqrt[4]{N_A N_B}$ and K'_B is replaced by K'.

From Equation 5 it can be seen that column efficiency has less effect than might be expected on resolution and a 2 × increase in efficiency only results in a 1.41 × increase in resolution. An increase in capacity factor, however, does have a marked effect on resolution. Capacity factor exerts its strongest effect on separation via the α term, which can also be termed the relative capacity factor. The simplest way to increase capacity factor is to change the solvent composition of the mobile phase in liquid chromatography or the temperature in gas chromatography.

Calculation example 10.1

A column has an efficiency of 14 000 theoretical plates. It has a t_o value of 1.3 min. Two analytes have retention times of 10.4 and 12.2. Calculate their resolution factor.

$$K'_A = \frac{10.4 - 1.3}{1.3} = 9.4$$

$$K'_B = \frac{12.2 - 1.3}{1.3} = 11.2$$

$$\alpha = \frac{11.2}{9.4} = 1.2$$

$$R_s = \frac{1}{4} \times \sqrt{14000} \times \frac{1.21}{1.2} \times \frac{11.2}{1 + (9.4 + 11.2)/2} = 5.0$$

Figure 10.8 shows the effect of decreasing the % of organic solvent in a reverse-phase chromatographic separation of two analytes A and B (see Chapter 12). The column has a t_o of 1.2 min; thus the change in the composition has changed the capacity factor for analyte A from 6.4 to 8.1 (% change = 26) and that for B from 7.0 to 10.0 (% change = 43). If the rate of change of capacity factor for two analytes with change of mobile-phase composition is different, then this indicates some difference in their retention mechanism. Often a simple change in organic solvent composition will be sufficient to give adequate resolution between two analytes; however, for critical separations involving a number of components, the selectivity of a method may need to be changed by using ternary mixtures of solvents or by changing the chromatographic column in order to change the α term in Equation 5.

Fig. 10.8

Effect of changing solvent composition on the capacity factor of two analytes on a reverse-phase column.
1. Water/acetonitrile 50:50.
2. Water/acetonitrile 52:48.

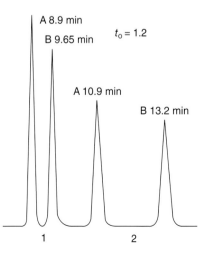

A 8.9 min

B 9.65 min

$t_0 = 1.2$

A 10.9 min

B 13.2 min

1   2

Peak asymmetry

Another situation which may lead to poor integrator performance is where peaks are tailing and thus have a high element of asymmetry. The expression used to assess this is:

$$\text{Asymmetry factor } (AF) = b/a$$

where a is the leading half of the peak measured at 10% of the peak height and b is the trailing half of the peak measured at 10% of the peak height (Fig. 10.9). This value should fall, ideally, in the range 0.95–1.15. Poor symmetry may be caused through loading too much sample onto the column, sample decomposition, the analyte adsorbing strongly onto active sites in the stationary phase, poor trapping of the analyte when it is loaded onto the column or too much 'dead volume' in the chromatographic system.

The peak in Figure 10.9A has an asymmetry factor of 0.97, and this is due to its tailing slightly at the front edge; this may be due to inefficient trapping of the sample at the head of the column as it is loaded. The peak in Figure 10.9B has an asymmetry factor of 1.77 and is thus tailing quite badly; the most common cause of tailing is due to adsorption of the analyte onto active sites in the chromatographic column.

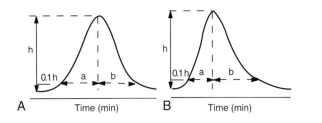

Fig. 10.9
Determination of peak asymmetry.

Data acquisition

An integrator, whether it is based on a microprocessor or PC software, simply measures the total amount of current which flows over the width of a chromatographic peak. To do this it measures the rate of increase of voltage approximately 30 times across the width of the peak. The parameter which indicates when measurement should start is the peak threshold, which determines the level that the voltage of the signal should rise to before accumulation of the signal will occur. To avoid storage of baseline drift the peak width parameter is linked to the peak threshold parameter, which indicates that if the signal rises above baseline the slope of the rise should have a certain steepness before it is regarded as a peak. A narrow peak width setting indicates that the expected slope should be steep and a wide peak width setting indicates that the expected slope should be relatively shallow. For good digital recording a peak should be sampled *ca* 30 times across its width. The setting relates to the estimated width at half-height of peaks in a chromatogram, e.g. a width setting of 0.4 min would cover many HPLC applications. There is quite a wide degree of tolerance in the peak width setting, although it should be set within ± 100% of the expected peak width at half-height to ensure accurate peak integration.

A factor which can cause a loss of precision in chromatographic quantification is the reproducibility of the way in which peaks are integrated. If peaks have good symmetry, are well resolved from neighbouring peaks and are well above baseline noise, integration is likely to be reproducible. The peak threshold (PT) setting has the greatest effect on peak area and it has to be set high enough for fluctuations in the baseline to be ignored. In the example shown in Figure 10.10, in the first case the threshold is set too low and a tail of baseline drift is attached to the peak during integration. In the second case, the threshold is set higher and the tail is ignored. The area of peak A determined with a peak threshold of 100 μV is only 94% of the area determined for peak A with tailing baseline included at a threshold of 10 μV. This could make a significant difference to the precision of the analysis, depending on how reproducibly the peak tail was integrated. This type of effect is only likely to be significant if the size of the peaks is low in relation to baseline fluctuations.

Fig. 10.10
The effect of the peak threshold setting.

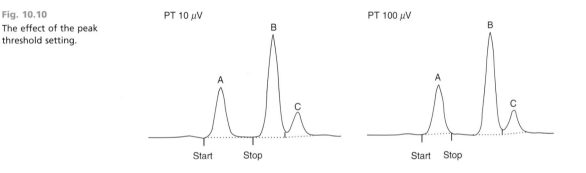

The two fused peaks shown in Figure 10.10 are not as affected by a change in the peak threshold setting; however, their areas can only be approximated because of their overlap. It is possible, by setting the integrator to produce a tangent skim, to change the way in which these peaks are integrated, as shown in Figure 10.11. (see Animation 10.1, Animation 10.2 and Animation 10.3) In this instance, where the peaks are almost resolved and are not vastly different in height, the integration method used in Figure 10.10 probably gives a better approximation of the areas.

Fig. 10.11
Tangent skimming of a peak on a tailing edge.

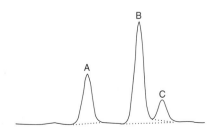

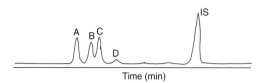

Fig. 10.12
Chromatographic trace with report
including system suitability tests.

Report generation

Computerised data handling systems will generate reports including a number of system suitability parameters. Figure 10.12 shows a chromatogram with a report form appended. In order for the report to be generated, the computer has to be given some information, e.g. the expected retention times of peaks for which resolution factors have to be measured and the retention time of an unretained peak, in order to determine capacity factor. With increasing dependence on computers, it is important to be able to guesstimate whether the computer is generating sensible data; the ability to calculate the various efficiency parameters from first principles is an important check on the performance of the integrator.

Component	Retention time	Area %	n per column	AF	$W_{1/2}$ min	R_s	K'
A	20.1	16.3	50 166	0.96	0.2	–	18.3
B	20.8	13.2	65 229	0.87	0.2	1.4	18.9
C	21.2	15.5	81 189	1.13	0.17	0.81	19.2
D	22.0	2.21	44 397	0.99	0.23	1.8	20.0
IS	25.7	37.9	64 316	0.75	0.23	–	23.4

Reference

1. Giddings JC. *Unified Separation Science*. Chichester: Wiley Interscience; 1991.

11

Gas chromatography

KEYPOINTS

Principles

A gaseous mobile phase flows under pressure through a heated tube either coated with a liquid stationary phase or packed with liquid stationary phase coated onto a solid support. The analyte is loaded onto the head of the column via a heated injection port, where it evaporates. It then condenses at the head of the column, which is at a lower temperature. The oven temperature is then either held constant or programmed to rise gradually. Once on the column, separation of a mixture occurs according to the relative lengths of time spent by its components in the stationary phase. Monitoring of the column effluent can be carried out with a variety of detectors.

(Continued)

> **KEYPOINTS** *(Continued)*
>
> **Applications**
> - The characterisation of some unformulated drugs, particularly with regard to detection of process impurities.
> - Limit tests for solvent residues and other volatile impurities in drug substances.
> - Sometimes used for quantification of drugs in formulations, particularly if the drug lacks a chromophore.
> - Characterisation of some raw materials used in synthesis of drug molecules.
> - Characterisation of volatile oils (which may be used as excipients in formulations), proprietary cough mixtures and tonics, and fatty acids in fixed oils.
> - Measurement of drugs and their metabolites in biological fluids.
>
> **Strengths**
> - Capable of the same quantitative accuracy and precision as high-pressure liquid chromatography (HPLC), particularly when used in conjunction with an internal standard.
> - Has much greater separating power than HPLC when used with capillary columns.
> - Readily automated.
> - Can be used to determine compounds which lack chromophores.
> - The mobile phase does not vary and does not require disposal and, even if helium is used as a carrier gas, is cheap compared to the organic solvents used in HPLC.
>
> **Limitations**
> - Only thermally stable and volatile compounds can be analysed.
> - The sample may require derivatisation to convert it to a volatile form, thus introducing an extra step in analysis and, potentially, interferants.
> - Quantitative sample introduction is more difficult because of the small volumes of sample injected.
> - Aqueous solutions and salts cannot be injected into the instrument.

Introduction (see Animation 11.1)

The use of gas chromatography (GC) as a quantitative technique in the analysis of drugs has declined in importance since the advent of high-pressure liquid chromatography (HPLC) and the increasing sophistication of this technique. However, it does still have a role in certain types of quantitative analyses and has broad application in qualitative analysis. Since HPLC currently dominates quantitative analyses in the pharmaceutical industry, the strengths of GC may be overlooked. Capillary GC is capable of performing much more efficient separations than HPLC, albeit with the limitation that the compounds being analysed must be volatile or must be rendered volatile by formation of a suitable derivative[1] and must also be thermally stable. GC is widely used in environmental science, brewing, the food industry, perfumery and flavourings analysis, the petrochemical industry, microbiological analyses and clinical biochemistry. Although packed column GC is still used in the pharmaceutical industry, this chapter will concentrate to a large extent on open tubular capillary GC, which is the more modern manifestation of GC.

Instrumentation

Figure 11.1 shows a schematic diagram of a GC system. The principles of the system are that:

(i) Injection of the sample may be made, manually or using an autosampler, through a re-sealable rubber septum.

Fig. 11.1
Schematic diagram of a
capillary gas chromatography
(GC) system.

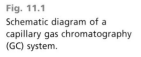

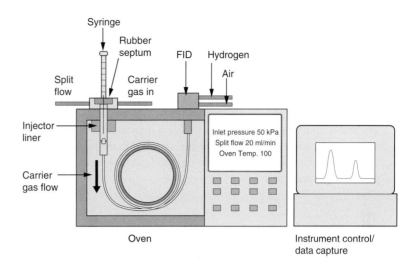

(ii) The sample is evaporated in the heated injection port area and condenses on the head of the column.

(iii) The column may be either a capillary or a packed column, which will be discussed in more detail later. The mobile phase used to carry the sample through the column is a gas – usually nitrogen or helium.

(iv) The column is enclosed in an oven which may be set at any temperature between ambient and *ca* 400°C.

(v) The most commonly used detector is the flame ionisation detector (FID).

Syringes

The volumes injected in GC are routinely in the range of 0.5–2 μl. The most commonly used type of syringe is shown in Figure 11.2; the usual syringe volumes are 5 and 10 μl. A recommended technique for injection into a capillary GC is to fill the syringe with about 0.5 μl of solvent and draw this solvent into the barrel slightly before filling with sample (see Animation 11.2). The sample is also drawn into the barrel to leave an air gap below it. The syringe needle can then be introduced into the injector and left for a couple of seconds to warm up before the plunger is depressed. The syringe is then withdrawn immediately from the injection port.

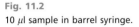

Fig. 11.2
10 μl sample in barrel syringe.

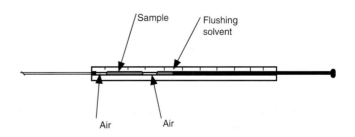

Injection systems

Packed column injections

Injection generally occurs through a re-sealable rubber septum. The injector port is held at 150–250° depending on the volatility of the sample and direct injection of 0.1–10 μl of sample is made onto the head of the column. The amount of sample injected onto a packed column is *ca* 1–2 μg per component. Injection into packed columns presents less of a problem than sample introduction into a capillary column, since all the sample is introduced into the packed column (Fig. 11.3). Thus, although packed columns do not produce high-resolution chromatography, this is their strength.

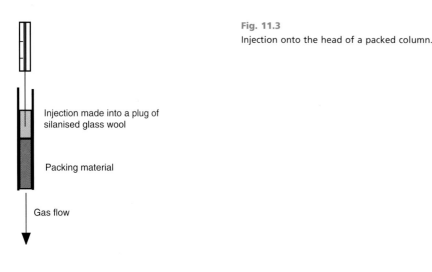

Fig. 11.3
Injection onto the head of a packed column.

Injection made into a plug of
silanised glass wool

Packing material

Gas flow

Split/splitless injection

This type of injector is used in conjunction with capillary column GC. Capillary columns commonly have internal diameters between 0.2 and 0.5 mm and lengths between 12 and 50 m. Injection takes place into a heated glass or quartz liner rather than directly onto the column.

In the split mode, the sample is split into two unequal portions, the smaller of which goes onto the column. Split ratios range between 10:1 and 100:1, with the larger portion being vented in the higher flow out of the split vent. This technique is used with concentrated samples. Figure 11.4 shows a chromatogram of a 4 mg/ml solution of the pharmaceutical excipient cetostearyl alcohol injected in a GC split and splitless mode. In splitless mode the peak shapes are poor due to overloading of the column with too much sample. In the splitless mode, all the sample is introduced onto the column and the injector purge valve remains closed for 0.5–1 min after injection.

The difficulty faced with split/splitless injection onto a capillary column is in obtaining good injection precision.[2]

Attention has to be paid to certain points:

(i)   Since injection is made at high temperatures into an injection port, a lack of precision resulting from decomposition of some of the components in a mixture before they reach the column has to be considered. Thus it

Fig. 11.4
Analysis of cetostearyl alcohol (4 mg/ml) in split and splitless mode A and splitless mode B 20:1 split (flow through column 1 ml/min flow out of split vent 20 ml/min). Column Rtx1 15 m × 0.32 mm i.d. × 0.5 μm film, programmed 100° (1 min) then 10°/min to 290°).

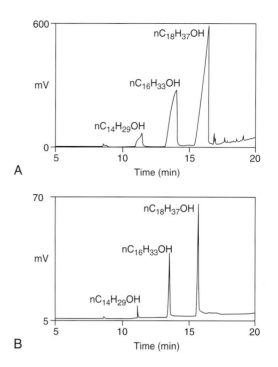

is important to ensure that the sample has minimal contact with metal surfaces during the injection process, since these can catalyse decomposition.

(ii)   If a split injection is used, care has to be taken that there is no discrimination between more and less volatile components in a mixture in terms of the proportion lost through the split vent (see Animation 11.3).

(iii) If a splitless injection is made, volumes have to be kept below *ca* 2 *μl* in case the sample backflashes through rapid expansion of the solvent in which it is dissolved, into either the gas supply lines or the purge lines. Each 1 *μl* of solvent expands greatly upon vapourisation, e.g. methanol *ca* 0.66 ml/*μl* or ethyl acetate *ca* 0.23 ml/*μl* at atmospheric pressure.

(iv) Even if an internal standard (p. 287) is used to compensate for losses, the possibility of its being randomly discriminated against through differences in either volatility or decomposition compared with the sample has to be considered.

(v)   In the splitless mode, the sample must be efficiently trapped at the head of the column. For this to occur, it must be sufficiently involatile, i.e. have a boiling point > *ca* 50°C higher than the column starting temperature. If the sample is relatively volatile, it has to be injected into the GC in a low-volatility solvent, which will condense at the head of the column, trapping the sample in the process. Figure 11.5 shows the effect of too high a starting temperature on the trapping of a volatile analyte resulting in misshapen peaks, which can be corrected by lowering the starting temperature and then programming the GC temperature to rise.

(vi) Sample transfer may be slow and it is important to take this into account when setting purge valve times, e.g. for a typical 1 ml/min flow of helium

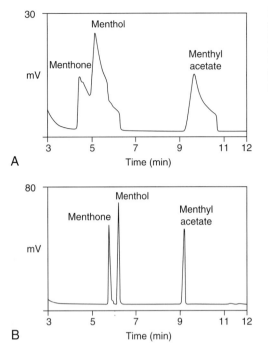

Fig. 11.5
(A) Gas chromatography (GC) trace for menthone, menthol and menthyl acetate under isothermal conditions, 110°C for 12 minutes. (B) 60°C (1 min) 30°C/min to 120°C for 9 minutes.

through a capillary column, about 0.5 min would be required to transfer a 2 μl injection volume of ethyl acetate onto the column.

(vii) Injection precision is greatly improved by the use of an autosampler to carry out injection since it can achieve much better precision in measuring volumes of *ca* 1 μl than a human operator.

Cool on-column injection

Direct on-column injection into the capillary column may be carried out in a manner analogous to injection into a packed column. This technique requires a syringe with a very fine fused-silica needle. The technique has the advantages of (1) reduced discrimination between components in mixtures, (2) no sample degradation in a hot injector and (3) no backflash, hence quantitative sample transfer. It also has the following disadvantages: (1) samples have to be clean otherwise residues will be deposited on the column; (2) the injector is mechanically more complex and requires more maintenance than a septum injection system and (3) the syringe needle may damage the head of the column.

Programmable temperature vapouriser (see Animation 11.4)

The programmable temperature vapouriser (PTV) is a recent innovation. This type of injector is designed to enable the injection of large volumes of sample onto capillary GC columns. Typically between 5 and 50 μl of sample are injected, with the injector being held at low temperature, e.g. 30°C. The solvent is then vented through a purge valve at high flow rate (e.g. 100 ml/min for 1 min). The less volatile, sample components are retained in the injection port; the purge valve is then closed and the injector temperature is ramped up rapidly (e.g. to 300°C at 700°C/min). This is possible because the liner is of narrow diameter (1 mm) compared with those in other types of injectors and is made of Silicosteel, which provides an inert surface but conducts heat much more rapidly than glass. The boiling point of the lowest boiling component in the sample should be at least 100°C greater than that of the solvent for this injector to work well. This injector provides one option for use in conjunction with fast GC. Fast GC utilises the high efficiency of capillary GC by using very short columns so that separations of complex mixtures may be achieved in less than a minute.

GC oven

GC ovens incorporate a fan, which ensures uniform heat distribution throughout the oven. They can be programmed to produce a constant temperature, isothermal conditions or a gradual increase in temperature. Oven programming rates can range from 1°C/min to 40°C/min. Complex temperature programmes can be produced involving a number of temperature ramps interspersed with periods of isothermal conditions, e.g. 60°C (1 min)/5°C/min to 100°C (5 min)/10°C/min to 200°C (5 min). The advantages of temperature programmes are that materials of widely differing volatilities can be separated in a reasonable time and also injection of the sample can be carried out at low temperature, where it will be trapped at the head of the column and then the temperature can be raised until it elutes.

Types of columns

Packed columns

The columns are usually made from glass which is silanized to remove polar silanol Si–OH groups from its surface, which can contribute to the peak tailing of the peaks of polar analytes. These columns have internal diameters of 2–5 mm. The columns are packed with particles of a solid support which are coated with the liquid stationary phase. The most commonly used support is diatomaceous earth (mainly calcium silicate). This material is usually acid washed to remove mineral impurities and then silanized as shown in Figure 11.6 to remove the polar Si–OH groups on the surface of the support, which can lead to tailing of the analyte peak.

The support can then be mechanically coated with a variety of liquid stationary phases. The mobile phase most commonly used in packed column GC is nitrogen, with a flow rate of *ca* 20 ml/min. Packed column GC affords a relatively low degree of resolution compared to capillary GC; typically 4000–6000 plates for a 2 m column compared to > 100 000 plates for a 25 m capillary column. The high temperature limit of packed columns is *ca* 280°C; beyond this temperature the liquid stationary phase evaporates at a rate which creates a large background signal. However, for many routine quality-control operations, they are quite adequate.

Fig. 11.6
Silanisation of free silanol groups.

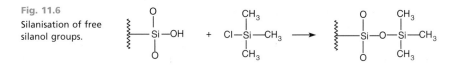

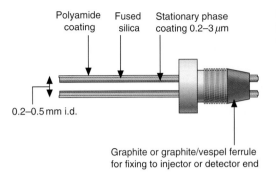

Fig. 11.7

Structure of a gas chromatography (GC) capillary column.

Polyamide coating Fused silica Stationary phase coating 0.2–3 μm

0.2–0.5 mm i.d.

Graphite or graphite/vespel ferrule for fixing to injector or detector end

Capillary columns

Capillary columns are made from fused silica, usually coated on the outside with polyamide to give the column flexibility (Fig. 11.7). Coating on the outside with aluminium has also been used for high-temperature (> 400°C) work. The internal diameter of the columns ranges between 0.15 and 0.5 mm. The wall of the column is coated with the liquid stationary phase, which may have a thickness between 0.1 and 5 μm. The most common type of coating is based on organo silicone polymers, which are chemically bonded to the silanol groups on the wall of the column, and the chains of the polymers are further cross-linked. These types of phases have more or less replaced the wall-coated open tubular (WCOT) and support-coated open tubular (SCOT) columns, which are reported in earlier literature, for most routine applications. SCOT columns are sometimes encountered in very high-temperature work. The wall-bonded phases are stable to at least 325°C and some types of coating will withstand temperatures of 370°C. The non-silicone-based polymers, e.g. carbowax, cannot be bonded onto the wall of the column in the same way and columns with these coatings are less temperature stable. For instance, the temperature limit for a carbowax capillary column is *ca* 240°C. The most commonly used carrier gas in capillary GC is helium and the flow rates used are between 0.5 and 2 ml/min. Since the flow rate from the end of the capillary column is low compared to the internal space of some detectors, 'make up' gas often has to be added to the gas flow post column in order to sweep the sample through the internal volume of the detector at a reasonable rate. Typically *ca* 100 ng per component is loaded onto a capillary column.

Selectivity of liquid stationary phases
Kovats indices and column polarity

Kovats indices (*I*-values) are based on the retention time of an analyte compared to retention times of the series of *n*-alkanes. For a particular GC phase, *I*-values are very reproducible from one column or from one GC to another. However, they are slightly affected by GC programming conditions. *n*-Alkanes have most affinity for non-polar phases and tend to elute more quickly from polar phases. In contrast, a polar analyte will elute more slowly from a polar phase and thus, relative to the *n*-alkanes, its retention time, and thus its *I*-value, will increase as the polarity of the GC phase increases. A measure of the polarity of a stationary phase is given by its McReynold's constant (Table 11.1), which is based on the retention times of benzene, *n*-butanol, pentan-2-one, nitropropane and pyridine

Table 11.1 McReynold's constants

Phase	Chemical type	McReynold's constant
Squalane	Hydrocarbon	0
Silicone OV-1	Methylsilicone	222
Silicone SE-54	94% methyl, 5% phenyl, 1% vinyl	337
Silicone OV-17	50% methyl, 50% phenyl	886
Silicone OV-225	50% methyl, 25% cyanopropyl, 25% phenyl	1813
Carbowax	Polyethylene glycol	2318

on a particular phase. The higher the McReynold's constant, the more polar the phase. Many stationary phases are described by an OV-number. The higher the number after the OV, the more polar the phase.

I-values provide a useful method for characterising unknown compounds, and tables of I-values have been compiled for a large number of compounds.[3] Under temperature programming conditions, where the GC temperature rises at a uniform rate, e.g. 10°C/min, a plot of the carbon numbers of n-alkanes (where 1 carbon = 100) against their retention times is a straight line. Under isothermal conditions, where the column is maintained at the same temperature throughout the analysis, a plot of carbon number against the logarithm of the retention times of the n-alkanes is a straight line. Such calibration curves can be used to convert the retention time of a compound into an I-value.

Examples of the separation of mixtures by GC
Analysis of peppermint oil on two GC phases
Figure 11.8 shows the structures of some of the major components in peppermint oil. The use of the retention index system is illustrated in Figures 11.8 and 11.9 for peppermint oil run in comparison with n-alkane standards on both a weakly polar OV-5-type column and a polar carbowax column.

Figure 11.9 indicates approximate I-values for some of the components in peppermint oil on a BPX-5 column; this column selects mainly on the basis of molecular weight and shape. For example, ß-pinene has the same molecular weight as limonene but has a more compact shape and thus a lower I-value. Menthyl acetate has a higher I-value than menthol because of its higher molecular weight.

A carbowax column is highly selective for polar compounds. As can be seen in Figure 11.10, the group of polar compounds including menthol and menthone is resolved more extensively on a carbowax column, with the alcohol menthol

Fig. 11.8
The structures of some components in peppermint oil.

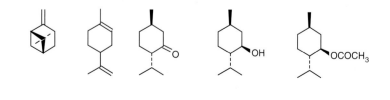

β-pinene   Limonene   Menthone   Menthol   Menthyl acetate

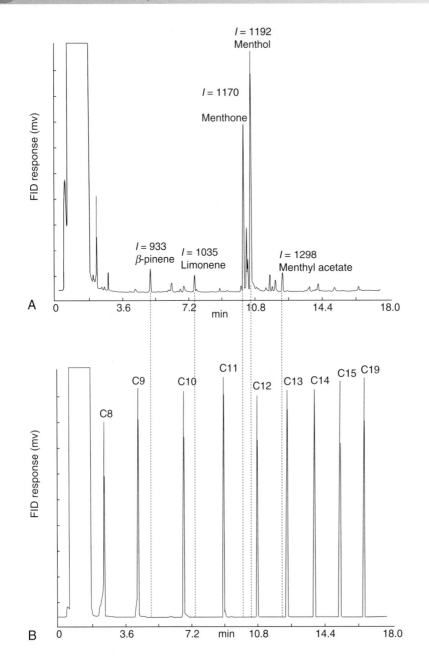

Fig. 11.9
(A) Peppermint oil analysed on a BPX-5 column (12 m × 0.25 mm i.d. × 0.25 μm film). Programmed 50°C (1 min), then 5°C/min to 70°C, then 10°C/min to 200°C. (B) *n*-alkanes C8-C16 chromatographed under the same conditions.

and a number of other minor alcohols eluting at around 12 min. In addition, the less polar ketone menthone and a number of minor ketones elute at around 10 min. Menthyl acetate, which on the non-polar BPX-5 column ran later than menthol, runs earlier than menthol on the carbowax column because its polar alcohol group is masked by the acetate and it thus has a lower polarity than menthol.

Fig. 11.10
(A) Peppermint oil analysed on a carbowax column (15 m × 0.25 mm i.d. × 0.5 μm film). Programmed 50°C (1 min), then 5°C/min to 70°C, then 10°C/min to 200°C. (B) *n*-alkanes C10-C18 chromatographed under the same conditions.

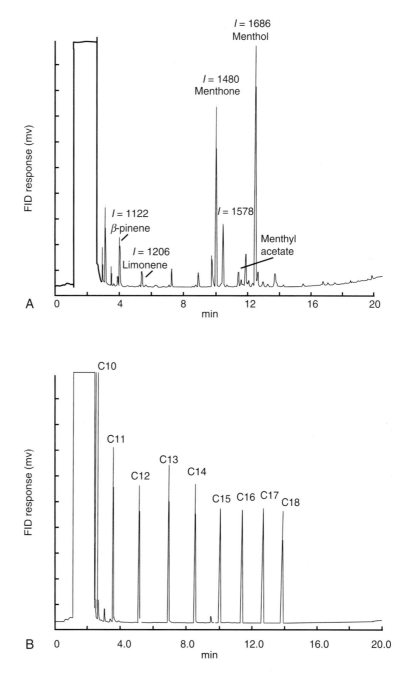

Self-test 11.1

Associate the following *l*-values obtained on an OV-1-type column with structures of the local anaesthetics shown below. *l*-values: 1555, 2018, 2323 and 2457. Note: Oxygen in an ether linkage is equivalent to *ca* 1 CH$_2$ unit.

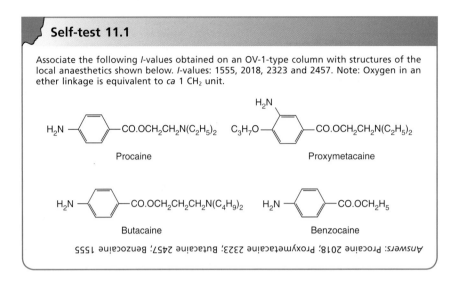

Procaine

Proxymetacaine

Butacaine

Benzocaine

Answers: Procaine 2018; Proxymetacaine 2323; Butacaine 2457; Benzocaine 1555

Analysis of the fatty acid composition of a fixed oil by GC

A very polar phase such as carbowax is generally only used for samples requiring a high degree of polar discrimination for adequate separation or retention. An example of this is in the analysis of fatty acids with differing degrees of unsaturation. On a non-polar column such as BPX-5, a series of C-18 acids such as stearic, oleic, linoleic and linolenic acids, which contain, respectively, 0, 1, 2 and 3 double bonds, overlaps extensively. However, on polar columns such as carbowax they are separated.

The BP monographs for many of the fixed oils contain a GC analysis to confirm the content of the fatty acids composing the triglycerides (fatty acid triesters of glycerol) present in the oil. The monograph for almond oil states the composition of the fatty acids making up the triglyceride should be:

- palmitic acid (16:0) 4.0–9.0%
- palmitoleic acid (16:1) < 0.6%
- margaric acid (17:0) < 0.2%
- stearic acid (18:0) 0.9–2.0%
- oleic acid (18:1) 62.0–86.0%
- linoleic acid (18:2) 7.0%–30.0%
- linolenic acid (18:3) < 0.2%
- arachidic acid (20:0) < 0.1%
- behenic acid (22:0) < 0.1%.

The first number in brackets, e.g. 16, refers to the number of carbon atoms in the fatty acid and the second number, e.g. 0, refers to the number of double bonds in the fatty acid. The percentage of each component is determined in relation to the sum of the areas of the chromatographic peaks of all the components listed above.

In order to determine the fatty acid composition of the triglycerides, they have to be first hydrolysed and the liberated fatty acids converted to their methyl esters, which have a good chromatographic peak shape compared to the free acids. A

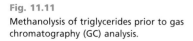

Fig. 11.11

Methanolysis of triglycerides prior to gas chromatography (GC) analysis.

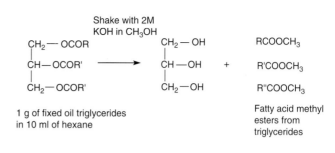

convenient method for achieving hydrolysis and methylation in one step is shown in Figure 11.11.

A GC trace of methanolysed almond oil is shown in Figure 11.12. It can be seen that the methyl esters stearic, oleic and linoleic acid are incompletely resolved on a BPX-5 column. The esters of the minor C-20 and C-22 acids are also incompletely separated. When a carbowax column is used, complete separation of oleic (18:1), linoleic (18:2), stearic (18:0) and a small amount of linolenic acid (18:3) in the sample is achieved.

The chromatogram obtained on the carbowax column gave the percentage of areas of the peaks in this particular sample of almond oil as follows: 16:0 (7.0%), 16:1 (0.4%), 17:0 (0.12%), 18:0 (1.5%), 18:1 (62.8%), 18:2 (28.4%), 18:3 (0.16%), 20:0 (0.09%), 22:0 (0.09%). Thus the almond oil is within the BP specification given above.

Chiral selectivity

An advanced type of column selectivity is chiral discrimination. Since enantiomers have identical physical properties, they are not separable on conventional GC columns. However, if chiral analytes are allowed to interact with a chiral environment, they will form transitory diastereomeric complexes, which results in their being retained by the column to a different extent. As increasing numbers of enantiomerically pure drugs are synthesised in order to reduce side effects, this type of separation will become increasingly important.

Chirasil Val was one of the first chiral GC phases; it has one chiral centre, as can be seen in its structure as shown in Figure 11.13.

A number of variations on this type of coating have been prepared and offer some improvement over the original phase. Figure 11.14 shows the volatile pentafluoropropionamide-trifluoroethyl ester (PFP-TFE) derivatives of *L* and *D* phenylalanine. Figure 11.15 shows the separation of PFP-TFE derivatives of the *D* and *L* enantiomers of the amino acids phenylalanine and *p*-tyrosine on a Chirasil Val column; the *D*(*R*)-enantiomers elute first. Chirasil Val generally performs best for the separation of enantiomers of amino acids; for many other compounds it is not as effective.

More recently, alkylated cyclodextrins have been developed as chiral phases. These phases are based on cyclodextrins, which are cyclic structures formed from 6, 7 or 8 glucose units. Alkylation of the hydroxyl groups in the structure of the cyclodextrins lowers their melting points and makes them suitable as GC phases. The cyclodextrins contain many chiral centres, and they separate enantiomers of drugs according to how well they fit into the chiral cavities of the cyclodextrin units (see Ch. 12, p. 351).

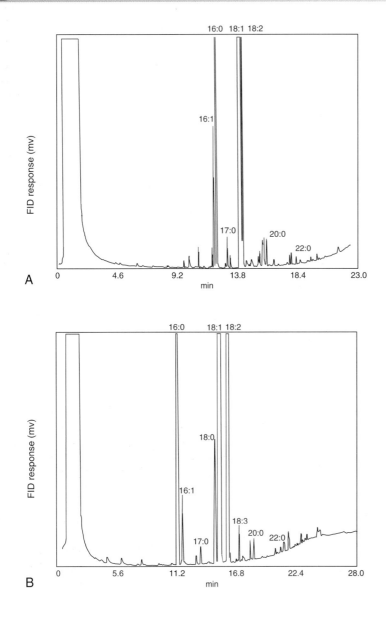

A

B

Fig. 11.12

(A) Separation of fatty acid methyl esters derived from almond oil on a BPX-5 column (12 m × 0.25 mm i.d. × 0.25 μm film). Programmed 100°C (1 min), then 10°C/min to 320°C. The major peaks are shown as offscale so that the minor peaks can be seen clearly. (B) The same sample separated on an HP Stabiliwax column (15 m × 0.25 mm × 0.5 μm film). Programmed 140°C (1 min), then 5°C/min to 250°C (5 min).

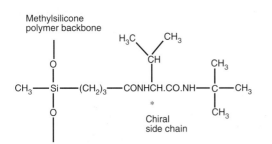

Methylsilicone polymer backbone

Chiral side chain

Fig. 11.13

The structure of Chirasil Val.

Fig. 11.14
Derivatives of *L* and *D* phenylalanine.

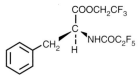
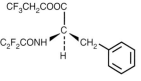

PFP–TFE derivative of *L* phenylalanine   PFP–TFE derivative of *D* phenylalanine

Fig. 11.15
Separation of the PFP-TFE derivatives of the *D* and *L* isomers of phenylalanine and *p*-tyrosine on a Chirasil Val column 25 m × 0.25 mm i.d. × 0.16 μm film. Programmed 120°C (1 min), then 3°C/min to 180°C.

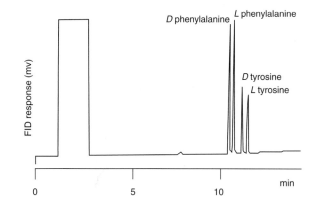

An alternative to buying expensive chiral columns in order to separate enantiomers is to use a chiral derivatisation agent. These reagents can be based on natural products which usually occur in an enantiomerically pure form. Chiral derivatising agents can often produce better separations than chiral columns, but if reaction conditions are too strong, there is a risk of small amounts of racemisation occurring in the analyte, i.e. chemical conversion of an enantiomer into its opposite. Reaction of an enantiomeric mixture with a chiral derivatising agent produces a pair of diastereoisomers which are separable by GC on non-chiral columns, e.g. the esters of menthol with (+) chrysanthemic acid.[4]

It can be seen in Figure 11.16 that, although the menthol portions of the esters are mirror images, addition of the chiral acylating reagent generates esters which are not mirror images but are diastereoisomers and thus have different physical properties.

Use of derivatisation in GC

Derivatisation has been mentioned above without fully indicating why it is necessary for conducting GC analysis. Derivatisation is generally required prior to GC

Fig. 11.16
(+) Chrysanthemyl esters of menthol.

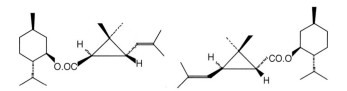

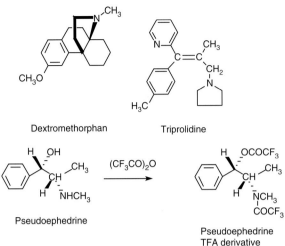

Dextromethorphan   Triprolidine

Pseudoephedrine   Pseudoephedrine
                       TFA derivative

(CF₃CO)₂O

Fig. 11.17
The components in a decongestant + derivatisation of
pseudoephedrine with trifluoroacetic anhydride (TFA).

if a compound is highly polar, so that good chromatographic peak shape can be achieved. A large number of derivatisation strategies are available.[2] In the following example, derivatisation is used to improve the peak shape of pseudoephedrine (Fig. 11.17).

A decongestant syrup was basified with ammonia and extracted into ethyl acetate, thus ensuring that the components extracted were in their free base forms rather than their salts, which is important for obtaining good chromatographic peak shape. Salts of bases will thermally dissociate in the GC injector port, but this process can cause a loss of peak shape and decomposition.

If the extract is run directly, the trace shown in Figure 11.18A is obtained. The free bases of triprolidine and dextromethorphan give good peak shape but pseudoephedrine, which is a stronger base and which has, in addition, a hydroxyl group in its structure, gives a poor peak shape. This can be remedied by masking the polar alcohol and amine groups of pseudoephedrine by reaction with trifluoroacetic anhydride TFA, resulting in the trace shown in Figure 11.18B. Treatment with TFA does not produce derivatives of the tertiary bases in the extract. This reagent is very useful because it is very reactive and boils at 40°C; thus excess reagent can be evaporated very easily prior to GC analysis and thus, unlike many reagents, it does not leave any residue. As outlined above, tertiary amines in their free base form give excellent GC peak shape.

Silylating reagents are another popular class of derivatisation reagents. Figure 11.19 shows the trimethylsilylation of glycerol and diethylene glycol (DEG) in order to improve GC peak shape by masking the hydroxyl groups in the structures and Figure 11.20 shows a GC trace of the separation of a mixture of glycerol and diethylene glycol in 20:1 ratio.

The pharmacopoeias utilise a GC test for DEG in glycerol. DEG is available in the form of anti-freeze, tastes sweet and has been used instead of glycerol to formulate syrups by unscrupulous manufacturers; it is, however, highly toxic. As can be seen in Figure 11.20 it is readily identified by using GC.

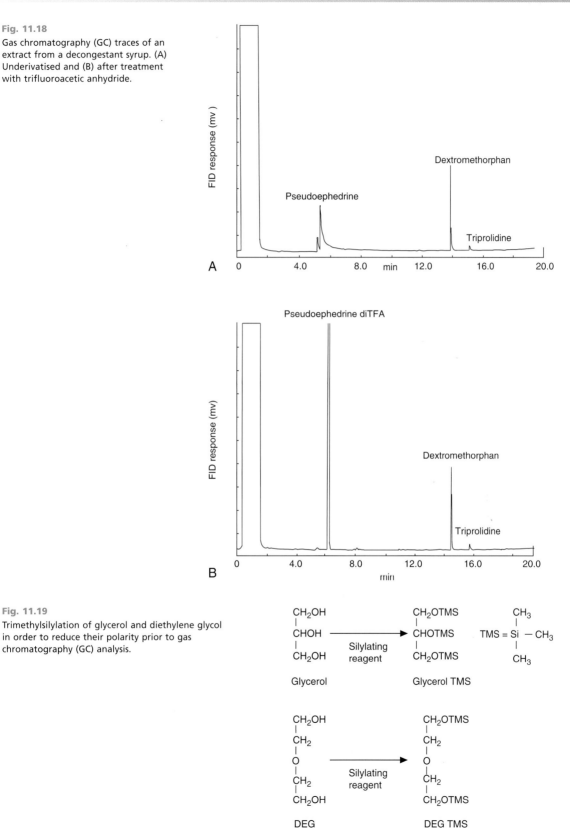

Fig. 11.18

Gas chromatography (GC) traces of an extract from a decongestant syrup. (A) Underivatised and (B) after treatment with trifluoroacetic anhydride.

Fig. 11.19

Trimethylsilylation of glycerol and diethylene glycol in order to reduce their polarity prior to gas chromatography (GC) analysis.

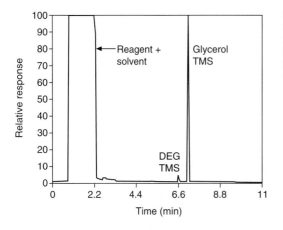

Fig. 11.20
Glycerol and diethylene glycol in
20:1 mixture separated on a
25 m × 0.32 mm i.d. × 0.5 μm film
DB5 column programmed 100°
(1 min), then 20°/min.

Self-test 11.2

A GC trace for bases A, B and C is shown below. Link the peaks to the structures.

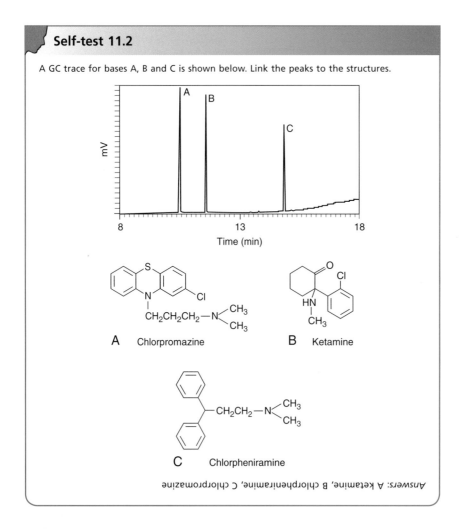

A   Chlorpromazine

B   Ketamine

C   Chlorpheniramine

Answers: A ketamine, B chlorpheniramine, C chlorpromazine

Summary of parameters governing capillary GC performance

Carrier gas type/flow

According to the Van Deemter equation, hydrogen and helium give higher efficiencies at high flow rates compared with nitrogen. For practical analysis times, hydrogen or helium is used in capillary GC and typical flow rates for hydrogen and helium are in the range of 30–50 cm/s; nitrogen has its optimum flow rate at 10–20 cm/s. Table 11.2 shows typical pressure settings to achieve optimal flow rate for three columns. The gas flow rate decreases with increasing temperature, and this may have an influence on column efficiency. Modern instruments have flow programming so that the flow can be set to remain constant as the temperature rises.

Table 11.2 Effect of temperature on flow rate at constant pressure

Column	Pressure	Temperature (°C)	T_o (s)	Flow rate	Temp (°C)	Flow rate	T_o (s)
25 m × 0.5 mm i.d.	22.2 KPa	100	83	30 cm/s	250	23.7 cm/s	106
25 m × 0.25 mm i.d.	91.1 KPa	100	83	30 cm/s	250	23.7 cm/s	106
12 m × 0.25 mm i.d.	42.8 KPa	100	40	30 cm/s	250	23.7 cm/s	51

Column temperature

As column temperature increases, the degree of resolution between two components decreases, because the degree of interaction with the stationary phase is reduced as the vapour pressure of the analytes increases. Lower temperatures produce better resolution.

Column length

The separating power of a column varies as the square root of its length. Thus, if a two-fold increase in resolution is required, a four-fold increase in column length would be required; this would result in a four-fold increase in analysis time. The increased resolution afforded by length can often be replaced with a decrease in temperature, ensuring that more interaction with the stationary phase occurs, especially if the stationary phase has characteristics that enable it to select one analyte more than another.

Film thickness phase loading

The greater the volume of stationary phase, the more a solute will partition into it. If the film thickness or loading of stationary phase doubles, then, in theory, the retention of an analyte should double. Thus thicker films are used for very volatile materials to increase their retention time and to increase resolution between analytes without increasing the column length.

Internal diameter

The smaller the internal diameter of a capillary column, the more efficient the column is for a given stationary-phase film thickness on the capillary wall. This is because the mass transfer characteristics of the column are improved, with the analyte being able to diffuse in and out of the mobile phase more frequently because of the shorter distance for transverse diffusion (Ch. 10, p. 258).

Self-test 11.3

A fixed temperature is used and the head pressure is adjusted so that the linear velocity of a helium carrier gas through the following capillary columns is 20 cm/s: (i) 30 m × 0.25 mm i.d. × 0.25 μm OV-1 film; (ii) 15 m × 0.15 mm × 0.2 μm OV-1 film; (iii) 12 m × 0.5 mm i.d. × 1.0 μm OV-1 film.

a. List the columns in the order in which they would increasingly retain a *n*-hexadecane standard.
b. List the columns in order of increasing efficiency.

Answers: a. (ii) (i) (iii); b. (iii) (i) (ii)

GC detectors (see Animation 11.5)

There are many GC detectors available, although the flame ionisation detector remains the most widely used and the most widely applicable to quality control of pharmaceutical products. However, newer detectors, such as the plasma emission detector for analysis of trace impurities or the GC-FTIR detector for the structural characterisation of components in mixtures, are becoming increasingly important. Selectivity in a detector is most often required for sensitive bioanalytical methods where trace amounts of compounds are being analysed in the presence of interferants, which are also present in the sample matrix. The properties of some commonly used detectors are summarised in Table 11.3.

Applications of GC in quantitative analysis

HPLC has more or less supplanted GC as a method for quantifying drugs in pharmaceutical preparations. Many of the literature references to quantitative GC assays are thus old, and the precision which is reported in these papers is difficult to evaluate based on the measurement of peak heights or manual integration. It is more difficult to achieve good precision in GC analysis than in HPLC analysis, and the main sources of imprecision are the mode of sample introduction, which is best controlled by an autosampler, and the small volume of sample injected. However, it is possible to achieve levels of precision similar to those achieved using HPLC methods. For certain compounds that lack chromophores, which are required for detection in commonly used HPLC methods, quantitative GC may be the method of choice for analysis of many amino acids, fatty acids and sugars. There are a number of assays in the BP, US Pharmacopoeia and European Pharmacopoeia, which are based on GC, but the selection of compounds analysed in this way appears to be rather random and many of the assays described could also be carried out by HPLC. The BP format for assays (for both HPLC and GC assays) is, most often, to run three samples. These are a calibration standard containing more or less equal amounts of a pure standard and an internal standard (Solution 1); an extract of the sample containing no internal standard to check for interference from the formulation matrix (Solution 2) and an extract from the sample containing the same amount of internal standard as Solution 1 (Solution 3). This is illustrated in Figure 11.21 for the analysis of methyltestosterone in a tablet formulation using testosterone as an internal standard (see p. 336).

Table 11.3 Commonly used gas chromatography (GC) detectors

Detector	Applications
Flame ionisation 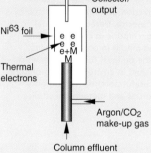	Compounds are burnt in the flame, producing ions and thus an increase in current between the jet and the collector. Detects carbon/hydrogen-containing compounds. Insensitive to carbon atoms attached to oxygen, nitrogen or chlorine. In combination with capillary GC it may detect as low as 100 pg–10 ng. Wide range of linear response *ca* 10^6
Electron capture 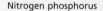 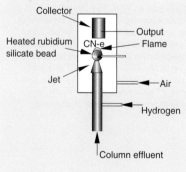	Compounds with a high affinity for electrons enter the detector and capture the electrons produced by the radioactive source, thus reducing the current to the collector. Highly halogenated compounds can be detected at the 50 fg–1 pg level. Has a large internal volume, therefore, some chromatographic resolution may be lost. Linearity of response is not as great as flame ionisation detector (FID), e.g. 10^3. Mainly used for analysis of drugs in body fluids. Has wide application in environmental monitoring, e.g. chlorofluoro-carbons in the atmosphere
Nitrogen phosphorus 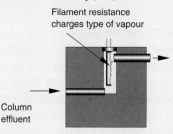	Nitrogen- and phosphorus-containing compounds react with the alkali metal salt in the detector to produce species such as CN^-, various phosphorus anions or electrons, all of which produce an increase in current which generates the signal. Detects phosphorus compounds at the pg level, nitrogen compounds at the low ng level. Highly selective for nitrogen- and phosphorus-containing compounds. Used mainly in the analysis of drugs and their metabolites in tissues and bodily fluids
Thermal conductivity (TCD)	Responds to cooling effect of the analyte passing over the filament. Relatively insensitive to organic compounds in comparison to FID. It is a universal detector which can be used to determine water vapour. It is also nondestructive, so analytes can be collected after detection, if required. Used to determine water in some BP assays, e.g. water in the peptides menotrophin, gonadorelin and salcatonin

(*Continued*)

Table 11.3 *(Continued)*

Detector	Applications
Radiochemical detector 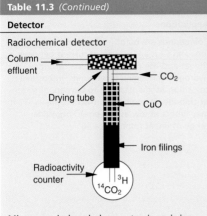	^{14}C and ^{3}H present in the molecule are respectively converted to $^{14}CO_2$ and $^{3}H_2$. Its sensitivity depends on the degree of radioactivity of the analyte. Useful for metabolic labelling studies, making metabolites of drugs easy to detect. The detector tends to work better with packed columns, since it has a large internal space
Microwave-induced plasma atomic emission 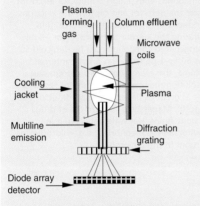	A hot plasma of argon is produced by heating to > 6000°C, which causes all the elements in the compound to produce emission spectra. The individual emission lines are passed through diffraction grating and detected by a diode array detector. Detects individual elements, e.g. chlorine in organochlorine pesticides and metals in organometallics. Sensitive to the pg level for some elements. Most widely used in environmental monitoring but also has useful potential for impurity profiling of drugs and metabolism studies
Fourier transform (FT) infrared (IR) detector 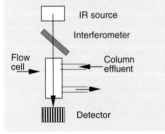	Essentially just an FT-IR instrument coupled to a GC, thus allowing IR spectra of compounds eluting from the GC column to be obtained. More useful for structure elucidation rather than quantitative studies. The detector is sensitive to the 10 ng level. Used as a tool for qualitative identification. There are some examples of quantitative applications, e.g. determination of propandiol in acyclovir cream[5]

Analysis of methyltestosterone in tablets

A calibration solution containing *ca* 0.04% w/v of methyltestosterone and *ca* 0.04% w/v testosterone in ethanol is prepared (Solution 1). A weight of tablet powder containing *ca* 20 mg of methyltestosterone is extracted with 50 ml of ethanol to prepare Solution 2. Solution 3 is prepared by dissolving tablet powder containing *ca* 20 mg of methyltestosterone in *exactly* 50 ml of ethanol containing *exactly* the same concentration of testosterone as Solution 1. In this example, 0.5 μl amounts of the solutions were injected into the GC in the splitless mode.

Fig. 11.21
Chromatograms of solutions 1, 2 and 3 prepared for the analysis of methyltestosterone tablets. RTX-1 column 15 m × 0.25 mm i.d. × 0.25 μm film. Programmed 150°C (1 min), then 10°C/min to 320°C (5 min).

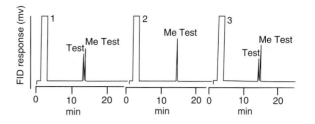

Solution 1 gives a response factor for the calibration solution as follows:

$$\frac{\text{area of methyltestosterone peak in calibration solution}}{\text{area of testosterone peak in calibration solution}}$$

Solution 3 gives a response factor for the sample as follows:

$$\frac{\text{area of methyltestosterone peak in sample solution}}{\text{area of testosterone peak in sample solution}}$$

The amount of methyltestosterone in the tablet powder can be calculated as follows:

$$\text{amount of methyltestosterone} = \frac{\text{response factor for sample}}{\text{response factor for calibration solution}}$$
$$\times \% \text{w/v of}$$

$$\text{methyltestosterone in calibration solution} \times \frac{\text{vol. sample solution}}{100}$$

Data from analysis of methyltestosterone tablets

- Weight of 5 tablets = 0.7496 g
- Stated content of methyltestosterone per tablet = 25 mg
- Weight of tablet powder taken for assay = 0.1713 g
- Solution 1 contains: 0.04% w/v methyltestosterone and 0.043% w/v testosterone
- Solution 3 contains: the methyltestosterone extracted from the powder taken for assay and 0.043% w/v testosterone
- Solution 1: Peak area testosterone = 216 268; Peak area methyltestosterone = 212 992
- Solution 3: Peak area testosterone = 191 146; Peak area methyltestosterone = 269 243.

Calculation example 11.1

$$\text{Response factor for Solution 1} = \frac{212\,992}{216\,268} = 0.9849$$

$$\text{Response factor for Solution 3} = \frac{269\,243}{191\,146} = 1.409$$

(Continued)

Calculation example 11.1 *(Continued)*

Amount of methyltestosterone in the tablet powder determined by analysis =

$$\frac{1.409}{0.9849} \times 0.04 \times \frac{50}{100} = 0.02861\,g = 28.61\,mg$$

Amount of methyltestosterone expected in tablet powder =

$$\frac{\text{weight of powder analysed}}{\text{weight of 5 tablets}} \times \text{stated content of 5 tablets} = \frac{0.1713}{0.7496} \times 5 \times 25$$

$$= 28.57\,mg$$

$$\text{Percentage of stated content} = \frac{28.61}{28.57} \times 100 = 100.1\%$$

A dilution factor may be incorporated into this calculation if the sample is first extracted and then diluted in order to bring it into the working range of the instrument. This approach to quantitation does not address the linearity of the method, but since the variation in the composition of formulations should be within ± 10% of the stated amount, there is some justification for using it. The precision of the method is readily addressed by carrying out repeat preparations of sample and calibration solutions.

Analysis of atropine in eyedrops

Another group which is used to mask polar groups in molecules in order to improve GC peak shape is the trimethylsilyl group. Atropine eyedrops BP are used to dilate the pupil prior to cataract surgery. The 1993 BP method for the analysis of atropine eyedrops BP uses derivatisation with a trimethylsilyl group to mask an alcohol group, as shown in Figure 11.22.

The method involves extraction of atropine and a homatropine internal standard from the aqueous phase, which is rendered alkaline by the addition of ammonia, followed by trimethylsilylation with *N,O*-bistrimethylsilyl acetamide (BSA).

In the calculation using the results of this experiment, it is better to use amount rather than concentration as a standard measure. The reason for this is, after the initial accurate volume, for the addition of the standard and internal standard to the calibration solution (Solution 1) and for the addition of the internal standard to a fixed volume of eyedrops, the volumes need only be measured approximately.

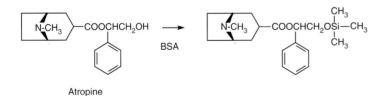

Atropine

Fig. 11.22
Trimethylsilylation of atropine.

Fig. 11.23
Chromatograms of solutions 1, 2 and 3 prepared for the analysis of atropine in eyedrops. RTX-1 column 15 m × 0.25 mm i.d. × 0.25 μm film. Programmed 140°C (1 min), then 10°C/min to 320°C (5 min).

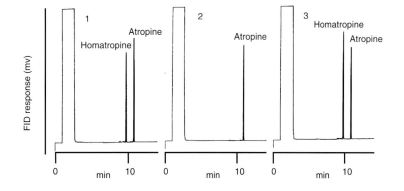

This is the advantage of using an internal standard (Fig. 11.23). The following formula is used:

amount of atropine in the eyedrop sample =

$$\frac{\text{response factor for sample}}{\text{response factor for calibration solution}} \times \text{amount of atropine in calibration solution}$$

Brief description of the assay

Solution 1 is prepared from *exactly* 5 ml of 0.4092% w/v atropine sulphate solution and *exactly* 1 ml of 2.134% w/v homatropine hydrobromide solution. The solution is basified and extracted; the solvent is removed and the residue is treated with 2 ml of BSA and then diluted to 50 ml with ethyl acetate. Solution 3 is prepared from *exactly* 2 ml of eyedrops and *exactly* 1 ml of 2.134% w/v homatropine hydrobromide solution. The solution is basified and extracted; the solvent is removed and the residue is treated with 2 ml of BSA and then diluted to 50 ml with ethyl acetate.

Data from analysis of eyedrop formulation

- Volume of eyedrops analysed = 2.0 ml
- Stated content of eyedrops = 1.0% w/v
- Solution 1: Peak area homatropine TMS = 118 510; Peak area atropine TMS = 146 363
- Solution 3: Peak area homatropine TMS = 145 271; Peak area atropine TMS = 117 964.

Calculation example 11.2

Amount of atropine sulphate in Solution 1 $= 0.4092 \times \dfrac{5}{100} = 0.02046$ g

Response factor for Solution 1 $= \dfrac{146\,363}{118\,510} = 1.2350$

(Continued)

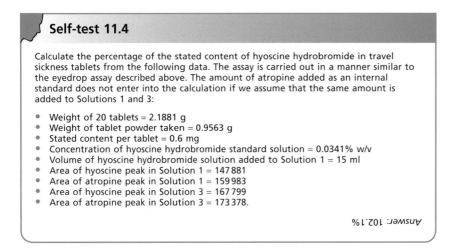

Calculation example 11.2 *(Continued)*

Response factor for Solution 3 $= \dfrac{117\,964}{145\,271} = 0.8120$

Amount of atropine sulphate in Solution 3 $= \dfrac{0.8120}{1.2350} \times 0.02046\text{ g} = 0.01345\text{ g}$

This was the amount originally present in 2 ml of eyedrops; therefore, percentage of w/v of atropine sulphate in eyedrops

$= 0.01345 \times \dfrac{100}{2} = 0.6725\%\text{ w/v}$

The amount determined in the eyedrops is well below the stated amount of 1% w/v, and this is because this sample of eyedrops was *ca* 10 years old and had probably suffered extensive degradation.

Self-test 11.4

Calculate the percentage of the stated content of hyoscine hydrobromide in travel sickness tablets from the following data. The assay is carried out in a manner similar to the eyedrop assay described above. The amount of atropine added as an internal standard does not enter into the calculation if we assume that the same amount is added to Solutions 1 and 3:

- Weight of 20 tablets = 2.1881 g
- Weight of tablet powder taken = 0.9563 g
- Stated content per tablet = 0.6 mg
- Concentration of hyoscine hydrobromide standard solution = 0.0341% w/v
- Volume of hyoscine hydrobromide solution added to Solution 1 = 15 ml
- Area of hyoscine peak in Solution 1 = 147 881
- Area of atropine peak in Solution 1 = 159 983
- Area of hyoscine peak in Solution 3 = 167 799
- Area of atropine peak in Solution 3 = 173 378.

Answer: 102.1%

Quantification of ethanol in a formulation

Gas chromatography provides a useful method for quantifying very volatile materials. In this case, columns are required which strongly retain volatile compounds. Ethanol is used in the preparation of tinctures and in disinfectant solutions. Typically ethanol may be quantified against a related alcohol. In the 1993 BP assay of chloroxylenol solution, ethanol is quantified against a propan-1-ol internal standard. The column used is packed with Porapak Q; Porapak is an example of a porous polymeric stationary phase which retains low-molecular-weight compounds strongly. These types of phases are also effective in separating gases such as CO_2, ammonia and acetylene. As an alternative to a Porapak column, a thick film (e.g. 5 μm film) GC capillary column may be used for this type of analysis.

Determination of manufacturing and degradation residues by GC

Determination of pivalic acid in dipivefrin eyedrops

GC provides a useful technique for estimating volatile degradation products. For example, the pivalic acid release from the hydrolysis of dipivefrin in an eyedrop preparation (Fig. 11.24) used for treating glaucoma may be estimated by GC.[6] Isovaleric acid, which is an isomer of pivalic acid, provides a suitable internal standard. Breakdown products of esters are more likely to occur in aqueous formulations such as eyedrops or injections.

Fig. 11.24
Breakdown of dipivefrin resulting in formation of pivalic acid.

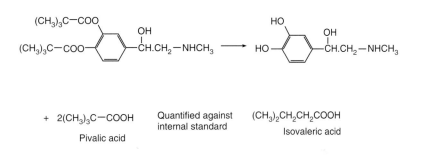

Determination of dimethylaniline in bupivacaine injection (Fig. 11.25)

Dimethylaniline is both a manufacturing impurity in bupivacaine and, since it is formulated in injections, a possible breakdown product, although hydrolysis of amides is much slower than hydrolysis of esters. The BP uses a spectrophotometric method to assay for this impurity, but GC provides a more sensitive and specific method for this determination.

The GC trace obtained from injection of a 10% w/v solution of bupivacaine free base extracted from an injection gave the trace shown in Figure 11.26. It is apparent from comparison with a standard for dimethylaniline that there is $\leq 0.1\%$ of the impurity present, although a number of other peaks due to excipients or impurities can be seen in the GC trace.

Determination of N,N-dimethylaniline in penicillins

Determination of N,N-dimethylaniline in penicillins is carried out by GC. In this case the dimethylaniline is present in the sample since it is used as a counter ion in the purification of the penicillins by recrystallisation. The aniline counter ion

Fig. 11.25
Bupivacaine and its degradation product.

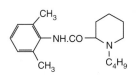

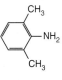

Bupivacaine

Dimethylaniline (manufacturing impurity and hydrolysis product)

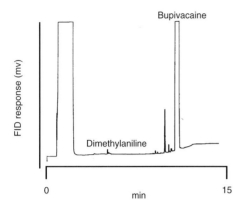

Fig. 11.26

Gas chromatography (GC) analysis of impurity residues in bupivacaine extracted from an injection. RTX-1 column 15 m × 0.25 mm i.d. × 0.25 μm film. Programmed 70°C (3 min), then 20°C/min to 320°C (5 min).

can be easily removed by mild basification and extraction. A pharmacopoeial limit test of 20 ppm is set for dimethylaniline using GC to analyse for the dimethylaniline residue. The penicillin is dissolved in 1 M NaOH, and the solution is extracted with cyclohexane containing naphthalene as an internal standard (Fig. 11.27). Then an aliquot of the cyclohexane layer is injected into the GC. Any peak obtained for N,N-dimethylaniline in the sample is compared with a peak obtained for a standard solution of dimethylaniline processed in the same way. The limit set by the BP for N,N-dimethylaniline in penicillins is 20 ppm.

Self-test 11.5

1.0512 g of ampicillin was dissolved in 5 ml of 1 M NaOH, and the solution was extracted into 1 ml of cyclohexane containing 50 μg/ml of naphthalene. 1 ml of a calibration sample containing approximately 20 μg/ml of N,N-dimethylaniline dissolved in 1 M HCL was mixed with 4 ml of 1 M NaOH and extracted into 1 ml of cyclohexane containing 50 μg/ml of naphthalene. The following data were obtained. Calculate the content of N,N-dimethylaniline in the sample in ppm:

Weight of N,N-dimethylaniline used to prepare calibration stock solution = 50.3 mg
Volume of calibration stock solution = 50 ml
Dilution of calibration stock solution= 5 ml to 250 ml
Peak area for dimethyl aniline obtained from calibration solution = 3521
Peak area obtained for naphthalene IS in calibration stock solution = 23616
Peak area for dimethyl aniline obtained from sample solution = 543
Peak area obtained for naphthalene IS in sample solution = 24773.

Answer: 2.81 ppm

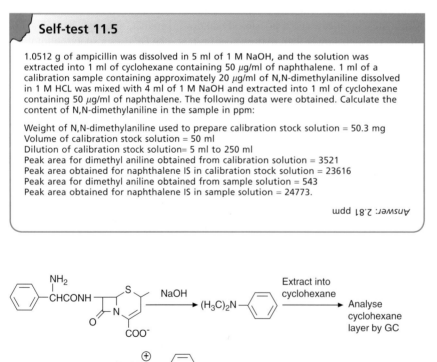

Dimethylaniline salt

Fig. 11.27

Process used to analyse N,N-dimethylaniline residues in penicillins.

Determination of a residual glutaraldehyde in a polymeric film

Sometimes derivatisation can provide a highly specific method of detecting impurities. In this example, the low-molecular-weight impurity glutaraldehyde, which is not stable to direct analysis by GC, is reacted with a high-molecular-weight derivatisating reagent pentafluorobenzyloxime; the reaction is shown in Figure 11.28. This reaction stabilises the analyte and increases its retention time into a region where it can be readily observed without interference from other components extracted from the sample matrix. The derivative is also highly electron capturing. In this example a GC method was found to be superior to an HPLC method using derivatisation with dinitrophenylhydrazine since the residues from the reagent produced less interference in the analysis.

The reaction is also useful for determining process residues such as formaldehyde and acetaldehyde, which occur as reaction residues in some plastic packaging materials.

The converse of this type of reaction has been used to determine hydrazine as a manufacturing impurity in the drug hydralazine by reaction of the hydrazine residue with benzaldehyde to form a volatile derivative for GC analysis.[7]

Fig. 11.28

Application of a selective derivatisation procedure used for the analysis of glutaraldehyde in a polymeric film.

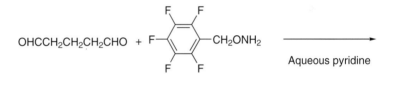

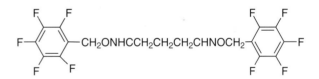

Determination of residual solvents
Typical BP procedures

The current BP methods for determination of solvent residues remaining from the manufacturing process in pharmaceuticals rely on direct injection of the sample dissolved in a suitable solvent (often water) and are based on packed column GC. Some examples are given in Table 11.4.

Table 11.4 Some BP procedures for the analysis of residual solvents

Drug	Residues	Gas chromatography conditions
Ampicillin sodium	Dichloromethane	10% polyethylene glycol 60°C
Ampicillin sodium	Dimethylaniline	3% OV-17 80°C
Colchicine	Ethyl acetate and chloroform	10% polyethylene glycol 75°C
Gentamycin sulphate	Methanol	Porapak Q 120°C
Menotrophin	Water	Chromosorb 102, 114°C, TCD
Warfarin sodium	Propan-2-ol	10% polyethylene glycol 70°C

Determination of residual solvents and volatile impurities by headspace analysis (see Animation 11.6)

A more refined method for determining residual solvents and volatile impurities is based on headspace analysis. The simplest method of sampling is to put the sample into a sealed vial and heat it as shown in Figure 11.29. The sample, either in solution or slurried with a relatively involatile solvent with little potential for interference, e.g. water or dimethylacetamide, is put into a sealed vial fitted with a rubber septum and heated and agitated until equilibrium is achieved. Then a fixed volume of headspace, e.g. 0.25 ml, is withdrawn. The sample is then injected into a GC in the usual way. If capillary column GC is used, a split injection has to be used to facilitate sample injection; a flow of 10 : 1 out of the split vent would ensure that a 0.25 ml sample could be injected in about 1.5 s with the flow through the column being 1 ml/min.

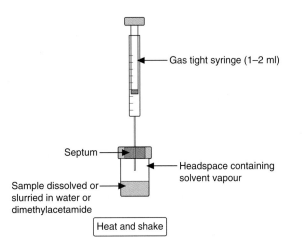

Gas tight syringe (1–2 ml)

Septum

Headspace containing solvent vapour

Sample dissolved or slurried in water or dimethylacetamide

Heat and shake

Fig. 11.29
Manual sampling of the headspace in a sealed vial with gas tight syringe.

Several points are important to note:

(i)   Partition equilibrium must be established by heating for an appropriate length of time and at an appropriate temperature.

(ii) A clean room is required away from all other sources of volatiles such as laboratory solvents; potential interference from rubber septa needs to be checked; reactive contaminants may react with the sample matrix at high temperatures (e.g. dichloromethane is an efficient alkylating reagent and may react with amines).

(iii) If the sample is ground and mixed in preparation for the headspace analysis care has to be taken that no volatiles are lost.

(iv) For best reproducibility the process should be automated, an automated system for direct injection is shown in Figure 11.30, and for quantitative accuracy it might be best to use the method of standard additions (Ch. 6).

(v) N,N-dimethylacetamide or diethylene glycol do not interfere in the analysis since they are much less volatile than the common solvent residues. Water is the ideal solvent since it does not show up at all with FID detection; however, recently it has become less popular, since hot water vapour can damage GC capillary columns.

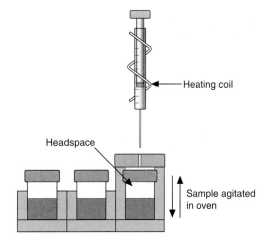

Fig. 11.30
Automated headspace sampling based on direct injection.

The European Pharmacopoeia has standardised on a phase composed of 6% cyanopropyl phenyl: 94% dimethylsiloxane (Fig. 11.31), e.g. DB-1301 or Rtx-1301. The film thickness used is generally 3 μm.

Figure 11.32 shows a chromatographic trace for some standard residual solvents dissolved in dimethyl acetamide, sampled using automated headspace sampling and separated on a Rtx-1303 column.

Self-test 11.6

Which of the following capillary columns would be most suitable for use in the determination of residual solvents by headspace analysis (consult Table 11.1)?

(i)   OV-1 column 12 m × 0.2 mm i.d. × 0.25 μm film
(ii) OV-17 column 15 m × 0.33 mm i.d. × 0.5 μm film
(iii) OV-225 column 30 m × 0.5 mm i.d. × 3 μm film
(iv) OV-1 column 25 m × 0.5 mm i.d. × 1 μm film.

Answer: (iii)

Processes such as automated residual solvent analysis or determination of residual volatile monomers in packaging materials (e.g. ethylene oxide or vinyl chloride) may now be carried out during the manufacturing process. Such real-time monitoring has been aided by the development of fast GC. Since GC

Fig. 11.31
The structure of Rtx-1301, a weakly polar phase.

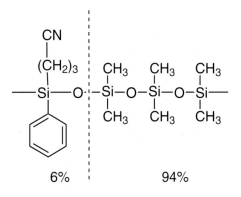

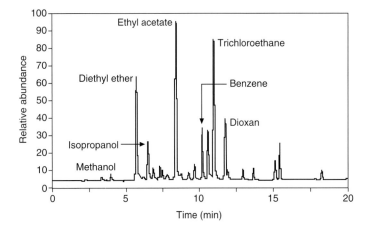

Fig. 11.32
Separation of a mixture of residual solvents on an Rtx 1303 column 30 m × 3 μm film. Sample dissolved in N,N-dimethylacetamide and headspace sampled. Flame ionisation detector.

columns have very high efficiencies, it is possible to reduce analysis times, in some cases to less than a minute, by using short columns with thin stationary-phase coatings in conjunction with rapid temperature programmes. Another advantage of short retention times is that detection limits are improved since the peaks produced are much narrower. In the case of a headspace analysis, improved detection limits mean that it is possible to inject a smaller volume of headspace in order to reduce injection time and make the injection compatible with a fast analysis time.

Purge trap analysis

Another form of headspace analysis uses a purge trapping device to trap volatile impurities. In this technique, a gas, e.g. helium, is bubbled through the sample, which is dissolved in suitable solvent (usually water), and the volatile impurities are thus 'stripped' from the solution and passed in the stream of gas through a polymeric adsorbant, where they become trapped and thus concentrated. The stream of gas is then switched so it passes in the reverse direction through the polymeric trap, which is heated to desorb the trapped volatiles, and the gas stream is then diverted into the GC. This type of procedure is used in environmental analysis to concentrate volatiles which are present at low levels in water.

Solid-phase microextraction (SPME) (see Animation 11.7)

Solid-phase microextraction (SPME) has developed rapidly over the past 10 years and has been applied quite widely in pharmaceutical analysis. It can be used to concentrate trace amounts of organic compounds either in the headspace of a sample or from an aqueous solution. SPME uses a fine fused-silica fibre coated with a polymer such as polydimethylsiloxane. The fibre is enclosed inside a metal needle so that it can pierce through a rubber septum into a vial. The fibre is then pushed out of the end of the metal needle and equilibrated with the sample while the sample is stirred and heated (Fig. 11.33). The fibre is then withdrawn into the needle and the needle is then pierced through the septum of a GC; the fibre is then pushed out of the metal needle again so that analytes can be thermally desorbed onto the GC column. Some GC autosamplers now offer the options of automatic injection from solution, headspace analysis and SPME all on the same instrument.

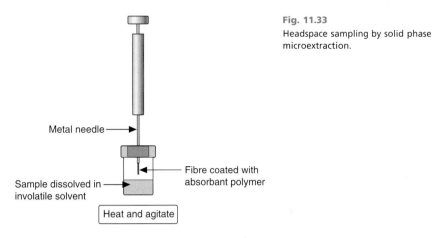

Fig. 11.33
Headspace sampling by solid phase microextraction.

Metal needle

Fibre coated with
absorbant polymer

Sample dissolved in
involatile solvent

Heat and agitate

Self-test 11.7

Suggest an analytical procedure based on gas chromatography for solving the following problems:

(i) Determination of residual solvents in a penicillin
(ii) Determination of the stability, in a formulation, of a drug with a propyl ester group
(iii) Determination of an amphetamine sulphate in tablet form
(iv) Determination of terbutaline in tablet form.

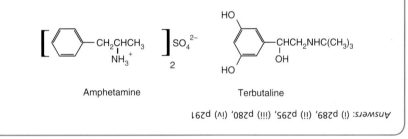

Amphetamine   Terbutaline

Answers: (i) p289, (ii) p295, (iii) p280, (iv) p291

Applications of GC in bioanalysis

In order to determine an optimum dosage regimen for a drug and to determine its mode of metabolism, methods for analysis of the drug and its metabolites in blood, urine and tissues have to be developed. Analysis of drugs in biological fluids and tissues by GC is quite common, although GC-MS (see Ch. 9) has replaced many GC methods which are reliant on less selective types of detectors.

A typical application of GC to the determination of a drug in plasma is in the determination of the anti-epileptic drug valproic acid[8] after solid-phase extraction (see Ch. 15) by GC with flame ionisation detection. In this procedure, caprylic acid, which is isomeric with valproic acid, was used as an internal standard. The limit of detection for the drug was 1 μg/ml of plasma. The trace shown in Figure 11.34 indicates the more extensive interference that occurs in bioanalysis, from background peaks extracted from the biological matrix, compared with the quality control of bulk materials.

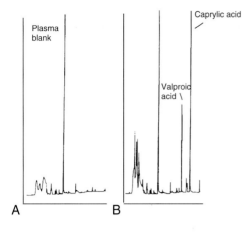

Fig. 11.34

(A) The gas chromatography (GC) trace of an extract of blank plasma obtained from a patient. (B) The GC trace of an extract of plasma obtained from the same patient after treatment with valproic acid (peak 1) to which caprylic acid (peak 2) has been added as an internal standard.

An example of the use of GC with nitrogen-selective detection is in the quantification of bupivacaine in plasma.[9] Bupivacaine contains two nitrogen atoms in its structure, which makes it a good candidate for this type of analysis. The limits of detection which can be achieved with a nitrogen-selective detector for this compound are much better than methods based on flame ionisation detection, which are much less selective.

Additional problems

1. Indicate the order of elution of the following compounds from an OV-1 column:
   1. Testosterone propionate
   2. Nandrolone
   3. Testosterone heptanoate
   4. Testosterone
   5. Methyltestosterone
   6. Nandrolone decanoate.

   Answer: 2, 4, 5, 1, 3, 6

2. The manufacturing residue chloropropandiol was determined in iohexol; 1.0673 g of iohexol were dissolved in 2 ml of water. The solution was extracted four times with 2 ml of methyl acetate, and the extracts were combined and concentrated to 2 ml. A calibration solution was prepared by dissolving 0.5378 g of chloropropandiol in 100 ml of methyl acetate and then diluting 1 ml of this solution to 100 ml with methyl acetate. 2 μl of each solution were injected into the GC. Calculate the amount of chloroprandiol in ppm, in the sample of iohexol from the following data:
Peak area for chloroprandiol in sample = 3276
Peak area for chloroprandiol in standard= 123452

   Answer: 2.67 ppm

3. A limit of 100 ppm methanol is set in ticlopidine. 0.2312 g of ticlopidine is dissolved in 1 ml of diethylene glycol (DEG) in a headspace vial. The calibration solution is prepared by dissolving 0.2023 g of methanol in 25 ml of DEG, then diluting 0.1 ml of this solution to 20 ml with DEG and finally transferring 0.5 ml of this dilution to a headspace vial and adding a further 0.5 ml of DEG. The solutions are then heated at 115°C for 15 minutes and then sampled and analysed by GC. Calculate the methanol content in the sample from the data below:
Peak area of methanol in ticlopidine sample = 1659
Peak area of methanol in calibration standard = 12432

   Answer: 13.35 ppm

References

1. Watson DG. Chemical derivatisation in gas chromatography. In: Baugh P, ed. *Gas Chromatography A Practical Approach*. Oxford: IRL Press; 1995:133-170.
2. Grob K. Injection techniques in capillary GC. *Anal Chem*. 1994;66:1009A-1019A.
3. Dawling S, Moffat AC, Osselton MD, Widdop B, eds. *Clarke's Analysis of Drugs and Poisons*. London: Pharmaceutical Press; 2004:425-499.
4. Brooks CJW, Gilbert MT, Gilbert JD. New derivatives for gas-phase analytical resolution of enantiomeric alcohols and amines. *Anal Chem*. 1973;45:896.
5. Gilbert AS, Moss CJ, Francis PL, Ashton MJ, Ashton DS. Combined gas chromatography infra-red spectroscopy for the determination of propanediol in acyclovir cream. *Chromatographia*. 1996;42:305-308.
6. Hall L. Quantitative-determination of pivalic acid in dipivefrin-containing ophthalmic solutions by gas-chromatography. *J Chromatogr*. 1994;679:397-401.
7. Gyllenhaal O, Grönberg L, Vessman J. Determination of hydrazine in hydralazine by capillary gas-chromatography with nitrogen-selective detection after benzaldehyde derivatization. *J Chromatogr*. 1990; 511:303-315.
8. Krogh M, Johansen K, Tnneson F, Rasmussen KE. *J Chromatogr*. 1995;673:299-305.
9. Leskot LJ, Ericson J. *J Chromatogr*. 1980;182:226-231.

Further reading

Cortes HJ, Winniford B, Luong J, Pursch M. Comprehensive two dimensional gas chromatography review. *J Sep Sci*. 2009;32:883-904.

Cruz-Hernandez C, Destaillats F. Recent advances in fast gas-chromatography: application to the separation of fatty acid methyl esters. *J Liq Chromatogr Relat Technol*. 2009;32:1672-1688.

Grant DW. *Capillary Gas Chromatography*. Chichester: Wiley Interscience; 1996.

Ioffe BV, Vitenberg AG, Manatov IA. *Headspace Analysis and Related Methods in Gas Chromatography*. Chichester: Wiley Interscience; 1984.

Li YT, Whitaker J, McCarty C. New advances in large-volume injection gas chromatography-mass spectrometry. *J Liq Chromatogr Relat Technol*. 2009;32:1644-1671.

McNair HM, Miller JM. *Basic Gas Chromatography*. Chichester: Wiley Interscience; 1997.

www.separationsnow.com

This site is the separations equivalent of the spectroscopy site. Less comprehensive with regard to separation science but under development.

www.agilent.com

Agilent are one of the premier manufacturers of GC systems. The site contains many applications of gas chromatography in pharmaceutical quality control.

www.restek.com

Website of one of the premier manufacturers of gas chromatography columns.

www.chromatographyonline.com

The website of LCGC magazine has many practical tips on chromatography and the latest advances in chromatographic techniques.

High-performance liquid chromatography

12

KEYPOINTS

Principles

A liquid mobile phase is pumped under pressure through a stainless steel column containing particles of stationary phase with a diameter of 3–10 μm (1.7 μm in ultra-high-performance liquid chromatography (UPLC)). The analyte is loaded onto the head of the column via a loop valve, and separation of a mixture occurs according to the relative lengths of time spent by its components in the stationary phase. It should be noted that all components in a mixture spend more or less the same time in the mobile phase in order to exit the column. Monitoring of the column effluent can be carried out with a variety of detectors.

Applications

- The combination of high-performance liquid chromatography (HPLC) with monitoring by UV/visible detection provides an accurate, precise and robust method for quantitative analysis of pharmaceutical products and is the industry standard method for this purpose.
- Monitoring of the stability of pure drug substances and of drugs in formulations, with quantitation of any degradation products.
- Measurement of drugs and their metabolites in biological fluids.
- Determination of partition coefficients and pKa values of drugs and of drug protein binding.

Strengths

- Easily controlled and precise sample introduction ensures quantitative precision.
- HPLC is the chromatographic technique which has seen the most intensive development in recent years, leading to improved columns, detectors and software control.
- The variety of columns and detectors means that the selectivity of the method can be readily adjusted.
- Compared to gas chromatography (GC) there is less risk of sample degradation because heating is not required in the chromatographic process.
- It is readily automated.
- With the advent of UPLC methods can be very rapid.

Limitations

- There is still a requirement for reliable and inexpensive detectors which can monitor compounds that lack a chromophore.
- Drugs have to be extracted from their formulations prior to analysis.
- Large amounts of organic solvent waste are generated, which are expensive to dispose of.

Introduction

High-performance liquid chromatography (HPLC) is the technique most commonly used for the quantitation of drugs in formulations (Fig. 12.1) (see Animation 12.1). Pharmacopoeial assays still rely quite heavily on direct UV spectroscopy but, in industry, detection by UV spectrophotometry is usually combined with a preliminary separation by HPLC. The theoretical background of HPLC has been dealt with in Chapter 10. There are many comprehensive books on this technique.[1–5]

Instrumentation (see Animation 12.2 and Animation 12.3)

A standard instrumental system for isocratic elution consists of:

(i)   a solvent reservoir

(ii)   a pump capable of pumping solvent up to a pressure of 4000 psi and at flows of up to 10 ml/min

(iii) a loop injector, which may be fitted with a fixed-volume loop of between 1 and 200 μl (20 μl is often used as standard)

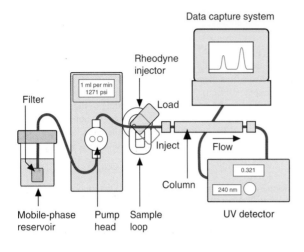

Data capture system

Rheodyne injector

Filter

1 ml per min
1271 psi

Load

Inject

Flow

Column

240 nm

0.321

Mobile-phase
reservoir

Pump
head

Sample
loop

UV detector

Fig. 12.1
Typical high-performance liquid chromatography (HPLC) system set to a flow rate of 1 ml/min producing a backpressure of 1271 psi and monitoring the column eluent at 240 nm.

(iv)　a column, which is usually a stainless steel tube packed, usually, with octadecylsilane-coated (ODS-coated) silica gel with an average particle diameter (3, 5 or 10 μm)

(v)　a detector, which is usually a UV/visible detector, although for specialist applications a wide range of detectors is available

(vi)　a data capture system, which may be a computing integrator or a PC with software suitable for processing chromatographic data

(vii)　the column is connected to the injector and detector with tubing of narrow internal diameter, *ca* 0.2 mm, in order to minimise 'dead volume', i.e. empty space in the system where chromatography is not occurring and band broadening can occur by longitudinal diffusion

(viii)　more advanced instruments may have automatic sample injection and a column oven and are capable of mixing two or more solvents in varying proportions with time to produce a mobile-phase gradient.

Stationary and mobile phases

There are two principal mechanisms which produce retardation of a compound passing through a column. These are illustrated in Figure 12.2 for silica gel, which is a straight-phase packing, where the mechanism of retardation is by adsorption of the polar groups of a molecule onto the polar groups of the stationary phase and for an ODS-coated silica gel, which is a reverse-phase packing, where the mechanism of retardation is due to partitioning of the molecule into the stationary phase according to its lipophilicity.

Silica gel and ODS silica gel are two of the most commonly used packings for straight- and reverse-phase chromatography applications, respectively, but there is a variety of straight- and reverse-phase packings available, most of which are based on chemical modification of the silica gel surface, although in recent years stationary phases which are based on organic polymers have become available. The extent to which a compound is retained will depend primarily upon its polarity, in the case of silica gel, and primarily upon its lipophilicity in the case of a reverse-phase packing such as ODS silica gel. Most drug molecules have both lipophilic and polar groups. The other factor to consider with regard to the degree of retention of a particular compound, apart from the stationary phase, is the nature of the mobile phase. The more polar a mobile phase, the more

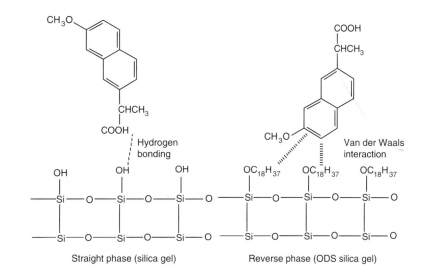

Fig. 12.2
Interaction of naproxen with the surfaces of silica gel and octadecylsilyl (ODS) silica gel high-performance liquid chromatography (HPLC) packings.

quickly it will elute a compound from a silica gel column, and the more lipophilic a mobile phase, the more quickly it will elute a compound from a reverse-phase column. Figure 12.3 shows the effect of increasing the % of organic solvent on the elution of a series of alkyl benzenes. In methanol/water mixture Dolan's rule of 3 applies where, in reverse-phase chromatography, a 10% decrease in methanol content produces a 3 times increase in capacity factor for an analyte. Taking the t_o value for both columns as 1.1 min then the capacity factors for propylbenzene can be calculated as follows:

In 80% methanol

$$K = \frac{5.6 - 1.1}{1.1} = 4.6$$

In 70% methanol

$$K = \frac{15.7 - 1.1}{1.1} = 13.3$$

thus supporting the rule of 3.

Self-test 12.1

Prednisolone (see Fig. 12.4 for the structure) is to be eluted from an ODS column. List the following solvent systems in order of decreasing rate at which they will elute prednisolone (i.e. in order of decreasing strength):

1. a. (i) methanol/water (20:80); (ii) methanol/water (80:20); (iii) methanol/water (50:50).
    b. (i) acetonitrile/water (50:50); (ii) methanol/water (50:50); (iii) acetonitrile/water/THF (50:40:10).

Prednisolone is to be eluted from a silica gel column.
List the following systems in order of decreasing rate at which they will elute prednisolone:

2. (i) hexane/isopropanol (90:10); (ii) hexane/dichloromethane (90:10); (iii) dichloromethane/methanol (90:10); (iv) dichloromethane/isopropanol (90:10); (v) dichloromethane/methanol (80:20).

Answers: 1. a. (ii), (iii), (i); b. (iii), (i), (ii); 2. (v), (iii), (iv), (i), (ii)

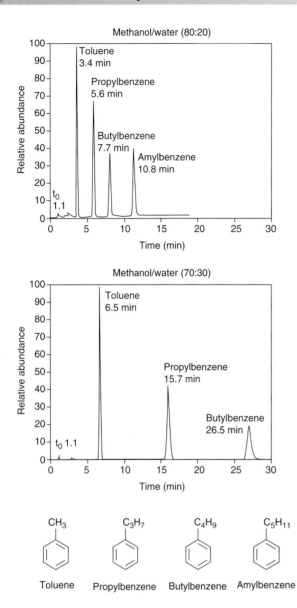

Fig. 12.3
Retention of a series of related compounds on a reversed phase high-performance liquid chromatography (HPLC) column (octadecylsilyl (ODS) 4.6 × 150 mm flow rate 1 ml/min) in methanol/water (80:20 v/v) and methanol/water (80:20). (see Animation 12.4, Animation 12.5 and Animation 12.6)

Structural factors which govern rate of elution of compounds from HPLC columns

Elution of neutral compounds

For a neutral compound it is the balance between its polarity and lipophilicity which will determine the time it takes for it to elute from an HPLC column; the pH of the mobile phase does not play a part. In the case of a reverse-phase column, the more lipophilic a compound is the more it will be retained. For a polar column such as a silica gel column, the more polar a compound is the more it will be retained. Polarity can often be related to the number and hydrogen-bonding strength of the hydroxyl groups present in the molecule; this is illustrated as follows for a series of corticosteroids shown in Figure 12.4. When these compounds are eluted from a reverse-phase column using a mobile phase containing

Fig. 12.4
The structures of some corticosteroids listed in order of their elution from an octadecylsilyl (ODS) column eluted with a methanol/water (75:25) mobile phase and below the chromatogram produced by the mixture.

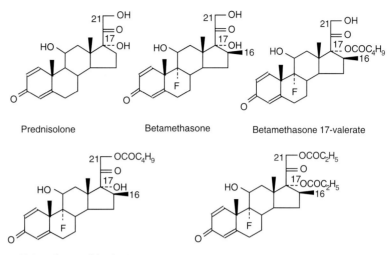

Fig. 12.4
The structures of some corticosteroids listed in order of their elution from an octadecylsilyl (ODS) column eluted with a methanol/water (75:25) mobile phase and below the chromatogram produced by the mixture.

methanol/water (75:25), the expected order of elution would be prednisolone, betamethasone, betamethasone 17-valerate, betamethasone 21-valerate and betamethasone dipropionate. Prednisolone should elute shortly before betamethasone since it lacks a lipophilic methyl group at position 16 (the fluorine group in betamethasone also contributes to its lipophilicity); the valerates both have large lipophilic ester groups masking one of their hydroxyl groups. The 21-hydroxyl group hydrogen bonds more strongly to the mobile phase, since it is an unhindered primary alcohol. Thus its conversion to an ester has a greater effect on the retention time of the molecule than esterification of the 17-hydroxyl group, which is a tertiary alcohol and is hindered with respect to hydrogen bonding to the mobile phase. Finally, the dipropionate of betamethasone has two lipophilic ester groups masking two hydroxyl groups, and this would mean that it would be most strongly retained by a lipophilic stationary phase. Figure 12.5 shows the chromatogram

Fig. 12.5
Prednisolone and betamethasone and their esters eluted from an octadecylsilyl (ODS) column (25 cm × 4.6 mm) with methanol/water (75:25) as mobile phase, UV detection at 240 nm.

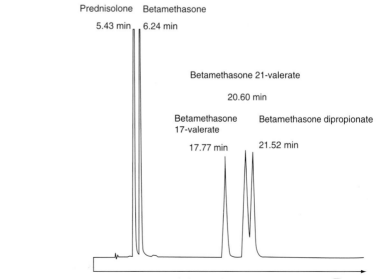

obtained from the mixture of corticosteroids using an ODS column with methanol/ water (75:25) as the mobile phase, indicating that the order of elution fits prediction. The lipophilicity of the steroids reflects their pharmaceutical uses since the more lipophilic esters are used in creams and ointments for enhanced penetration through the lipophilic layers of the skin. The order of elution of these steroids would be more or less reversed on a polar silica gel column, although chromatographic behaviour is usually more predictable on reverse-phase columns. Considering the chromatogram shown in Figure 12.5 in more detail, the resolution between the betamethasone 21-valerate and the betamethasone dipropionate is incomplete. Increasing the water content of the mobile phase would result in longer retention times for these two components and better separation; however, increasing the water content would also give very long retention times. In the case of a formulation containing both the 21-valerate and 17,21-dipropionate, another type of column might be chosen to effect separation of these two components within a reasonable length of time, e.g. a silica gel column. If the betamethasone dipropionate were absent from this mixture, a different separation strategy could be adopted to bring the valerate esters closer to betamethasone and prednisolone. It would not be possible to add more methanol to the mobile phase without losing resolution between betamethasone and prednisolone, but, after these two compounds had eluted, if an HPLC system with a binary or ternary gradient system were used, the instrument could be programmed to gradually increase the methanol content in the mobile phase to expedite the elution of the later-running valerates (see Animation 12.7). For example, a suitable solvent programme might be as follows: methanol/water (75:25) for 7 min, then ramping the solvent composition to methanol/water (85:15) up to 17 min. This type of programme would greatly reduce the retention times of the valerates.

Self-test 12.2

Predict the order of elution, from first to last, of the following steroids from an ODS column with methanol/water (70:30) as the mobile phase.

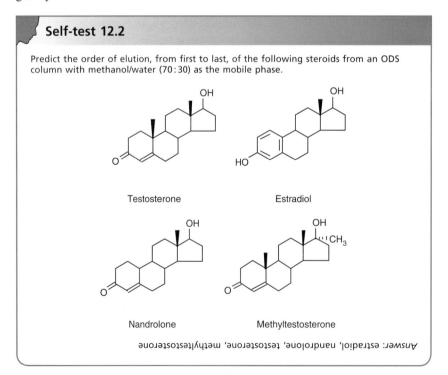

Testosterone

Estradiol

Nandrolone

Methyltestosterone

Answer: estradiol, nandrolone, testosterone, methyltestosterone

Control of elution rate of ionisable compounds by adjustment of pH of mobile phase

This area is not often considered in any detail in books on HPLC; however, pharmacists generally have a good grasp of the concept of pKa, and it is worth devoting some space to its effects in relation to HPLC. An additional factor which can be used to control the solvent strength of the mobile phase is pH; pH control is employed mainly in reverse-phase chromatography. However, mobile-phase conditions may be selected in straight-phase chromatography where the ionisation of the analytes is suppressed, and basic compounds are run in a basic mobile phase and acidic compounds are run with an acidic mobile phase. Control of the rate of elution via the pH of the mobile phase is, of course, only applicable to compounds in which the degree of ionisation is dependent on pH, but this covers a majority of commonly used drugs. The pH of the mobile phase can only be set within the range of *ca* 2–8.5 pH units because of the tendency for extremes of pH to dissolve silica gel and break the bonds between silane-coating agents and the silica gel support. This pH range is gradually being extended with the advent of stabler coatings. The effects of pH on retention time, surprisingly, are as yet not fully understood. The following examples give an approximation of the effect of the pH of the mobile phase on the retention time of drugs on a reverse-phase HPLC column, which provides a starting point for considering the effect of pH on retention time. In fact many drugs are still retained by lipophilic stationary phases to some degree even when they are fully ionised; in this case the drug is probably partitioning into the reverse phase as a lipophilic ion pair. The greatest effects of alteration of pH in the mobile phase are observed within 1 pH unit either side of the pKa value of the drug, i.e. where the partition coefficient of the partially ionised drug varies between 90% and 10% of the partition coefficient of the un-ionised drug (see Ch. 2, p. 31).

The same type of calculation as shown in Calculation example 12.1 can be carried out for basic drugs. Figure 12.6 shows the structures of some local anaesthetic drugs with their pKa values.

Figure 12.7 shows the effect of the pH of the mobile phase on the four local anaesthetics shown in Figure 12.6. The largest effects of pH are on bupivacaine

Fig. 12.6

The structures of some local anaesthetic bases.

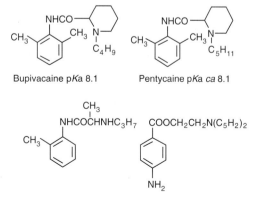

Bupivacaine pKa 8.1

Pentycaine pKa ca 8.1

Prilocaine pKa 7.9

Procaine pKa 9.0

Calculation example 12.1

The effect of pH on the HPLC retention time of an ionisable acidic drug.

Ibuprofen, an acidic drug, which has a pKa of 4.4, is analysed by chromatography on ODS silica gel with a mobile phase consisting of acetonitrile/0.1 M acetate buffer pH 4.2 (40:60).

The t_o for the column at a mobile-phase flow rate of 1 ml/min is 2.3 min. The retention time of ibuprofen at pH 4.2 is 23.32. If K'app is the apparent capacity factor of the partially ionised drug, then:

$$K'\text{app at pH } 4.2 = 23.32 - 2.3/2.3 = 9.14$$

Using the expression introduced in Chapter 2 for the effect of pH on partition coefficient of an acid, it is possible to predict approximately the effect of pH on retention time, since the effect of pH on partition coefficient will reflect its effects on capacity factor and in theory:

$$K'\text{app} = K'/1 + 10^{\text{pH}-\text{p}Ka}$$

Using the observed K' app at pH 4.2: $9.14 = K'/1 + 10^{4.2-4.4} = K'/1.63$

$$K' = 9.14 \times 1.63 = 14.90$$

If ibuprofen is analysed using the same ODS column with the mobile phase now composed of acetonitrile/0.1 M acetate buffer at pH 5.2 (40:60), the partition coefficient will now be lowered as follows:

$$K'\text{app at pH } 5.2 = K'/1 + 10^{5.2-4.4} = 14.9/7.3$$

$$K'\text{app at pH } 5.2 = 2.04$$

$$\text{Retention time} = t_o + t_o \times K'\text{app} = 2.3 + 2.3 \times 2.04 = 7.0 \text{ min}$$

Experimentally, the retention time of ibuprofen was found in fact to be 12.23 min. This reflects the fact that the pKa of the drug may not be exactly as given in the literature under the conditions used for chromatography and the fact that the low dielectric constant of the mobile phase in comparison with water suppresses ionisation so that the drug is less ionised than predicted. However, the calculation gives a reasonable approximation of the behaviour of ibuprofen.

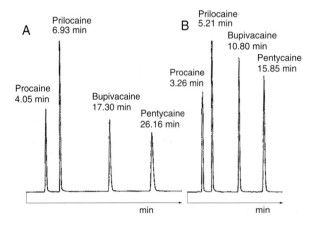

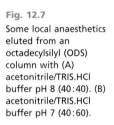

Fig. 12.7
Some local anaesthetics eluted from an octadecylsilyl (ODS) column with (A) acetonitrile/TRIS.HCl buffer pH 8 (40:40). (B) acetonitrile/TRIS.HCl buffer pH 7 (40:60).

Calculation example 12.2

The effect of pH on the HPLC retention time of an ionisable basic drug. Bupivacaine, which has a pKa of 8.1, is analysed by chromatography on ODS silica gel with a mobile phase consisting of acetonitrile/TRIS buffer pH 8.4 (40:60) at a flow rate of 1 ml/min. The t_o for the column at a mobile-phase flow rate of 1 ml/min is 2.3 min. The retention time of bupivacaine at pH 8.4 is 17.32. If $K'app$ is the apparent capacity factor of the partially ionised drug, then for a base:

$$K'\mathrm{app} = K'/1 + 10^{\mathrm{p}Ka - \mathrm{pH}}$$

The $K'app$ at pH $8.4 = 17.82 - 2.3/2.3 = 6.75$

$$6.75 = K'/1 + 10^{8.1 - 8.4} = K'/1.5$$

$$K' = 6.75 \times 1.5 = 10.13$$

If the drug were analysed using acetonitrile/TRIS buffer pH 7.4 (40:60) at a flow rate of 1 ml/min using the same column, the retention time can be estimated as follows:

$$K'\mathrm{app} \text{ at pH } 7.4 = K'/1 + 10^{8.1 - 7.4} = 10.13/6.01$$

$$K'\mathrm{app} \text{ at pH } 7.4 = 1.69$$

$$\text{Retention at pH 7.4 time} = t_o + t_o \times K'\mathrm{app} + 2.3 + 1.69 \times 2.3 = 6.18 \text{ min}$$

Experimentally, the retention time was found to be 10.80 min. The deviation from the theoretical value was probably due to the factors discussed earlier for ibuprofen.

and pentycaine, which are very close in structure; the pH adjustment made in the example is within ± 1 pH unit of their pKa values. The least effect is on procaine, which has a higher pKa (9.0) than the other drugs and is thus already 80% ionised at pH 8.4; for this reason, the lowering of the pH has a less marked effect on its retention time. The effect of pH on prilocaine might initially appear somewhat less than expected, but this is because it is closer to t_o than the other drugs; the decrease in its retention time observed at the lower pH is, in fact, in line with the decreases observed for bupivacaine and pentycaine. In chromatogram B, the procaine peak has lost some of its integrity due to its proximity to the solvent front; this results in poor trapping of the analyte at the head of the column. The effect of the organic content of the mobile phase on the pKa of analytes is given some additional consideration in Box 12.1.

Self-test 12.3

The retention time of the acidic drug naproxen on an ODS column with a t_o of 2.3 min in a mixture containing acetonitrile/0.05 M acetate buffer pH 5.2 (40:60) is 9.07 min. The pKa of naproxen is 4.2; what would be the effect of reducing the pH of the mobile phase to 4.2?

Answer: In theory, the retention time would be 39.47 min (in practice it was found to be 19.78 min. The pKa of this drug is probably lower than the literature value under the mobile-phase conditions used or it is less ionised at pH 5.2 than expected in the mobile phase, which has a lower dielectric constant than water)

Figure 12.8 shows the effect of pH on the retention of a series of acidic non-steroidal anti-inflammatory drugs shown in Figure 12.9.

Box 12.1 Additional consideration of mobile-phase pH

A major factor that is often ignored in preparing mobile phases is the effect of the addition of organic solvent to the buffer. The effect of addition of acetonitrile on the pifa value of acetic acid has been calculated to be as follows:[6]

Percentage of w/w acetonitrile:	0	10	30	40	50
pKa value of acetic acid:		4.75	5.0	5.6	6.0	6.4

The addition of organic solvent thus suppresses the ionisation of the acid, reducing the $[H^+]$ in solution, and the overall effect is an increase in pH. The same effect can be observed for other buffers such as phosphate and citrate, and with 50% organic solvent the effective pH of the mobile phase may be 1–1.5 units higher than the measured pH of the buffer before mixing.

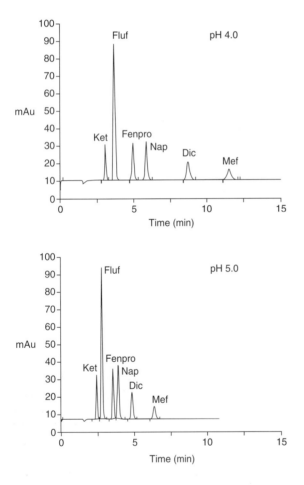

Fig. 12.8
Effect of pH on the retention of non-steroidal anti-inflammatory drugs (ketoprofen, flufenamic acid, fenoprofen, naproxen, diclofenac, mefenamic acid). Reversed phase column with methanol/0.05 M acetate buffer pH 5 (70:30) as the mobile phase 4 (60:40) and (B) acetonitrile/TRIS.HCl buffer pH 7.4 (60:40).

Fig. 12.9
Structures of
fenoprofen,
naproxen,
diclofenac and
mefenamic acid.

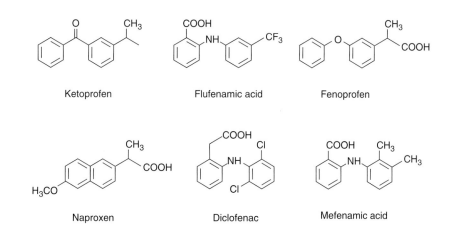

Ketoprofen

Flufenamic acid

Fenoprofen

Naproxen

Diclofenac

Mefenamic acid

More advanced consideration of solvent selectivity in reverse-phase chromatography

The simplest selectivity factor that can be varied in reverse-phase chromatography is solvent composition. Lowering the amount of organic solvent in the mobile phase during reverse-phase chromatography increases the retention time. Dolan's rule of 3 states that a 10% decrease in the organic phase produces a threefold increase in capacity factor, this only really applies to methanol in the case of acetonitrile the increase in capacity factor is approximately 2 for a 10% reduction in organic component. The three common solvents used in reverse-phase chromatography are methanol, acetonitrile and tetrahydrofuran. Another approximate rule is that 40% methanol = 33% acetonitrile = 23% tetrahydrofuran. Apart from eluting power these three solvents also differ in the way that they interact with analytes. Selectivity is important in the impurity profiling of drug substances. Impurities closely related to the drug may elute with very similar retention times. The selection of an optimal solvent system is thus important, and in such cases mixtures of three or four solvents may be used. Figure 12.10 shows the effect of using mixtures of three solvents on the separation of hydrocortisone and the closely related steroid cortisone (Fig. 12.11). The cortisone is present in the mixture at 5% of the concentration of hydrocortisone. In chromatogram A, separation was obtained between the two peaks with acetonitrile/water (30 : 70). In chromatogram B, a mixture of acetonitrile/methanol/water (15 : 15 : 70) does not produce a separation, even though the introduction of methanol produces a longer retention time. In chromatogram C, a mixture of acetonitrile/THF/water (15 : 15 : 70) causes a reversal in the elution order of hydrocortisone and cortisone. The elution of the smaller, potential impurity, peak for cortisone earlier than the hydrocortisone is more desirable, since even slight tailing of the large peak for the major component can cause closely eluting later-running peaks to be obscured. Such a hit and miss approach for achieving an optimal solvent system for separating out minor impurities could be time consuming. A less hit and miss approach uses log K' plots to predict retention times. Table 12.1 shows the data obtained

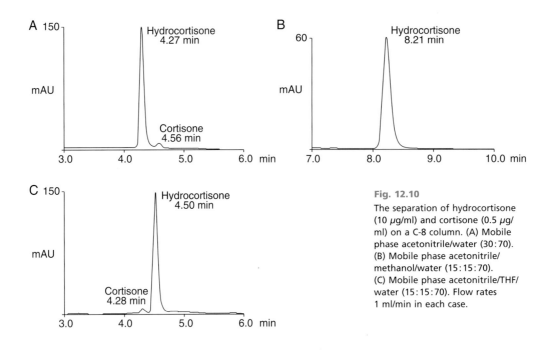

Fig. 12.10

The separation of hydrocortisone (10 µg/ml) and cortisone (0.5 µg/ml) on a C-8 column. (A) Mobile phase acetonitrile/water (30:70). (B) Mobile phase acetonitrile/methanol/water (15:15:70). (C) Mobile phase acetonitrile/THF/water (15:15:70). Flow rates 1 ml/min in each case.

Table 12.1 Data used plot log K' against % MeOH (t_0 for column 1.8 min)

Compound	tr 60% MeOH min	K' 60% MeOH	Log K' 60% MeOH	tr 50% MeOH min	K' 50% MeOH	Log K' 50% MeOH
Cortisone	4.01	1.22	0.09	8.58	3.78	0.58
Hydrocortisone	5.03	1.77	0.25	11.01	5.11	0.71
Ketoprofen	7.95	3.44	0.53	21.49	10.9	1.04
Sulindac	8.28	3.61	0.56	27.57	14.3	1.16

for the analysis of two steroidal and two non-steroidal anti-inflammatory (Fig. 12.12) drugs on a reverse-phase column in mobile phase consisting of methanol and 0.1% v/v aqueous formic acid. The capacity factors for the four drugs can be calculated, and from just two runs log K' plots can be constructed (Fig. 12.13) based on the assumption that plots of log K' against percentage of organic solvent is linear where simple reverse-phase partitioning is occurring.

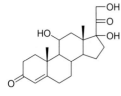

Hydrocortisone

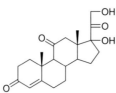

Cortisone

Fig. 12.11

Hydrocortisone and cortisone.

Fig. 12.12
Ketoprofen and sulindac.

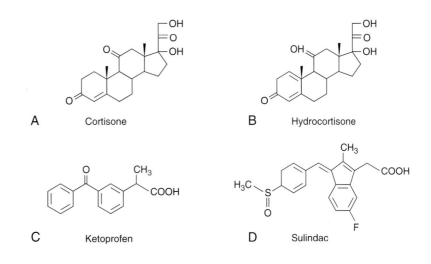

A   Cortisone   B   Hydrocortisone

C   Ketoprofen   D   Sulindac

As can be seen in Figure 12.13, according to the log K′ plots there is an opportunity to produce a method with a short run time since the plots for sulindac and ketoprofen cross over when the percentage of methanol is high. Practical application of this information produced the chromatogram shown in Figure 12.14 where fast separation has been produced with sulindac eluting earlier than ketoprofen.

Software packages such as Drylab® can provide an automated approach to prediction of retention times based on log K′ plots and also model the effects of stationary phase particle size, column length and column diameter changes. A popular method for modelling retention times is based on a 2 gradient run. Figure 12.15 shows acebutolol and its impurities which are listed in the EP. Figure 12.16 shows the separation of acebutolol and its impurities using two different solvent gradient methods.

From the retention times obtained in the runs shown in Figure 12.16, Drylab® was asked to predict the mobile-phase conditions required for a rapid separation based on a 30 × 2.1 mm column. Figure 12.17 shows the rapid separation of acebutolol from its impurities spiked at the 0.1% w/w reporting level.

Fig. 12.13
Log K′ plots based on the data shown in Table 12.1.

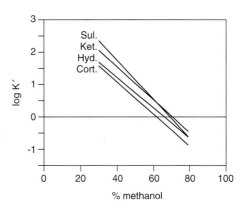

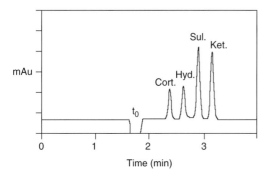

Fig. 12.14
Separation of cortisone, hydrocortisone, ketoprofen and sulindac in 0.1% formic acid/ methanol (25:75) flow rate 1 ml/min on an ACE C18 5 μm column 150 × 4.6 mm (t_0 = 1.8 min.) with UV detection at 220 nm.

Effect of temperature on HPLC

Temperature can also be used to change retention behaviour since capacity factor decreases with an increase in temperature according to the van't Hoff equation. In addition mass transfer effects are reduced at higher temperatures, and thus peak efficiency is better. Returning to the model mixture of cortisone, hydrocortisone, sulindac and ketoprofen, Figure 12.18 shows that increasing temperature both reduces retention times and changes selectivity. Drylab® can be used to model the effects of temperature as well.

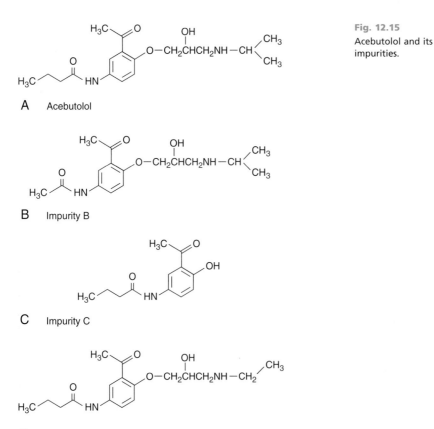

Fig. 12.15
Acebutolol and its impurities.

Fig. 12.16
Two gradient run for acebutolol (Ace) and its impurities (B, I and C). Gradient: 95% tris buffer pH 7.0:5% acetonitrile to 100% acetonitrile in 20 and 60 minutes on an ACE C18 column 4.6 × 150 mm × 5 μm particle size.

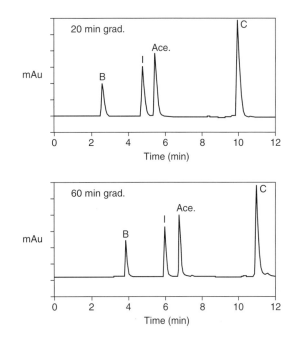

Summary of stationary phases used in HPLC

The intention of this book is to focus mainly on applications of techniques to pharmaceutical analysis. Detailed discussions of stationary phases and detectors can be found elsewhere.[1,2,4,5] Table 12.2 summarises some of the stationary phases which are used in HPLC. Currently, ODS silica gel or related phases such as octyl silica gel are used for > 80% of all pharmaceutical analyses, as judged from a comprehensive survey of the literature;[3] other phases are only used where special selectivity is required, such as for very water-soluble compounds or for bioanalytical separations which may be difficult because the sample matrix produces many interfering peaks. In recent years polymeric phases have become available for certain specialist applications; the surface chemistries of these phases are similar to those of the silica-gel-based phases. Advantages of the polymeric phases are stability to extremes of pH and the lack of secondary

Fig. 12.17
Separation of acebutolol (1 mg/ml) from its manufacturing impurities at a concentration of 0.001 mg/ml using 87.5% tris buffer:12.5% acetonitrile at 1 ml/min on an ACE C18 column 2.1 mm × 30 mm × 5 μm particle size.

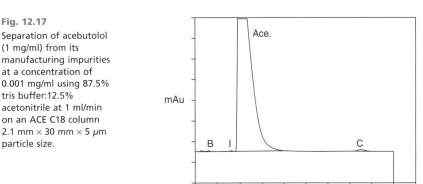

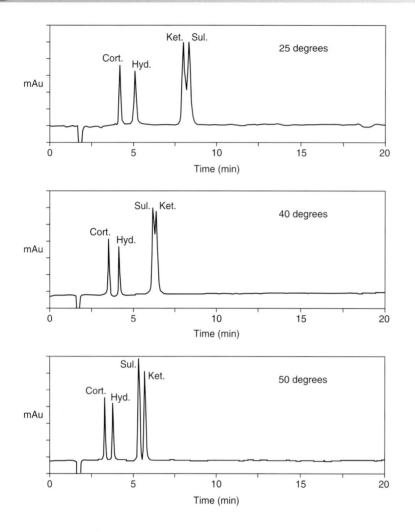

Fig. 12.18
Retention of cortisone, hydrocortisone, sulindac and ketoprofen eluted with 0.1% formic acid: methanol (40:60) at 1 ml/min on an ACE C18 column 4.6 × 150 mm × 5 μm particle size at different temperatures.

interactions of analytes with uncapped silanol groups. Disadvantages include expense and a tendency to swell when in contact with highly lipophilic mobile phases, which can destroy them. Such phases are best used with predominantly aqueous-based mobile phases. In the past 10 years the use of hydrophilic interaction chromatography (HILIC) has increased, and in the case of very polar molecules it provides an alternative to ion pair chromatography. However, there are still some doubts whether or not it is sufficiently robust for routine chromatographic methods.

A more advanced consideration of reverse-phase stationary phases

All reverse-phase chromatography columns are not equivalent. There are big differences between stationary phases obtained from different manufacturers. Recently, definitive work has been carried out on the classification of reverse-phase stationary phases.[8] Six variables that affected the performance of reverse-phase stationary phases were assessed:

Table 12.2 Some commonly used high-performance liquid chromatography (HPLC) stationary phases

Stationary phase	Applications/comments
Octadecylsilyl (ODS) silica gel	The most commonly used phase, applicable to most problems in analysis of pharmaceutical formulations. Early phases gave problems with strongly basic compounds because of low purity silica gels and incomplete endcapping of silanol (Si-OH) groups. Amines adsorb strongly onto free silanol groups not covered by the stationary phase. Fully endcapped phases and phases with low metal content are now available, which enable the analysis of strongly basic compounds that formerly tended to produce tailing peaks. ODS silica gel can even be applied to the analysis of peptides, where wide-pore packings are used to improve access of these bulky molecules to the internal surface of the packings
Octyl silane and butyl silane silica gels	Useful alternatives to ODS phases. The shorter hydrocarbon chains do not tend to lead to shorter retention times of analytes since the carbon loading on the surface of the silica gel may be higher for these phases and retention time is also dependent on how much of the stationary phase is accessible to partitioning by the analyte[7]
Phenyl silane silica gel	Useful for slightly more selective analyses of compounds containing large numbers of aromatic rings, e.g. propranolol and naproxen, where π-π interactions can occur with the phenyl groups on the stationary phase if the analyte is deficient π electrons, e.g. nitro compounds. These interactions are, however, very subtle
Silica gel	Often used in the past for problematical compounds but, with gradual improvement of reverse phases, increasingly less used. Useful for chromatography of very lipophilic compounds such as in the separation of different classes of lipids and in the analysis of surfactants, which tend to form micelles under the conditions used for reverse-phase chromatography
Aminopropyl silica gel	A moderately polar phase often used for the analysis of sugars and surfactants. In the case of sugars the chromatographic interactions are due to hydrophilic interactions (see below)
Cyanopropyl silica gel	A moderately polar phase applicable to the analysis of surfactants. Some of its selectivity is due to dipole–dipole interactions
Strong cation exchanger (SCX)	Usually based on ion pairing of the analyte with sulfonic acid groups on the surface of the stationary phase. Useful for analysis of very polar compounds such as aminoglycosides and other charged sugar molecules and polar bases such as catecholamines
Strong anion exchanger (SAX)	Usually based on ion pairing of the analyte with quaternary ammonium groups on the surface of the stationary phase. Useful for the separation of polar compounds with anionic groups such as nucleotides and anionic drug metabolites such as sulphates or glucuronides

(i)   Retention factor for the lipophilic compound pentylbenzene, k_{PB}

This test provides a measure of how completely the surface of the silica gel is covered with reverse-phase coating and of the area of the surface that is available for interaction with the analyte. The higher K_{PB} for a column, the greater the surface coverage and available surface area of the stationary phase (mobile phase methanol/water (80:20)). Different ODS columns give a wide range of K_{PB} values.

(ii) Hydrophobic selectivity $\alpha_{CH2} = k_{PB}/k_{BB}$

This is measured by the ratio of the capacity factors for pentylbenzene (K_{PB}) and butylbenzene (K_{BB}) and gives a measure of the surface coverage of the silica gel with the bonded phase. The higher α_{CH2}, the greater the surface coverage; this factor varies much less than K_{PB} between different reverse-phase columns (mobile phase methanol/water (80:20)).

(iii) Shape selectivity $\alpha_{T/O} = k_T/k_O$

This is based on the ratio of the capacity factors for triphenylene and *o*-terphenyl, which have very similar structures, but *o*-terphenyl is less rigid than triphenylene and thus has a more three-dimensional structure (Fig. 12.19). Retention of a molecule via lipophilic interactions depends on the size of molecular surface that interacts with the stationary phase. This means for a surface with large lipophilic groups less of the *o*-terphenyl molecule will be in contact with the surface, whereas the flat triphenylene molecule can contact a uniform surface more fully. Triphenylene, because of its flatness, is less sensitive to the surface of the stationary phase. Stationary phases with smaller alkyl chains attached to the surface, such as octyl, phenyl or butyl, often do not discriminate between *o*-terphenyl and triphenylene as strongly as octadecyl phases (mobile phase methanol/water (80:20)).

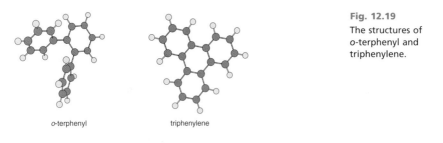

o-terphenyl   triphenylene

Fig. 12.19
The structures of *o*-terphenyl and triphenylene.

(iv) Hydrogen bonding capacity $\alpha_{C/P} = k_C/k_P$

Hydrogen bonding capacity may be measured as the ratio of the capacity factors for phenol (k_P) and caffeine (k_C). The smaller the value for $\alpha_{C/P}$ the higher the hydrogen bonding capacity, since phenol can hydrogen bond whereas caffeine cannot. The term measures the level of free silanol (Fig. 12.20), or other groups with hydrogen-bonding capacity, in the phase (mobile phase methanol/water (30:70)).

uncapped silanol

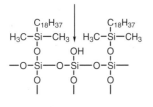

Fig. 12.20
Uncapped silanol group.

(v) Total ion exchange capacity $a_{B/P} = k_B/k_P$ (pH 7.6)

This term gives a measure of the total silanol group activity and is based on the ratio of the capacity factors for benzylamine (k_B) and phenol (k_P) when analysed using a mobile phase with a pH of 7.6, where most of the uncapped silanol groups (Fig. 12.17) in a silica-gel-based chromatographic phase will be ionised. The benzylamine interacts strongly with negatively charged silanol groups and is thus more strongly retained on phases where there are a high number of silanol groups. The higher the value of $\alpha_{B/P}$, the greater the ion exchange capacity of the phase.

(vi) The acidic ion exchange capacity $a_{B/P} = k_B/k_P$ (pH 2.7)

This term gives a measure of the activity of the most acidic silanol groups in the stationary phase and is based on the ratio of the capacity factors for benzylamine (k_B) and phenol (k_P) when analysed using a mobile phase with a pH of 2.7, where only the most acidic (isolated) uncapped silanol groups in a silica-gel-based chromatographic phase will be ionised.

Table 12.3 shows the specification details of some Hypersil columns taken from the manufacturer's literature along with some Tanaka test measurements.[8]

Table 12.3 Data for four different reverse-phase Hypersil columns[8]

Column	%C	EC*	Silica**	K_{PB}	$\alpha_{B/P}$ pH 7.6	$\alpha_{B/P}$ pH 2.7
C18 HS 100	16	Y	UP	7.66	1.01	0.25
C18 BDS	11	Y	AW	4.5	0.19	0.17
C18 HyPurity	13	Y	HP	3.2	0.29	0.1
C8 HyPurity	8	Y	HP	1.59	0.3	0.11

*EC = endcapped
**UP = unpurified, AW = acid washed, HP = high purity

The C18 HS 100 column has a high carbon load and thus has the greatest retention factor of pentyl benzene. It is also made from unpurified silica gel, so that it strongly retains benzylamine relative to phenol due to strong ion exchange interactions. This column would not be useful for the analysis of many basic compounds. The C18 BDS column has a lower carbon load and so retains pentyl-benzene less than the HS column; it does not show strong retention for benzylamine because the acid washing process has removed many of the trace metals from the silica gel used to prepare it, making it more suitable for the analysis of bases. The HyPurity C18 phase shows a lower retention factor for pentylbenzene despite having higher carbon load than the BDS phase; this is not immediately easy to explain but may relate to the surface areas of the phases since the HyPurity phase has a larger surface area per gram. The HyPurity C8 has a lower retention factor for pentylbenzene, which would be expected from its lower carbon load. This is not always the case for C8 phases; some have a carbon load closer to that of a C18 phase and thus a retention factor not much lower than the C18 phase. The use of column characterisation parameters enables selection of similar columns based on their performance according to the Tanaka tests. The data obtained by Euerby and Peterson[8] has been converted into column selection software which is available as a free download from ACD Labs at http://www.acdlabs.com/products/adh/chrom/chromproc/.

Table 12.4 shows some examples of recent developments in the chemistry of reverse-phase packings.

Self-test 12.4

Go to the ACD site and download column selector and associated software (this process takes about 30 minutes by the time the software is downloaded and installed, but it is useful software and free!!). Use the software to select the column most similar to the ACE C18 column. List the Tanaka parameters for the ACE C18 column and the most closely related column in the list.

Table 12.4 Some examples of modern reverse-phase chemistry

Stationary phase	Comments
Endcapped and high-purity phases	The biggest source of variation in modified silica gel is the quality of the base silica supporting the alkyl coating. The latest generation of base deactivated phases is made from high-purity silica formed by the hydrolysis of tetramethoxysilane. Reaction of uncapped silanols with a non-polar end-capping group such as trimethylsilane also reduces unwanted interaction with basic compounds
	Polar embedded groups increase the penetration of water into the stationary phase, through its being able to hydrogen bond to a group such as an amide group. These phases give stronger retention of polar analytes
	Altered bonding such as bidentate attachment of ligands gives greater deactivation and stability so that the stationary phase can be used up to pH 11.0
	Base silica gel particles can be engineered to contain alkyl groups, making a more inert and stable gel

Summary of detectors used in HPLC

For the majority of analyses of drugs in formulations, variable wavelength UV or diode array UV detectors are used. A typical UV detector has a narrow cell about 1 mm in diameter with a length of 10 mm, giving it an internal volume of about 8 μl. The linear range of such detectors is between 0.0001 and 2 absorbance units, and samples have to be diluted sufficiently to fall within the range. Although the exact concentration of a sample passing through the flow cell is not known, a suitable concentration can be approximated as shown in Calculation example 12.3.

Selective detectors tend to be employed where the analyte is present in small amounts in a complex matrix such as in bioanalytical procedures, where components extracted from the biological matrix along with the analyte can cause

Calculation example 12.3

A typical elution volume of chromatographic peak volume is 400 μl. If 20 μl (0.02 ml) of a solution containing paracetamol at a concentration of 1 mg/100 ml is injected into an HPLC system with a flow cell with a pathlength of 10 mm:

Amount of paracetamol injected = 1 mg × 0.02/100 = 0.0002 mg

Mean concentration of paracetamol in the peak volume = 0.0002 × 100/0.4 = 0.05 mg/100 ml

The A(1%, 1 cm) value for paracetamol at 245 nm is 668.

The absorbance of a 0.05 mg (0.00005 g) solution = 0.00005 × 668 = 0.0334.

The mean absorption across the peak would be 0.00334.

If the peak has a Gaussian shape, the maximum absorption for the peak would be *ca* 1.5 times the mean absorption, i.e. in this case 0.05 or 50 milliabsorbance units (mAU).

interference. Some formulated compounds have only very poor chromophores – these include sugars, lipids, surfactants, amino acids and some classes of drugs, e.g. a number of anticholinergic drugs lack chromophores. In these cases an alternative to UV detection has to be employed.

Performance of a diode array detector

Table 12.5 summarises the detectors commonly used in HPLC analyses (see also Animation 12.8). Sometimes it is not possible to be completely confident that an HPLC has chromatographically resolved all the compounds in a sample, and it might be suspected that a particular chromatographic peak might be due to more than one component. The DAD has developed into a tool of some sophistication for determining the purity of chromatographic peaks eluting from an HPLC column. Since a whole UV/visible spectrum is acquired several times across the width of a peak, this provides a means of checking the purity of the peak by checking for variations in the shape of the absorption spectrum across the chromatographic peak. Figure 12.21 illustrates four methods for looking at the purity of a peak using the information acquired by a DAD.

In the example illustrated in Figure 12.21, the spectrum of the apex of the peak (A) (where interference by impurities is likely to be the least) is compared with a spectrum from the leading edge of the peak (B). Comparison of individual spectra from anywhere across the width of the peak may also be made with a spectrum produced by combining each spectrum taken across the chromatographic peak to produce a composite spectrum for the peak. The four methods used are:

(i) Spectrum A and spectrum B are normalised to get the best possible overlay and are then correlated by plotting their absorbances at *ca* 1 nm intervals across the spectra against each other. The correlation coefficient of best-fit line through the resultant points can be determined (Ch. 1, p. 16). A good correlation between the spectra should give $r^2 > 0.995$, and the r^2 for such a plot is multiplied by 1000 to give a similarity factor, which is quoted as a measure of peak purity when the spectra of leading

Table 12.5 Some detectors commonly used in high-performance liquid chromatography (HPLC)

Detector	Applications
Variable wavelength UV detector 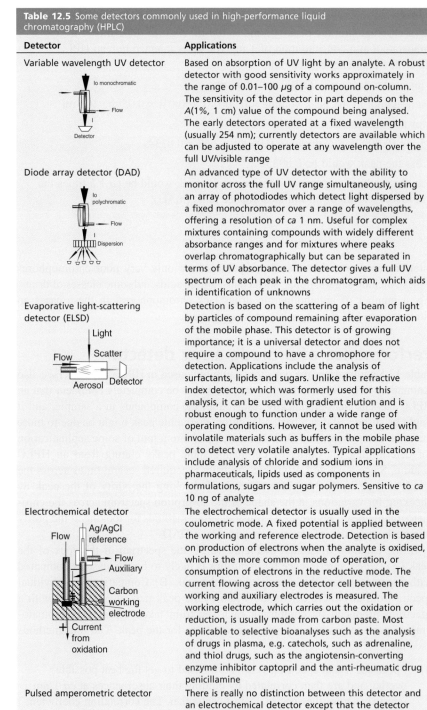	Based on absorption of UV light by an analyte. A robust detector with good sensitivity works approximately in the range of 0.01–100 μg of a compound on-column. The sensitivity of the detector in part depends on the A(1%, 1 cm) value of the compound being analysed. The early detectors operated at a fixed wavelength (usually 254 nm); currently detectors are available which can be adjusted to operate at any wavelength over the full UV/visible range
Diode array detector (DAD)	An advanced type of UV detector with the ability to monitor across the full UV range simultaneously, using an array of photodiodes which detect light dispersed by a fixed monochromator over a range of wavelengths, offering a resolution of *ca* 1 nm. Useful for complex mixtures containing compounds with widely different absorbance ranges and for mixtures where peaks overlap chromatographically but can be separated in terms of UV absorbance. The detector gives a full UV spectrum of each peak in the chromatogram, which aids in identification of unknowns
Evaporative light-scattering detector (ELSD)	Detection is based on the scattering of a beam of light by particles of compound remaining after evaporation of the mobile phase. This detector is of growing importance; it is a universal detector and does not require a compound to have a chromophore for detection. Applications include the analysis of surfactants, lipids and sugars. Unlike the refractive index detector, which was formerly used for this analysis, it can be used with gradient elution and is robust enough to function under a wide range of operating conditions. However, it cannot be used with involatile materials such as buffers in the mobile phase or to detect very volatile analytes. Typical applications include analysis of chloride and sodium ions in pharmaceuticals, lipids used as components in formulations, sugars and sugar polymers. Sensitive to *ca* 10 ng of analyte
Electrochemical detector	The electrochemical detector is usually used in the coulometric mode. A fixed potential is applied between the working and reference electrode. Detection is based on production of electrons when the analyte is oxidised, which is the more common mode of operation, or consumption of electrons in the reductive mode. The current flowing across the detector cell between the working and auxiliary electrodes is measured. The working electrode, which carries out the oxidation or reduction, is usually made from carbon paste. Most applicable to selective bioanalyses such as the analysis of drugs in plasma, e.g. catechols, such as adrenaline, and thiol drugs, such as the angiotensin-converting enzyme inhibitor captopril and the anti-rheumatic drug penicillamine
Pulsed amperometric detector	There is really no distinction between this detector and an electrochemical detector except that the detector has arisen largely as part of ion chromatography and tends to be used in the amperometric mode, where

(Continued)

Table 12.5 *(Continued)*	
Detector	**Applications**
	conduction of current between two electrodes by an ionic analyte is measured rather than current changes resulting from oxidation or reduction of the analyte. The working electrode in this detector is usually gold rather than carbon paste. Highly sensitive to ionic compounds, the detector is used in ion chromatography for the analysis of inorganic ions such as phosphate and sulphate. Typical pharmaceutical applications include the analysis of cardenolides and aminoglycoside antibiotics which do not have chromophores. Sensitivity is typically down to 1 ng of analyte. Widely used in glycobiology for the analysis of sugar residues derived from glycoproteins. In the pulsed mode, the polarities of the electrodes are alternated in order to keep the electrode surfaces clean
Refractive index detector (RI)	Detection is based on changes of refractive index when the analyte passes through the sample cell (Samp.) in the detector, the reference cell (Ref.) being filled with the mobile phase. Like the ELSD, the RI detector is a universal detector with even less selectivity than the ELSD. It is very sensitive to mobile-phase composition and temperature, making it non-robust. It is still used as a universal detector since it is cheaper than an ELSD. Sensitive to *ca* 1 µg of compound
Fluorescence detector	Detection is based on fluorescent emission following excitation of a fluorescent compound at an appropriate wavelength. A robust and selective detector applicable to compounds exhibiting fluorescence and to fluorescent derivatives. Most useful for selective bioanalyses. Sensitive to below the ng level for highly fluorescent compounds. Normally uses a xenon lamp for excitation but instruments with high-intensity deuterium lamps are available for excitation of short-wavelength absorption bands
Corona® charged aerosol detector (CAD)	The CAD detector is increasing in importance. It is a universal detector like RI and ELSD detectors but is much more sensitive than these detectors. Detection is based on nebulisation of the HPLC eluent, and then the nebulised analyte particles pass a platinum corona discharge pin which imparts a positive electrostatic charge to them. The charge is then finally collected and measured. The detector response is largely independent of the chemical structure of the analyte, unlike most other detectors, which makes it very useful for mass balance studies. The detector has a dynamic range $> 10^4$.

and tailing ends of the peak are compared to the spectrum of the apex. A perfect match is $r^2 = 1.000$.

(ii) Spectra can be correlated to the apex spectrum or to a composite spectrum at several points across the width of the chromatographic peak, giving rise to a similarity curve. The threshold curve gives an indication of the contribution from noise to spectral differences, which is greatest at the ends of the peak, where spectra are weak in comparison with background noise from the mobile phase, etc. An impurity is detected

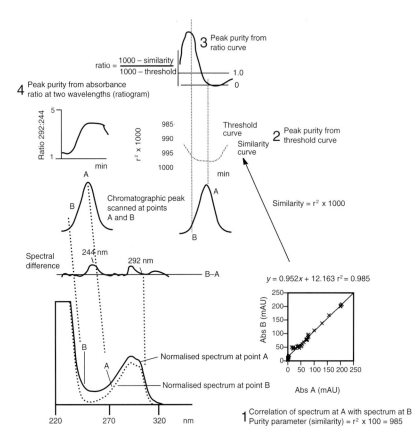

Fig. 12.21
Applications of diode
array detection to peak
purity determination.

Self-test 12.5

Rank the following detectors in order of decreasing: a. Selectivity b. Robustness c. Sensitivity:

(i)   Variable wavelength UV detector
(ii)   Evaporative light scattering detector (ELSD)
(iii) Refractive index (RI) detector
(iv) Electrochemical detector

Answers: Selectivity: electrochemical detector, variable wavelength UV detector, ELSD, RI detector. Robustness: variable wavelength UV detector, ELSD, electrochemical detector, RI detector. Sensitivity: electrochemical detector, variable wavelength UV detector, ELSD, RI detector

---

when the similarity curve rises above the threshold curve. In the example illustrated the major impurity in the peak is around point B.

(iii) For a very minor impurity, spectral differences across the peak can be amplified by plotting the values for 1000 − similarity/1000 − threshold across its width.

(iv) If it is possible to determine the wavelength where the impurity absorbs strongly relative to the analyte, a ratiogram can be constructed. This is obtained by plotting the ratio of a wavelength where the sample absorbs strongly and the impurity absorbs weakly against a wavelength where the impurity absorbs intensely. If the peak is impure, the ratio will fall around where the impurity elutes. A pure peak will exhibit a fairly constant ratio across the width of the peak.

Applications of HPLC to the quantitative analysis of drugs in formulations

The majority of applications of HPLC in pharmaceutical analysis are to the quantitative determinations of drugs in formulations. Such analyses usually do not require large amounts of time to be spent optimising mobile phases and selecting columns and detectors so that analyses of complex mixtures can be carried out. A standard joke is that most quality-control applications can be carried out with an ODS column and with methanol:water (1:1) as a mobile phase. Analyses of formulations are not quite that simple but, compared to analysis of drugs in biological fluids or elucidation of complex drug degradation pathways, they present fewer difficulties. The main potential interferants in analysis of a formulation are preservatives, colourants (see Ch. 15) and possible degradation products of the formulated drug. Some formulations contain more than one active ingredient, and these may present more of an analytical challenge since the different ingredients may have quite different chemical properties and elute at very different times from an HPLC column. In this case, achieving a short analysis time may be difficult. Since the emphasis in pharmaceutical analysis is on quantitative analysis of formulations, this will be considered first.

Analyses based on calibration with an external standard

HPLC assays of formulated drugs can often be carried out against an external standard for the drug being measured. The instrumentation itself is capable of high precision, and in many cases drugs are completely recovered from the formulation matrix. If complete recovery can be guaranteed, then the area of the chromatographic peak obtained from a known weight of formulation can be compared directly with a calibration curve constructed using a series of solutions containing varying concentrations of a pure standard of the analyte. The use of a single point of calibration can also be justified since, in quality control applications, the content of the formulation is unlikely to vary by > ± 10% from the stated content. The Food and Drug Administration (FDA) have suggested that for an assay of the active ingredients in a formulation, calibration should be carried within a range of ± 20% of the expected concentration in the sample extract. The steps required in a quantitative HPLC assay based on the use of an external standard are summarised as follows:

- Weigh accurately an analytical standard for the analyte, and dissolve it in a precise volume of solvent to prepare a stock solution.
- Prepare appropriate dilutions from the stock to produce a calibration series of solutions so that (1) appropriate amounts of analyte are injected into the instrument giving consideration to its operating range and (2) the concentration of analyte which is expected in a diluted extract from the sample is at

approximately the mid-point of the range of concentrations prepared in the calibration series.
- Inject the calibration solutions into the HPLC system starting with the lowest concentration and finishing with a blank injection of the mobile phase to check for carryover.
- Prepare the formulation for extraction, e.g. powder tablets, and weigh accurately portions of the prepared material.
- Extract the formulation with a solvent which is likely to give good extraction recovery and make up to a precise volume.
- Filter if necessary and take a precise aliquot of the sample extract and dilute this until its concentration falls at approximately the mid-point of the calibration series prepared using the analytical standard.
- Inject the diluted sample solution into the HPLC system. Replicates of the sample preparation and of the injection of the sample into the HPLC may be carried out; sample preparation procedures are more likely to give rise to imprecision than instrumental variation.
- Plot a calibration curve for the area of the peaks obtained in the calibration series against the concentrations of the solutions. The peak areas given by integrators are in arbitrary units and may be to seven or eight figures. Assays are not usually precise beyond four significant figures; thus it may be appropriate to only consider the first five figures from the integrator output to be of any significance, e.g. 78993866 might be better considered as being 78994000.
- Check the linearity of the calibration curve, i.e. r > 0.99. Determine the concentration of the diluted sample extract from the calibration curve by substituting the area of its chromatographic peak into the equation for the calibration line.

Analysis of paracetamol tablets using a calibration curve

Tablets

Tablets contain paracetamol 500 mg, phenylpropanolamine 5 mg.

Explanation of the assay

Even without chromatographic resolution the small amount of phenylpropanolamine present in the formulation could be disregarded since its $A(1\%, 1\ cm)$ value at the wavelength 243 nm used for monitoring paracetamol is *ca* 4 compared to an $A(1\%, 1\ cm)$ of 668 for paracetamol. An ODS column retains paracetamol adequately if the amount of water in the mobile phase is high. Thus the mobile phase used is 0.05 M acetic acid/acetonitrile (90:15); the weakly acidic mobile phase ensures there is no tendency for the phenol group in paracetamol (pKa 9.5) to ionise. The tablet extract has to be diluted sufficiently to bring it within the range of the UV detector. Figure 12.22 shows the chromatographic traces obtained for an extract from paracetamol tablets and a paracetamol standard (1.25 mg/100 ml) run using the system described above.

Assay

(i)   Weigh out 125 ± 10 mg of the paracetamol standard, transfer it to a 250 ml volumetric flask made up to volume with acetic acid (0.05 M) and shake well (stock solution).

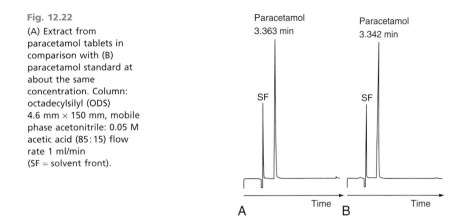

Fig. 12.22
(A) Extract from paracetamol tablets in comparison with (B) paracetamol standard at about the same concentration. Column: octadecylsilyl (ODS) 4.6 mm × 150 mm, mobile phase acetonitrile: 0.05 M acetic acid (85 : 15) flow rate 1 ml/min (SF = solvent front).

(ii)   Prepare a series of solutions containing 0.5, 1.0, 1.5, 2.0 and 2.5 mg/100 ml of paracetamol from the stock solution.

(iii)   Weigh and powder 20 tablets.

(iv)   Weigh out tablet powder containing 125 mg ± 10 mg of paracetamol.

(v)   Shake the tablet powder sample with *ca* 150 ml of acetic acid (0.05 M) for 5 min in a 250 ml volumetric flask, and then adjust the volume to 250 ml with more acetic acid (0.05 M).

(vi)   Filter *ca* 50 ml of the solution into a conical flask, then transfer a 25 ml aliquot of the filtrate to 100 ml volumetric flasks and adjust the volume to 100 ml with acetic acid (0.05 M).

(vii)   Take 10 ml of the diluted extract, transfer to a further 100 ml volumetric flask and make up to volume with 0.05 M acetic acid.

(viii)   Analyse the standards and the extract using the chromatographic conditions specified earlier.

Data obtained

- Weight of 20 tablets = 12.1891 g
- Weight of tablet powder taken = 150.5 mg
- Weight of paracetamol calibration standard = 126.1 mg
- Area of paracetamol peak extracted from tablets = 45 205.

Calculate the percentage of the stated content of paracetamol in the tablet powder analysed.

The graph shown in Figure 12.23 is obtained from the data given in Table 12.6; it is linear with r = 1.000.

The equation of the line can be used to calculate the amount of paracetamol in the diluted extract of the tablet powder.

Assay of paracetamol and aspirin in tablets using a narrow-range calibration curve

Tablets

Tablets contain paracetamol 250 mg, aspirin 250 mg, codeine phosphate 6.8 mg.

Explanation of the assay

This problem is slightly more difficult than that posed by paracetamol tablets since there are two major active ingredients in the formulation. The codeine

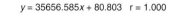

$y = 35656.585x + 80.803$ $r = 1.000$

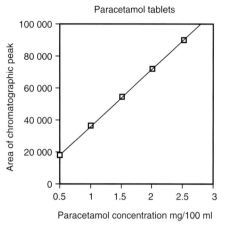

Fig. 12.23
Calibration curve for the determination of paracetamol in tablets obtained from high-performance liquid chromatography (HPLC) analysis of calibration standards.

Table 12.6 Data obtained from the analysis of paracetamol standard solutions by high-performance liquid chromatography (HPLC)

Concentration of paracetamol standard solution mg/100 ml	Area of chromatographic peak
0.5044	17 994
1.009	36 109
1.513	54 121
2.018	71 988
2.522	89 984

Calculation example 12.4

Substituting the area obtained for the paracetamol peak obtained from the analysis of the tablet powder extract into the equation for the line:

$$45205 = 35656x + 80$$

Solving for x gives the concentration of the extract in mg/100 ml.

Concentration of paracetamol in diluted tablet extract $= \dfrac{45205 - 80}{35656} = 1.266$ mg/100 ml

Dilution steps

The dilution steps used were:

- 25 ml into 100 ml ($\times 4$)
- 10 ml into 100 ml ($\times 10$)
- Total $= \times 40$.

Concentration of paracetamol in undiluted tablet extract

$$1.266 \text{ mg/100 ml} \times 40 = 50.64 \text{ mg/100 ml}$$

(Continued)

Calculation example 12.4 *(Continued)*

Amount of paracetamol in undiluted tablet extract

- The volume of the undiluted tablet extract = 250 ml
- Amount of paracetamol in 100 ml of the extract = 50.64 mg
- Amount of paracetamol in 250 ml of extract = 250/100 × 50.64 mg = 126.6 mg
- Amount of paracetamol found in the tablet powder assayed = 126.6 mg.

Amount of paracetamol expected in the tablet powder taken for assay

- Weight of 20 tablets = 12.1891 g
- Weight of one tablet = 12.1891/20 = 0.6094 g = 609.5 mg
- Stated content per tablet = 500 mg
- Amount of paracetamol expected in the weight of tablet powder taken for assay = 150.5/609.5 × 500 mg = 123.5 mg.

Percentage of stated content

- Percentage of stated content = 126.6/123.5 × 100 = 102.5%.

Self-test 12.6

Calculate the percentage of stated content in paracetamol tablets using the calibration curve given above and the following data:

Data

- Weight of 20 tablets = 12.2243 g
- Weight of tablet powder taken = 152.5 mg
- Stated content per tablet = 500 mg
- Initial extraction volume = 200 ml.

Dilution steps

- 20 ml into 100 ml
- 10 ml into 100 ml
- Area of chromatographic peak for paracetamol extracted from the tablets = 44 519.

Answer: 99.8%

---

phosphate cannot be determined using the chromatographic system described here since it elutes from the column in the void volume and is obscured by the solvent front. Again an ODS column is quite suitable, and since aspirin is ionised extensively above pH 4.0, the pH of the mobile phase can be manipulated to move it to a region of the chromatogram where it can be run in the same mobile phase as paracetamol without its retention time being inconveniently long. Figure 12.24 shows the effect of mobile-phase pH on the elution time of aspirin; the pKa of paracetamol is much higher than that of aspirin, and it is unaffected by the adjustment in pH of the mobile phase. The mobile phase which resulted in chromatogram B is preferred for the analysis.

Brief outline of the assay

The assay is more or less the same as that described for the paracetamol tablets except that the tablets are extracted with 0.05 M sodium acetate buffer pH 4.4.

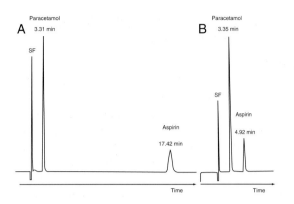

Fig. 12.24
(A) A tablet extract containing paracetamol and aspirin run at a pH of *ca* 3.7 in 0.05 M acetic acid/acetonitrile (85:15) (150 mm × 4.6 mm octadecylsilyl (ODS) column, flow rate 1 ml/min). (B) Shows the tablets extract run at pH 4.4 in 0.05 M sodium acetate buffer/acetonitrile (85.15). ODS column 150 mm × 4.6 mm, flow rate 1 ml/min. UV detection at 243 nm.

The calibration standard solutions are prepared so that they contain both aspirin and paracetamol in 0.05 M sodium acetate buffer pH 4.4 in the concentration range 1.0–1.5 mg/100 ml.

Data obtained

- Weight of 20 tablets = 11.2698 g
- Weight of tablet powder taken = 283.8 mg
- Weight of paracetamol standard = 125.5 mg
- Weight of aspirin standard = 127.3 mg.

Mean area of chromatographic peaks for a duplicate analysis of the tablet extract:

- Aspirin: 15 366
- Paracetamol: 44 535.

The equations for the calibration lines obtained were as follows:

- Aspirin: $y = 12\,136\,x + 139$
- Paracetamol: $y = 35\,374\,x - 35$.

Dilution of sample

- Initial volume in 250 ml.

Diluted:

- 25 to 100 ml
- 10 to 100 ml.

Self-test 12.7

Calculate the percentage of the stated content of aspirin and paracetamol in the tablet powder analysed using the data obtained above.

Answers: Paracetamol = 100.1% of stated content; aspirin = 99.7%

Assay of active ingredients in an anaesthetic gel using a single-point calibration curve

Content per 100 g of gel

Lidocaine (lignocaine).HCl 2 g/100 g, chlorhexidine digluconate solution* 0.25% v/v and morphine sulphate 0.1 g/100 g. Specific gravity of gel = 1.03.

In addition to illustrating the use of ratios of chromatographic peaks in calculating content this example illustrates the importance of paying attention to the salt forms of a drug used in a formulation. In the case of lidocaine and morphine the salt forms used to calibrate the method are the same as those in the formulation, but in the case of chlorhexidine the standard is in the form of the free base. The salt form in the formulation is the gluconate which cannot be stored as a crystalline salt since it absorbs water so rapidly and thus is available as a 20% w/v solution.

Explanation of the assay

This assay is altogether more difficult since three active ingredients are involved and several excipients potentially could interfere in the analysis. In addition, the active ingredients are bases, which have a tendency to interact with any uncapped silanol groups in the stationary phase, and it is essential to use a column which is deactivated with respect to the analysis of basic compounds. The three active ingredients are all at different concentrations in the formulation so attention has to be paid to selection of a detection wavelength at which each component can be detected. In this particular assay a DAD would be useful.

Brief outline of the assay

One gram of the morphine sulphate in Instillagel admixture was removed from a syringe and weighed into a 50 ml volumetric flask; 10 ml of methanol was added and, finally, the volume was made up to 50 ml with water. Samples were then transferred to an auto-sampler vial, and 20 μl of the solution was injected.

A chromatogram obtained from the analysis of the sample is shown in Figure 12.25:

Fig. 12.25
Separation of components in Instillagel/Morphine Admixture. ACE C18 column (150 × 4.6 mm i.d.). Buffer pH 3 (A) and acetonitrile (B). The solvent programme used was as follows: 0 min, 95% A/5% B; 27 min, 55% A/45% B; 30 min, 95% A/5% B; 35 min, 95% A/5% B.

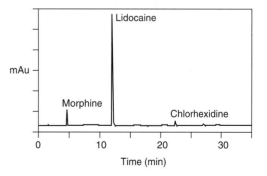

*Chlorhexidine digluconate solution contains 20% w/v.

- The concentrations of the calibration standards, the peak areas obtained for the calibration standards and the corresponding compounds in the sample are shown in Table 12.7.
- Weight of gel analysed = 1.0513 g
- Final volume of extract = 50 ml
- Calculate the percentage of stated content for the lidocaine. HCl in the formulation.

Table 12.7 Peak area data obtained for analysis of in Instillagel/morphine admixture

Standard + concentration	Area of peak in standard	Area of peak in sample
Morphine sulphate 2.132 mg/100 ml	15763	15967
Lidocaine (lignocaine).HCl 40.02 mg/100 ml	614757	633713
Chlorhexidine 0.5731 mg/100 ml	4107	4448

Calculation example 12.5

From a simple ratio:

$$\text{Concentration of morphine sulphate in extract} = 2.132 \times \frac{15967}{15763} = 2.160 \text{ mg/100ml.}$$

The sample was dissolved in 50 ml.

Amount of morphine sulphate in 50 ml = 1.080 mg

Thus, 1.080 mg was extracted from 1.0513 g of gel.

Morphine sulphate in formulation = 0.1 g/100 mg = 100 mg/100 g = 1 mg/g

$$\text{Expected content in 1.0513 g of gel} = 1 \times \frac{1.0513}{1.03} = 1.021 \text{ ml}$$

$$\text{Percentage of stated content} = \frac{1.080}{1.0513} \times 100 = 102.7\%$$

The calculation for the % of stated content of the chlorhexidine gluconate is more complicated. The gel is stated to contain 0.25% v/v (0.25 ml/100 ml) of chlorhexidine gluconate solution which contains 20% w/v chlorhexidine gluconate. Thus to be completely accurate the volume of gel analysed has to be calculated by dividing by its specific gravity.

$$\text{Volume of gel analysed} = \frac{1.0513}{1.03} = 1.021 \text{ ml}$$

There are 0.25 ml chlorhexidine gluconate solution per 100 ml of gel. Thus in 1.021 ml the

$$\text{volume of solution} = \frac{0.25}{100} \times 1.021 = 0.002553 \text{ ml.}$$

The chlorhexidine gluconate solution contains 20% w/v, or 20 g per 100 ml.

The expected content of chlorhexidine gluconate in the gel = 0.002553 × 0.2 = 0.0005105 g = 0.5105 mg.

(Continued)

Calculation example 12.5 *(Continued)*

From the HPLC data content of chlorhexidine =

$$0.5173 \times \frac{4448}{4107} = 0.5603 \text{ mg/100 ml} = 0.2801 \text{ mg/50 ml}.$$

Thus 0.2801 mg of chlorhexidine was extracted from 1.0513 g of gel.

However, the chlorhexidine content is stated in terms of its digluconate salt. The MW of chlorhexidine is 505.5 and the MW of its digluconate is 897.8.

Thus the content of chlorhexidine digluconate $= \dfrac{897.8}{505.5} \times 0.2801 = 0.4975 \text{ mg}$

% of stated content $= \dfrac{0.4975}{0.5105} \times 100 = 97.5\%.$

Self-test 12.8

Calculate the percentage of stated content of lidocaine in the gel.

Answer: 98.1%

Assays using calibration against an internal standard

If the recovery in an assay is good and the instrumentation used for measurement of the sample is capable of high precision, the use of an internal standard (Box 12.2) is not necessary. HPLC instrumentation is usually capable of high precision, but for certain samples, recoveries prior to injection into the HPLC may not be accurate or precise. Examples of formulations in which recoveries may not be complete include ointments and creams, which require more extensive extraction prior to analysis. Problems of recovery are also typical of advanced drug delivery systems, which may be based on polymeric matrices in which a drug is dispersed. An internal standard is a compound related to the analyte (the properties required for an internal standard are summarised later), which is ideally added to the formulation being analysed prior to extraction. Quantification is achieved by establishing a response factor for the analyte relative to the internal standard, i.e. a ratio for the areas of the chromatographic peaks obtained for equal amounts of the analyte and internal standard; ideally this should be close to 1 for equal amounts of analyte and internal standard. The response factor may be based

---

Box 12.2 Properties of an internal standard

- Ideally should be closely related in structure to the analyte
- Should be stable
- Should be chromatographically resolved from the analyte and any excipients present in the chromatogram of the formulation extract
- Should elute as close as possible to the analyte with the restrictions above
- For a given weight should produce a detector response similar to that produced by the analyte

on a single-point calibration or a full calibration curve may be constructed; all the BP assays of this type are based on single-point calibrations. Once a response factor has been established, the sample is extracted with a solution containing the *same* concentration of internal standard as was used in determining the response factor (or a solution which after dilution will yield an extract in which the internal standard is at the same concentration as in the calibration solution). Provided the solution containing the fixed concentration of internal standard is added to the sample in a precisely measured volume, any subsequent losses of sample are compensated for, since losses of the analyte will be mirrored by losses of the internal standard (see Animation 12.9). The example given in Box 12.3 is typical of a BP assay incorporating an internal standard.

Box 12.3 Response factors

Assays based on the use of an internal standard use response factors to compare the sample solution with the calibration solution. In this case a simple one-point calibration is used. The concentration of betamethasone can be ignored since it is the same in Solutions 1 and 3; it should usually be the case that the same concentration of internal standard is present in the calibration and sample solutions. If this is the case, then for the assay described above:

Response factor for Solution 1 (calibration solution)

$$= \frac{\text{area of hydrocortisone peak in Solution 1}}{\text{area of betamethasone peak in Solution 1}}$$

Response factor for Solution 3 (sample solution)

$$= \frac{\text{area of hydrocortisone peak in Solution 3}}{\text{area of betamethasone peak in Solution 3}}$$

The amount of hydrocortisone in the cream can be calculated as follows: Concentration of hydrocortisone in Solution 3 =

$$\frac{\text{Response factor for Solution 3}}{\text{Response factor for Solution 1}} \times \text{concentration of hydrocortisone in Solution 1}$$

$$\times \frac{\text{volume of Solution 3}}{100}$$

Assay of hydrocortisone cream with one-point calibration against an internal standard

Explanation of the assay

Excellent separations of corticosteroids can be achieved on an ODS column with a suitable ratio of methanol/water as an eluent. In this assay hydrocortisone is quantified using betamethasone as an internal standard. The structure of beta-methasone is close to that of hydrocortisone but since it is more lipophilic it elutes from the ODS column after hydrocortisone (Fig. 12.26). The assay is a modification of the BP assay for hydrocortisone cream. In the assay described here, the internal standard is added at the first extraction step rather than after extraction has been carried out, in order to ensure that any losses in the course of sample preparation are fully compensated for. Extraction is necessary in the case of a cream because the large amount of oily excipients in the basis of the cream would soon clog up the column if no attempt was made to remove them. The corticosteroids are sufficiently polar to remain in the methanol/water layer as they have a low solubility in hexane, while the oily excipients are removed by

Fig. 12.26
Chromatogram from the analysis of hydrocortisone cream with betamethasone as an internal standard on an octadecylsilyl (ODS) column (25 cm × 4.6 mm) with methanol/water (70:30) as the mobile phase. (A) Calibration standard (Solution 1). (B) Cream extract + internal standard (Solution 3). (C) Cream extract without the addition of internal standard (Solution 2).

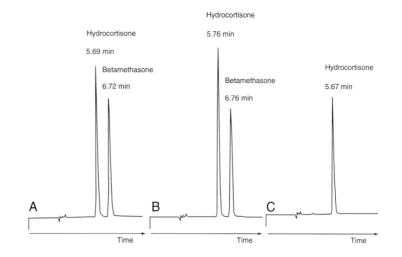

extraction into hexane. The sodium chloride (NaCl) is included in the sample extraction solution to prevent the formation of an emulsion when the extract is shaken with hexane. Solution 2, where the internal standard is omitted, is prepared in order to check that there are no excipients in the sample which would interfere with the peak due to the internal standard.

Brief outline of the assay

(i)   Prepare a mixture of methanol/15% aqueous NaCl solution (2:1).
(ii) Prepare Solution 1 as follows:
   - Mix together 10 ml of a 0.1% w/v solution of hydrocortisone and add 10 ml of a 0.1% w/v solution of betamethasone in methanol (internal standard solution).
   - Add 20 ml of methanol and then add water to dilute the solution to 100 ml.

(iii) Prepare Solution 2 as follows:
   - Disperse cream containing *ca* 10 mg of hydrocortisone in 30 ml of the methanol/NaCl solution + 10 ml of methanol.
   - Extract the dispersed cream with warm hexane (50 ml).
   - Remove the lower layer (methanol/water layer) and wash the hexane layer with 2 × 10 ml of the methanol/NaCl solution, combining the washings with the original extract.
   - Dilute the extract to 100 ml with water.

(iv) Prepare Solution 3 as follows:
   - Repeat the procedure used in preparing Solution 2 except, in the initial step, use 30 ml of methanol/NaCl solution + 10 ml of the betamethasone internal standard solution.
   - Analyse the solutions using a mobile phase containing methanol/water (70:30) and an ODS column.
   - Set the UV detector at 240 nm.

The calculation carried out from the data obtained in the assay described above uses response factors for the sample and standard (Box 12.3).

Data obtained

- Stated content of hydrocortisone cream = 1% w/w
- Weight of hydrocortisone cream used to prepare solution 3 = 1.173 g
- Area of hydrocortisone peak in Solution 1 = 103 026
- Area of betamethasone peak in Solution 1 = 92 449
- Area of hydrocortisone peak in Solution 3 = 113 628
- Area of betamethasone peak in Solution 3 = 82 920
- Concentration of hydrocortisone in the solution used in the preparation of Solution 1 = 0.1008% w/v
- Concentration of betamethasone used in preparation of Solutions 1 and 3 = 0.1003% w/v.

Calculation example 12.6

Solution 1 is prepared by diluting 10 ml of a 0.1008% w/v solution of hydrocortisone to 100 ml. Dilution × 10.

Concentration of hydrocortisone in Solution 1 $= \dfrac{0.1008}{10} = 0.01008\%$ w/v.

Response factor for Solution 1 $= \dfrac{103026}{92449} = 1.1144$

Response factor for Solution 3 $= \dfrac{113628}{82920} = 1.3703$

Concentration of hydrocortisone in Solution 3 =

$$\dfrac{1.3703}{1.1144} \times 0.01008 = 0.01239\% \text{ w/v} = 0.01239 \text{ g/100 ml}$$

Amount of hydrocortisone in Solution 3 $= \dfrac{\text{volume of Solution 3}}{100} \times \text{weight of hydrocortisone/100 ml}$

The volume of Solution 3 = 100 ml

Amount of hydrocortisone in Solution 3 $= \dfrac{100}{100} \times 0.01239 = 0.01239$ g

Weight of hydrocortisone cream analysed = 1.173 g

Percentage of w/w of hydrocortisone in cream $= \dfrac{0.01239}{1.173} \times 100 = 1.056\%$ w/w

Stated content of hydrocortisone in the cream = 1% w/w

Percentage of stated content $= \dfrac{1.056}{1} \times 100 = 105.6\%$

The cream conforms to the BP requirement that it should contain between 90 and 110% of the stated content.

Assay of miconazole cream with calibration against an internal standard over a narrow concentration range

Explanation of the assay

In this case the selective extraction of oily excipients from the cream is made somewhat easier by the fact that the miconazole (pKa 6.5) is almost fully ionised at pH 4.0; the econazole internal standard used differs from miconazole by only one chlorine atom (Fig. 12.27). Thus a preliminary extraction can be made with hexane to remove much of the basis of the ointment, and then the sample can be simply diluted with mobile phase, filtered and analysed.

Brief outline of the assay

A chromatographic mobile phase consisting of acetonitrile/0.1 M sodium acetate buffer pH 4.0 (70:30) is prepared. Separate stock solutions in 250 ml of chromatographic mobile phase containing miconazole nitrate (200 ± 20 mg) and econazole nitrate (200 ± 20 mg) (internal standard) are prepared. 25 ml of econazole nitrate stock solution is transferred to five 100 ml volumetric flasks, and varying amounts of miconazole stock solution (15, 20, 25, 30 and 35 ml) are

Fig. 12.27
The structures of miconazole and econazole.

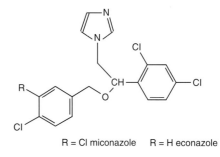

R = Cl miconazole   R = H econazole

Self-test 12.9

Betamethasone valerate is analysed in a sample of ointment used for treating haemorrhoids; the related steroid beclomethasone dipropionate is used as an internal standard. The following data were produced:

- Stated content of betamethasone valerate in ointment = 0.05% w/w
- Weight of ointment analysed = 4.3668 g
- Area of betamethasone valerate peak in Solution 1 (calibration solution) = 89 467
- Area of beclomethasone dipropionate in Solution 1 = 91 888
- Area of betamethasone valerate peak in Solution 3 = 87 657
- Area of beclomethasone dipropionate peak in Solution 3 = 90 343
- Concentration of betamethasone valerate present in the calibration solution = 0.004481% w/v
- Concentration of beclomethasone dipropionate in the calibration solution and in the sample extract solution = 0.00731% w/v (Note: if this is the same in both the calibration and sample solutions, it can be ignored)
- Volume of sample extract = 50 ml.

Calculate the %w/w of betamethasone valerate in the cream.

Answer: 0.051113% w/w

added to the five flasks. The flasks containing the calibration series are diluted to volume with mobile phase. A sample of cream containing 20 mg miconazole nitrate is shaken with 25 ml of the stock solution of econazole nitrate for 5 min. The sample is then extracted with 50 ml of hexane, and the hexane layer is removed and discarded. Nitrogen gas is then blown through the solution for a few minutes to remove residual hexane, and the solution is then transferred to a 100 ml volumetric flask, diluted to volume with mobile phase and a portion (20 ml) is filtered prior to analysis. The detection wavelength used is 220 nm since miconazole and econazole lack strong chromophores. On a 15 cm × 4.6 mm ODS column at a flow rate of 1 ml/min, econazole elutes at *ca* 6 min and miconazole elutes at *ca* 10 min; the extra chlorine atom in the structure of miconazole increases its lipophilicity considerably.

Data obtained

- Weight of miconazole used to prepare stock solution = 201.5 mg
- Weight of cream taken for assay = 1.0368 g
- Area of miconazole peak obtained from sample = 119 923
- Area of econazole peak obtained from sample = 124 118.

Table 12.8

Concentration of miconazole in calibration solution mg/100 ml	Area of miconazole peak	Area of econazole peak	In 80% methanol $K = \dfrac{5.6 - 1.1}{1.1} = 4.6$ In 70% methanol $K = \dfrac{15.7 - 1.1}{1.1} = 13.3$
12.09	70 655	123 563	0.5718
16.12	96 218	125 376	0.7674
20.15	119 793	126 783	0.9449
24.18	151 310	127 889	1.183
28.21	166 673	125 436	1.329

The equation of the line obtained from the data shown in Table 12.8 is $y = 0.048\,x - 0.006$; r = 0.998.

Self-test 12.10

Calculate the percentage of w/v of miconazole in the cream from the data obtained above.

Answer: 1.954% w/v

Assays involving more specialised HPLC techniques

Although more than 80% of all separations by HPLC utilise reverse-phase chromatography, there are certain analytes which require more specialised chromatographic methods. A few examples are given in the following section.

Assay of adrenaline injection by chromatography with an anionic ion-pairing agent

Explanation of the assay

Injections of local anaesthetics often contain low concentrations of adrenaline in order to localise the anaesthetic for a time by constricting blood vessels in the vicinity of the injection. Adrenaline can be analysed by straight-phase chromatography, for instance on silica gel, but this generally requires strongly basic conditions, under which the catechol group in adrenaline is unstable. Adrenaline is not retained by reverse-phase columns and elutes in their void volume. A commonly used technique for the analysis of adrenaline and other highly water-soluble amines is ion pair chromatography. This can be viewed essentially as the generation of an ion exchange column in situ. The process is illustrated in Figure 12.28, where sodium octanesulphonic acid (SOSA) is added to the mobile phase (e.g. 0.1 M sodium phosphate buffer/methanol 9:1 containing 0.02% SOSA); the SOSA partitions into the lipophilic stationary phase and saturates it. The stationary phase is then able to retain adrenaline by electrostatic interaction. Elution occurs by a combination of displacement of adrenaline from its ion pair by sodium ions and by migration of the ion pair itself in the mobile phase. An additional benefit of using an ion-pairing reagent, rather than resorting to straight-phase chromatography, is that the organic solvent content in the mobile phase can be kept low, thus enabling the use of an electrochemical detector, which works best in mobile phases with a low content of organic solvent and which is highly selective for the readily oxidised catechol groups of adrenaline.

Assay of ascorbic acid by chromatography with a cationic ion-pairing agent and electrochemical detection

Ascorbic acid is highly polar and is not retained by reverse-phase columns. One technique for retaining it on a reverse-phase column is to use a cationic

Fig. 12.28
Interaction of adrenaline with an ion-pairing agent coated onto an octadecylsilyl (ODS) stationary phase.

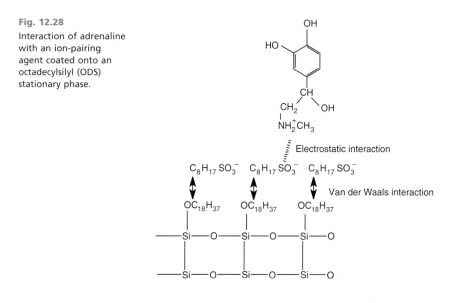

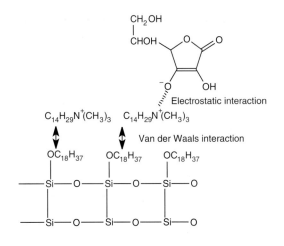

Electrostatic interaction

Van der Waals interaction

Fig. 12.29
Interaction of ascorbic acid with an ion-pairing agent coated onto the surface of an octadecylsilyl (ODS) column.

ion-pairing reagent. In the example given in Figure 12.29, cetrimide is used as the ion-pairing reagent in the mobile phase (e.g. 0.1 M sodium acetate buffer pH 4.2/acetonitrile 95 : 5 containing 0.03 M cetrimide). Again the low organic solvent content of the mobile phase enables monitoring with an electrochemical detector. Selectivity is important in the determination of ascorbic acid because it is often present in multivitamin formulations and as a preservative in pharmaceutical formulations containing other components in large amounts.

Assay of ascorbic acid by hydrophilic interaction chromatography

The hydrophilic interaction mechanism was first proposed by Alpert in 1990.[9] There are a number of HILIC phases. The simplest kinds are based on the use of bare silica, but the most popular is the ZIC-HILIC phase, the structure of which is shown in Figure 12.30. The mobile phase used is generally acetonitrile mixed with water or aqueous buffer. In this mode of chromatography the water associated with the surface of the stationary phase is regarded as acting as a pseudostationary phase. The phase thus works in the opposite way to a reverse phase. (1) The more polar or the lower the partition coefficient of a compound the more

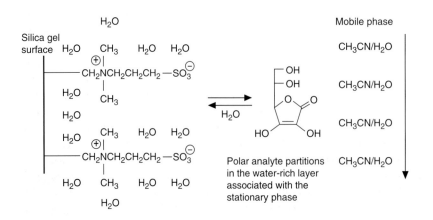

Polar analyte partitions in the water-rich layer associated with the stationary phase

Fig. 12.30
The structure and proposed mode of action of the zwitterionic hydrophilic interaction liquid chromatography (ZIC-HILIC) stationary phase illustrated by its interaction with ascorbic acid.

strongly it is retained. (2) The higher the water content in the mobile phase, the more quickly compounds elute. There is also the possibility of ion exchange interactions which can occur in the case of strongly acidic and basic compounds.

Figure 12.31 shows chromatograms obtained on a ZICHILIC phase for two important physiological antioxidants, ascorbic acid and glutathione (GSH), and for oxidised glutathione (GSSG), which forms as a result of oxidative stress. The chromatographic peaks were detected using mass spectrometry. None of these molecules would be retained by a reverse-phase column even in 100% water.

Fig. 12.31

Chromatograms for ascorbic acid, glutathione (GSH) and oxidized glutathione (GSSG) analysed on a zwitterionic hydrophilic interaction liquid chromatography (ZIC-HILIC) column 150 × 4.6 mm with a gradient between 0.1% formic acid/acetonitrile (10:90) and 0.1% formic acid/ acetonitrile (80:20).

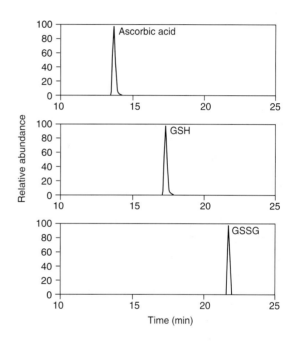

Assay of hyaluronic acid by size-exclusion chromatography (see Animation 12.10)

Polymeric materials have a number of pharmaceutical applications. Hyaluronic acid is a high-molecular-weight polymeric carbohydrate (Fig. 12.32) which has excited much interest in recent years because properties such as the promotion of wound healing are attributed to it. It is also used as a surgical aid during surgery to remove cataracts. In recent years, high-performance gel filtration columns containing rigid beads of porous polymers have become available for determination of high-molecular-weight analytes. The retention mechanism in size-exclusion or gel-permeation chromatography (GPC) is based on the extent to which an analyte enters pores within the stationary phase (Fig. 12.33). The largest molecules are completely excluded from the internal space of the column and elute from the column first. Columns with varying pore sizes are available, and for hyaluronic acid a large pore size is required since the polymer has a molecular weight $> 10^6$ Daltons. In order to determine molecular weights, such columns are

Self-test 12.11

The chromatograms below obtained on a ZICHILIC column are for various amino acids. Link the peaks to the amino acid structures shown below.

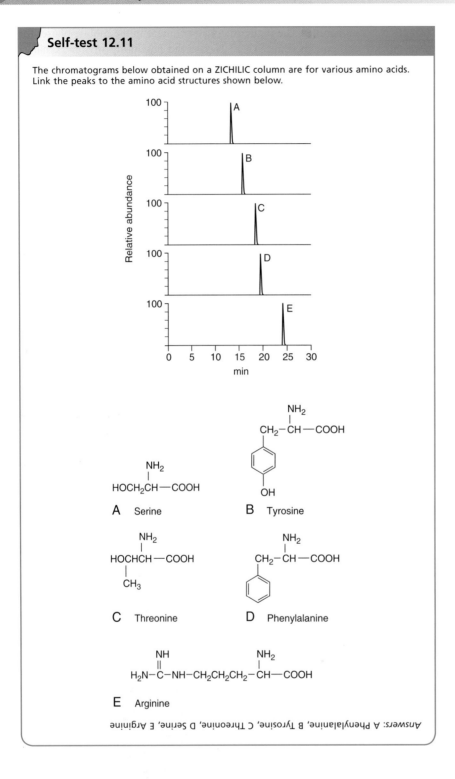

A Serine

B Tyrosine

C Threonine

D Phenylalanine

E Arginine

Fig. 12.32
The hyaluronic acid
polymer.

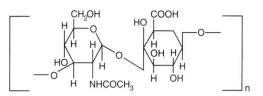

calibrated with polymeric standards of known molecular weight. Although corrections related to the viscosity of the analyte are made when a column used for determining the molecular weight of one type of polymer is calibrated using a different type of polymer, because of differences in three-dimensional shape.

Typically such an assay can be carried out using a column packed with an aqueous compatible porous polymer with a mobile phase consisting of, for example, 0.05 M sodium sulphate solution. Hyaluronic acid exhibits some weak UV absorption due to its *N*-acetyl groups at short wavelengths, and UV monitoring of the eluent can be carried out at *ca* 215 nm. Alternatively a refractive index detector or an ELSD can be used to monitor the eluent for polymers exhibiting no UV absorption at all. GPC of lipophilic polymers can be conducted in the same way using polymeric phases which are compatible with organic solvents.

Methods used for the assay of proteins by HPLC

For large molecules such as peptides, chromatographic packings with wide pores have to be used to facilitate partitioning of the large structures into the stationary phase. Typically ODS packings with 0.0003 μm pores are used. The chromophores in proteins are usually not particularly strong so UV detectors are set at short wavelengths. The mobile phases used are similar to those used for chromatography of small molecules on ODS columns. The mobile phase used in the EP analysis of insulin is composed of a mixture of phosphate buffer pH 2.3 and acetonitrile, and detection is carried out with the wavelength of the UV detector

Fig. 12.33
The mechanism
governing the analysis of
high-molecular-weight
analytes by gel permea-
tion chromatography
(GPC).

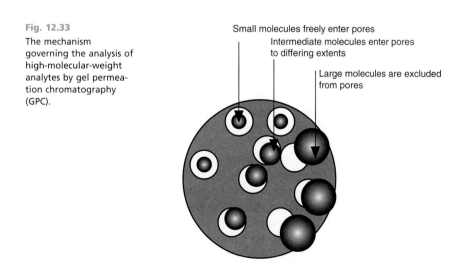

Small molecules freely enter pores

Intermediate molecules enter pores
to differing extents

Large molecules are excluded
from pores

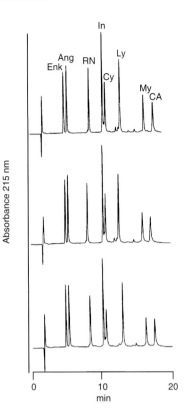

Fig. 12.34
Separation of a mixture of
proteins on three lots of the
same wide-pore (300 Å)
octadecylsilyl (ODS) packing.
Solvent A: $H_2O/CH_3CN/$
trifluoroacetic acid (95:5:0.1
v/v/v). Solvent B: $H_2O/CH_3CN/$
trifluoroacetic acid (5:95:0.085
v/v/v). Gradient 85% A + 15%
B to 47% A + 53% B over
20 min. Proteins: Leucine
enkephalin (Enk), angiotensin
(Ang), Rnase (RN), insulin (In),
cytochrome C (Cy), lysozyme
(Ly), myoglobin (My) and
carbonic anhydrase (CA).
*(Reproduced with permission
from Journal of Pharmaceutical
and Biomedical Analysis.)*[10]

set at 214 nm. Peptide drugs may be contaminated with closely related peptides, which may differ by only one or two amino acids from the main peptide but may have high biological potency even when they are present in small amounts. The BP assay of human insulin includes a test for the presence of porcine insulin, which differs from human insulin by only one amino acid out of 30. The monograph stipulates that there should be a resolution of at least 1.2 between the peaks for human and porcine insulin when a test solution containing equal amounts of the two insulins is run.

Proteins may differ widely in lipophilicity depending on their amino acid composition. In the literature example shown in Figure 12.34, the reproducibility of three batches of a 300 Å ODS packing for the separation of a mixture of proteins was studied.[10] The mobile phase used was the popular system for protein analysis, utilising gradient elution with aqueous trifluoroacetic acid and acetonitrile with gradually increasing acetonitrile content. Under these conditions the most lipophilic proteins elute last.

With the increasing importance of drugs produced using biotechnology, which are mainly proteins, the pharmacopoeias have adopted a number of chromatographic methods specific to protein characterisation. To detail these methods in full would require a whole chapter; however, Table 12.9 summarises the main HPLC methods used in the quality control of protein drugs.

Table 12.9 The main high-performance liquid chromatography (HPLC) methods used in the quality control of protein drugs

Method	Description	Examples
Determination of protein impurities in bulk protein	Size exclusion chromatography using diol-modified silica gels. Proteins partition in the pores within the silica gel and high-molecular-weight (MW) species elute first	Control of high-MW proteins in somatropin, erythropoietin, aprotinin, alteplase, human and porcine insulins, size distribution in monoclonal antibodies and factor VIII. Control of low-MW heparins*
Analysis of tryptic and other proteolytic digests providing a unique fingerprint identity of the protein	Trypsin is the most widely used protease and breaks the protein down in low-MW peptides by cleaving at the C-terminus side of lysine or arginine residues, proteases with other specificities are used. The peptides are separated by reverse-phase chromatography	Fingerprint id of alteplase, somatropin, molgramostin, interferon-gamma 1b, erythropoietin, human, porcine and bovine insulins, insulin lispro, glucagon
Automated Edman degradation	The Edman degradation removes one amino acid at each cycle from the N-terminus. Separation of the amino acid derivatives is carried out by reverse-phase chromatography	Identification of the first 15 amino acids at the N-terminal of erythropoietin, alteplase and molgramostin

*Carbohydrate molecules.

Analysis of non-ionic surfactants with an evaporative light scattering detector and gradient elution

Non-ionic surfactants are used in formulations to solubilise drugs with poor water solubility; these compounds consist, in their simplest form, of an alkyl group attached to a polyethylene glycol chain. Non-ionic surfactants are usually mixtures, e.g. Cetomacrogol 1000, which has the general formula:

$$CH_3(CH_2)_m(OCH_2CH_2)_nOH$$

where m is 15 or 17 and n is 20 to 24. These compounds are amphiphilic and have affinity for water and organic solvents. Their analysis by HPLC requires a universal detector which does not require substances to have a chromophore in order to detect them. Formerly RI detectors were used for this type of analysis, but the ELSD allows gradient elution to be used, which is advantageous where complex mixtures contain compounds with widely different lipophilicities or polarities. For example, mixtures similar to Cetomacrogol 1000 have been separated on a polar aminopropyl column using a gradient between hexane/chloroform/methanol (76:19:5) and hexane/chloroform/methanol (56:14:30) over 30 min with ELSD monitoring of the eluent,[11] as shown in Figure 12.35. The methanol content of the mobile phase is gradually increased with time so that the more polar (longer chain) components elute within a reasonable time.

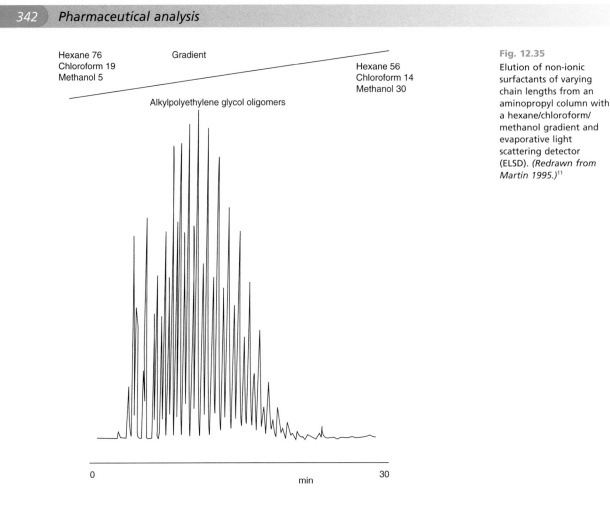

Hexane 76
Chloroform 19
Methanol 5

Gradient

Hexane 56
Chloroform 14
Methanol 30

Alkylpolyethylene glycol oligomers

0

min

30

Fig. 12.35
Elution of non-ionic surfactants of varying chain lengths from an aminopropyl column with a hexane/chloroform/methanol gradient and evaporative light scattering detector (ELSD). *(Redrawn from Martin 1995.)*[11]

Derivatisation in HPLC analysis

Derivatisation in pharmaceutical analysis is most often used to improve the selectivity of bioanalytical methods. However, in some cases it is necessary to detect compounds which lack a chromophore. The analysis of aminoglycoside antibiotics is difficult because of complete absence of a chromophore and in addition the antibiotics are usually mixtures of several components. The BP assay of neomycin eyedrops carries out an identity check on the neomycin B and neomycin C components in the eyedrops by derivatising them so that they are detectable by UV monitoring (Fig. 12.36). The polarity of the highly polar amino sugars is reduced in some degree by the derivatisation so that they can be run on a silica gel column in a mobile phase composed of chloroform and ethanol. The advantage of using silica in this case is that the excess non-polar fluorodinitrobenzene derivatising agent will elute from the column well before the polar derivatised glycosides. Derivatisation reactions have also been extensively used in the analysis of amino acids. The literature on derivatisation for HPLC is extensive, but generally the use of a suitable detector would be preferred instead of resorting to derivative formation. In recent years pulsed amperometric detection has been increasingly applied to the analysis of aminoglycosides.

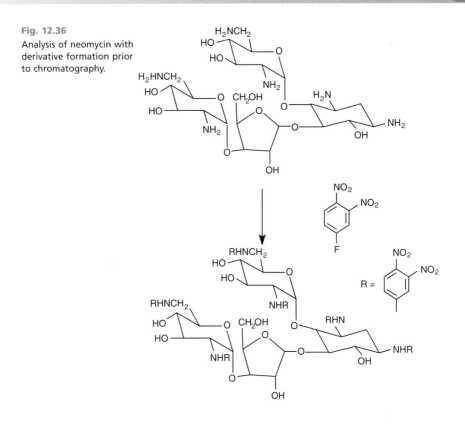

Fig. 12.36
Analysis of neomycin with derivative formation prior to chromatography.

Separation of enantiomers by chiral HPLC

Although about 40% of drugs are chiral compounds, only about 12% of drugs are administered as pure single enantiomers. This situation is gradually changing as a number of companies have now started to move toward producing enantiomerically pure forms of established drugs. Thus chromatographic separation of enantiomers is important from the point of view of quality control of enantiomerically pure drugs and also in bioanalytical studies, where the pharmacokinetics of two enantiomers may be monitored separately.

The basis of separation in chiral HPLC is the formation of temporary diastereomeric complexes within the chiral stationary phase. This causes enantiomers, which normally exhibit identical partitioning into a non-chiral stationary phase, to partition to a different extent into the stationary phase. Separation is due to the fact that enantiomers cannot interact with the three points of contact on a chiral surface in the same way. This is shown in Figure 12.37 where enantiomer 1 interacts with groups A, B and C. Its mirror image, enantiomer 2, is unable to interact in the same way with more than two of the groups on the chiral stationary phase, no matter how it is positioned.

There are numerous chiral stationary phases available commercially, which is a reflection of how difficult chiral separations can be, and there is no universal phase which will separate all types of enantiomeric pairs. Perhaps the most versatile phases are the Pirkle phases, which are based on an amino acid linked to aminopropyl silica gel via its carboxyl group and to (a-naphthyl)ethylamine via

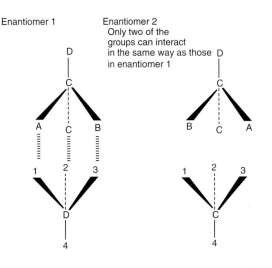

Enantiomer 1

Enantiomer 2
Only two of the groups can interact in the same way as those in enantiomer 1

Fig. 12.37
The three points of attachment model for the separation of enantiomers on chiral stationary phase.

its amino group; in the process of the condensation, a substituted urea is generated. There is a range of these types of phases. As can be seen in Figure 12.38 the interactions with phase are complex but are essentially related to the three points of contact model. Figure 12.39 shows the separation of the two pairs of enantiomers (RR, SS, and RS, SR) present in labetalol (see Ch. 2, p. 47) on Chirex 3020.

Another popular chiral HPLC phase is based on cyclodextrins anchored onto the surface of silica gel. Cyclodextrins consist of 6, 7 or 8 glucose units linked together into a ring. They adopt a barrel-like shape, and the hydrophobic portion of an analyte fits into the cavity. For good separation, the chiral centre in the molecule must be level with the chiral 2 and 3 positions of the glucose units, which are arranged around the barrel rim, and which carry hydroxyl groups that can interact with the groups attached to the chiral centre through three-point contact. Figure 12.40 shows the β-blocker propranolol included within the cyclodextrin cavity.

Other chiral phases include those based on proteins, cellulose triacetate, amino acids complexed with copper and chiral crown ethers.

Two other strategies for producing separations of enantiomers involve the addition of chiral modifiers to the mobile phase (e.g. chiral ion-pairing reagents), which can bring about separation on, for instance, an ordinary ODS column and the formation of derivatives with chirally pure reagents that produce different

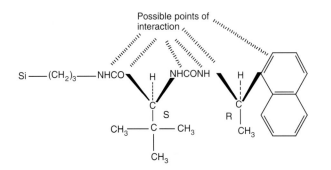

Possible points of interaction

Fig. 12.38
Potential points for asymmetric interaction with a Pirkle-type chiral high-performance liquid chromatography (HPLC) phase. Pirkle type: Chirex 3020.

Fig. 12.39
'Separation of the four
enantiomers of labetalol on
Chirex 3020. Mobile phase
hexane/1,2-dichloroethane/
ethanol (containing one part
in 20 of trifluoroacetic acid)
(60:35:5). *(Reproduced
with permission from
Phenomenex Inc., technical
document download
TN-1015, file:///C:/Users/
ConnF/Downloads/
TN-1015%20Chiral%20
HPLC%20of%20
Antimalarials.pdf Fig 1.)*

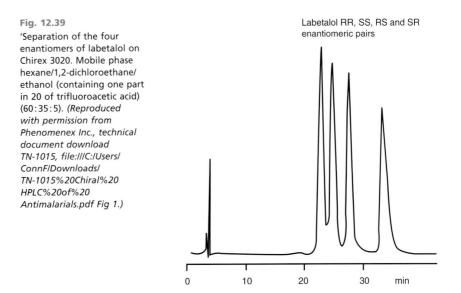

Labetalol RR, SS, RS and SR
enantiomeric pairs

diastereoisomers when reacted with opposite enantiomers of a particular compound (see GC example, Ch. 11, p. 280).

Ion chromatography

Pharmaceutical formulations usually contain a range of anions and cations in addition to the active ingredient. In order to ensure the quality of a product, tests should be carried out for these inactive components in the formulation. The columns used in this type of analysis are packed with either anion or cation exchange resins. The resins are polymeric with anionic or cationic groups on the surface that can interact with analyte ions. Typical interactions between ions and the surfaces of the resins are shown in Figure 12.41. Typical mobile phases consist of aqueous methane sulphonic acid for cation exchange and aqueous sodium hydroxide for anion exchange. Figures 12.42A and B show separations of anions and cations in two formulations. In example A, the anions are present in the

Fig. 12.40
Mechanism for chiral
separation on a
cyclodextrin phase.

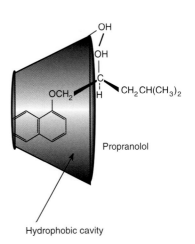

OH

OH

$CH_2CH(CH_3)_2$

OCH$_2$

Propranolol

Hydrophobic cavity

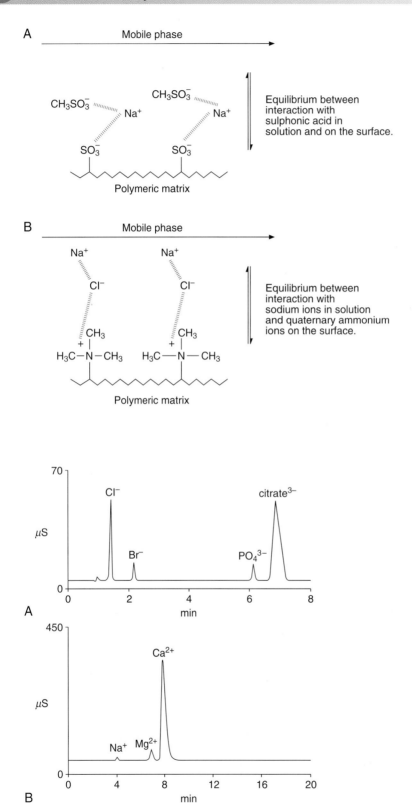

Fig. 12.41
Interactions in ion
chromatography.

Fig. 12.42
(A) Analysis of anionic counter
ions in a decongestant
formulation, mobile phase
sodium hydroxide gradient.
(B) Analysis of cationic counter
ions to excipients present in a
decongestant/antihistamine
tablet. μS = microsiemens (the
units of conductivity are
siemens). *(Reproduced with
permission from © Dionex Ltd.
from Ion Chromatography in
the Pharmaceutical Industry
Application Note 106, http://
www.dionex.com/en-us/
webdocs/4642-AN106_
LPN0660.pdf fig 9 and fig 10.)*

formulation as counter ions for the bases in the mixture, and in the tablet formulation, in example B, the cations are counter ions to commonly used excipients such as calcium phosphate, which is used as a diluent, and magnesium stearate, which is used as a mould-release agent. The greater the charge of an anion or cation, the longer its elution time, e.g. Ca^{2+} elutes after Na^+. Also, the greater the ionic radius the longer the elution time, so the larger Ca^{2+} elutes after Mg^{2+}. A conductivity detector is used for detection of anions and cations. In this type of electrochemical detection, the conductivity of the mobile phase is measured as it passes through the detector. When an anion or cation passes through the detector, conductivity increases. In order for conductivity to be measured, the anions and cations used in the mobile phase (e.g. methane sulphonic acid and sodium) are removed, prior to detection, using a chemical suppressor device that replaces them with water. This leaves the anions or cations present in the sample as the main conducting species present in solution.

Ultra-high-performance liquid chromatography

As outlined in Chapter 10 (p. 256) the column efficiency is inversely proportional to the square root of the particle size of the stationary phase. The main factor that held back the use of very small particles was the very high pressures required to pump solvent through a column packed with such particles. In recent years ultra-high-pressure pumps which can pump up to 600 bar or more have been developed, and thus particle sizes down to 1.7 μm can be used. In Figure 12.43 a van Deemter plot is shown for propranolol run on a 5 μm and a 1.7 μm column. The reduction in the contribution for the mass transfer terms and the eddy diffusion terms resulting from lower particle size results in a plot where the value for H is less affected by flow rate and the column efficiency is higher. From the plot shown in Figure 12.43 the optimum point in the van Deemter plot for the 1.7 μm column is at 3.4 times the flow rate and twice the efficiency compared with the optimum for the 5 μm column. Thus UPLC can be used to produce comparable separations to HPLC but with much shorter run time.

UPLC also produces narrower peaks, meaning that the limits of detection are lower than with HPLC. Figure 12.44 shows a comparison between analysis of a steroid cream on a 5 μm C18 column and a 1.7 μm C18 column. It can be seen

Fig. 12.43

Van Deemter plots for propranolol analysed on a 5 μm column and a 1.7 μm column. *(Redrawn with permission from Wren SAC, Tchelitcheff P. Use of ultra-performance liquid chromatography in pharmaceutical development.* J Chromatogr A *2006;1119:140–6.)*

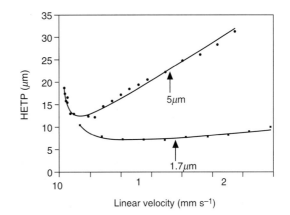

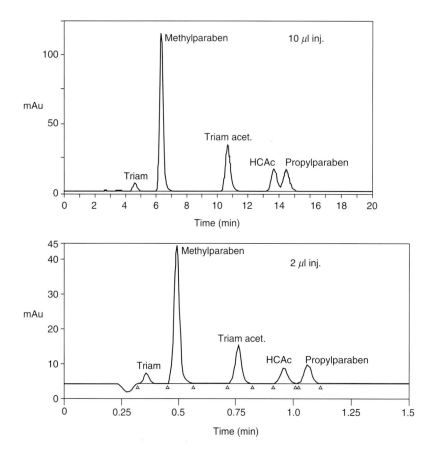

Fig. 12.44
Separation of triamcinolone acetonide in a cream from its excipients and related substances (Triam. = Triamcinolone, Triam. acet. = Triamcinolone acetonide, HCAc = hydrocortisone acetate–internal standard) by ultra-performance liquid chromatography (UPLC) and high-performance liquid chromatography (HPLC). *(Redrawn with permission from Wren SAC, Tchelitcheff P. Use of ultra-performance liquid chromatography in pharmaceutical development. J Chromatogr A 2006;1119:140–6.)*

that separation of the drug and the excipients in the cream occurs in a much shorter time on the UPLC column. Thus for new registrations of drug products it is likely that UPLC methods will become standard.

Additional problems

1. Some non-steroidal anti-inflammatory drugs (NSAIDs) were found to have the following capacity factors in a particular mobile on a reverse-phase column: aspirin 0.4, naproxen 3.6, ibuprofen 14.5, diclofenac 10.4, paracetamol 0.2. Given that the column had a t_o of 2 min, determine the retention times of the NSAIDs.

   Answers: aspirin 2.8 min; naproxen 9.2 min; ibuprofen 31 min; diclofenac 22.8 min; paracetamol 2.4 min.

2. Predict the order of elution from first to last of the following steroids from an ODS column in methanol/water (60:40) as a mobile phase (Fig. 12.32).

   Answers: triamcinolone, prednisolone, methylprednisolone, fluorometholone, fluoromethalone acetate, progesterone.

3. Predict the order of elution from first to last of the following morphinane compounds from an ODS column in an acetonitrile/buffer mixture pH 8.0 (10:90). Assume the pKa values of the bases are all similar (Fig. 12.33).

   Answer: normorphine, morphine, codeine, ethylmorphine, thebaine, benzylmorphine

   (Continued)

Additional problems (Continued)

4. An analysis is carried out on codeine linctus stated to contain 0.3% w/v of codeine phosphate. The mobile phase consists of 0.1 M acetic acid/methanol (40:60) and 0.01 M octane sulphonic acid, and chromatography is carried out on a reverse-phase column with UV monitoring at 285 nm. A one-point calibration was carried out against a calibration standard containing *ca* 0.06% w/v codeine phosphate. The following data were obtained:
   - Weight of linctus analysed = 12.7063 g
   - Density of linctus = 1.25 g/ml
   - The linctus is diluted to 50 ml with water prior to analysis
   - Area of codeine peak obtained by analysis of the linctus = 86 983
   - Area of codeine phosphate calibration peak = 84 732
   - Percentage of w/v of codeine phosphate in calibration standard = 0.06047.

   Why is the octane sulphonic acid included in the mobile phase?
   Calculate the percentage of w/v of codeine phosphate in the linctus.

   Answer: 0.3053% w/v

5. Analysis is carried out on tablets containing naproxen 100 mg and aspirin 250 mg per tablet. A narrow-range calibration curve is constructed within ± 20% of the expected concentration of the diluted tablet extract. UV monitoring of the column effluent is carried out at 278 nm. Suggest a column and mobile phase for this analysis; both aspirin and naproxen are discussed earlier in this chapter. The following data were obtained for the analysis:
   - Weight of 20 tablets = 10.3621 g
   - Weight of tablet powder assayed = 257.1 mg
   - Volume of initial extract = 250 ml.

   Dilution steps:
   - 10 to 100 ml
   - 20 to 100 ml
   - Calibration curve for naproxen $y = 174\,040\,x + 579$, r = 0.999
   - Calibration curve for aspirin $y = 54\,285\,x + 1426$, r = 0.999 where x is in mg/100 ml
   - Area of peak obtained for naproxen in diluted sample extract = 72 242
   - Area of peak obtained for aspirin in diluted sample extract = 54 819.

   Calculate the percentage of stated content for naproxen and aspirin.

   Answers: naproxen 103.7%; aspirin 99.1%

6. Analysis is carried out on a cream stated to contain 2% w/w of both miconazole and hydrocortisone. An ODS column is used with a mobile phase consisting of acetonitrile/acetate buffer pH 4.0 (70:30) and the eluent is monitored at 220 nm. A narrow-range calibration curve, within ± 20% of the expected concentration of each analyte in the sample extract, was prepared for each analyte by plotting the ratio of the areas of the analyte peaks against fixed amounts of the internal standards for both analytes. The internal standards used were econazole and hydrocortisone 21-acetate, for miconazole and hydrocortisone, respectively.

   How would the retention time of hydrocortisone compare in the mobile phase used in this assay with a mobile phase containing methanol/acetate buffer pH 4.0 (70:30), and why do you think hydrocortisone 21-acetate is used as an internal standard rather than the betamethasone used in the assay discussed earlier in this chapter?

   Suggest a suitable extraction procedure for extracting the analytes from the cream and for removing oily excipients, and indicate any other preparation which might be required prior to analysis.

   The following data were obtained:
   - Weight of cream taken for assay = 1.0223 g
   - Final volume of extract from cream = 100 ml
   - Equation of line for miconazole $y = 0.044\,x - 0.013$, r = 0.999
   - Equation of line for hydrocortisone $y = 0.048\,x - 0.024$, r = 0.999

   where x is in mg/100 ml
   - Area of hydrocortisone peak in sample extract = 62 114
   - Area of hydrocortisone acetate peak in sample extract = 64 452
   - Area of miconazole peak in sample extract = 35 557
   - Area of econazole peak in sample extract = 38 385.

   Calculate the percentage of w/v of miconazole and hydrocortisone in the cream.

   Answers: hydrocortisone 2.013% w/w; miconazole 2.088% w/w

References

1. Meyer VR. *Practical High Performance Liquid Chromatography*. Chichester: J. Wiley and Sons; 1994.
2. Robards K, Haddad PR, Jackson PE. *Principles and Practice of Modern Chromatography*. London: London Academic Press Inc; 1994.
3. Lunn G, Schmuff N. *HPLC Methods for Pharmaceutical Analysis*. Chichester: Wiley Interscience; 1997.
4. Riley CM, Lough WJ, Wainer IW. *Pharmaceutical and Biomedical Applications of Liquid Chromatography*. Amsterdam: Elsevier; 1994.
5. Snyder LR, Kirkland JJ. *Practical HPLC Method Development*. Chichester: Wiley Interscience; 1997.
6. Barbosa J, Sanznebot V. Standard pH values in non-aqueous mobile phases used in reversed-phase liquid chromatography. *Anal Chim Acta*. 1993;283:320-325.
7. Kaibara A, Hirose M, Nakagawa T. Retention characteristics of octadecylsilyl silica, trimethylsilyl silica and phenyldimethylsilyl silica in reversed-phase liquid chromatography. *Chromatographia*. 1990;30:99-104.
8. Euerby MR, Petersson P. Chromatographic classification and comparison of commercially available reversed-phase liquid chromatographic columns using principal component analysis. *J Chromatogr*. 2003;994:13-36.
9. Alpert AJ. Hydrophilic-interaction chromatography for the separation of peptides, nucleic acids and other polar compounds. *J Chromatogr*. 1990;499:177.
10. Ricker RD, Sandoval LA, Permar BJ, Boyes BE. Improved reversed-phase high performance liquid chromatography columns for biopharmaceutical analysis. *J Pharm Biomed Anal*. 1995;14:93-105.
11. Martin N. Analysis of nonionic surfactants by HPLC using evaporative light scattering detector. *J Liquid Chromatogr*. 1995;18:1173-1194.

Further reading

Christodoulou EA. An overview of HPLC methods for the enantiomer separation of active pharmaceutical ingredients in bulk and drug formulations. *Curr Org Chem*. 2010;14:2337-2347.

De Brabander HF, Noppea H, Verheyden K, et al. Residue analysis: future trends from a historical perspective. *J Chromatogr A*. 2009;1216:7964-7976.

Guillarme D, Ruta J, Rudaz S, Veuthey JL. New trends in fast and high-resolution liquid chromatography: a critical comparison of existing approaches. *Anal Bioanal Chem*. 2010;397:1069-1082.

Jandera P. Stationary and mobile phases in hydrophilic interaction chromatography: a review. *Anal Chim Acta*. 2011;692:1-25.

Kupiec T, Slawson M, Pragst F, Herzler M. *Clarke's Analysis of Drugs and Poisons*. London: Pharmaceutical Press; 2004:500-534.

Liu DQ, Sun M, Kord AS. Recent advances in trace analysis of pharmaceutical genotoxic impurities. *J Pharma Biomed Anal*. 2010;51:999-1014.

Pieters S, Dejaegher B, Heyden YV. Emerging analytical separation techniques with high throughput potential for pharmaceutical analysis, Part I: stationary phase and instrumental developments in LC. *Comb Chem High Throughput Screen*. 2010;13:510-529.

Wren SAC, Tchelitcheff P. Use of ultra-performance liquid chromatography in pharmaceutical development. *J Chromatogr A*. 2006;1119:140-146.

www.agilent.com

One of the premier manufacturers of HPLC equipment. Many application notes on the use of HPLC in pharmaceutical analysis.

www.dionex.com

Contains a lot of information on ion chromatography.

www.separationsnow.com

A fairly new website containing much background material on various separation techniques.

www.chromatographyonline.findanalytichem.com.

13

Thin-layer chromatography

KEYPOINTS

Principles

- An analyte migrates up or across a layer of stationary phase (most commonly silica gel), under the influence of a mobile phase (usually a mixture of organic solvents), which moves through the stationary phase by capillary action. The distance moved by the analyte is determined by its relative affinity for the stationary vs the mobile phase.

Applications

- Used to determine impurities in pharmaceutical raw materials and formulated products.
- Often used as a basic identity check on pharmaceutical raw materials.
- Potentially useful in cleaning validation, which is part of the manufacture of pharmaceuticals.

Strengths

- Detection by chemical reaction with a visualisation reagent can be carried out, which means that more or less every type of compound can be detected if a suitable detection reagent is used.
- Robust and cheap.
- In conjunction with densitometric detection, it can be used as a quantitative technique for compounds which are difficult to analyse by other chromatographic methods because of the absence of a chromophore.
- Since all the components in the chromatographic system can be seen, there is no risk, as is the case in gas chromatography (GC) and HPLC analyses, that some components are not observed because they do not elute from the chromatographic system.
- Batch chromatography can be used to analyse many samples at once, increasing the speed of analysis, and can be automated.
- The method is flexible since thin-layer chromatography (TLC) plates can be simply treated with a variety of chemicals, thus imparting a wide range of properties to the stationary phase.

(Continued)

> **KEYPOINTS** *(Continued)*
>
> **Limitations**
> - The number of theoretical plates available for separation is limited in routine TLC systems, although high-performance TLC (HPTLC) plates can offer nearly the same efficiency in a 10 cm distance as an HPLC column of the same length.
> - Sensitivity is often limited.
> - Not suitable for volatile compounds.
> - Requires more operator skill for optimal use than HPLC.

Introduction

Thin-layer chromatography (TLC) has developed into a very sophisticated technique for identification of compounds and for determination of the presence of trace impurities. Since it was one of the earliest chromatographic techniques, a huge array of TLC-based tests is available and pharmacopoeial monographs reflect the extent to which this technique has been developed as a fundamental quality control technique for trace impurities. The reason for its prominence in this regard is due to its flexibility in being able to detect almost any compound, even some inorganic compounds. Following TLC, the entire chromatogram can be seen, and thus there is no doubt over whether or not components in a sample have failed to elute from a chromatographic system, as is the case with HPLC and GC and even capillary electrophoresis (CE). In this short chapter it would be impossible to outline all of the tests that can be used; comprehensive reviews of the technique have been written.[1,2] Even the most advanced form of TLC, high-performance TLC (HPTLC), remains essentially a simple technique. The sophistication in the application of the technique derives from the broad choice of stationary phases, mobile phases and the wide range of spray reagents which can be used for visualising the chromatogram.

The advances in the technology of the technique have been recently reviewed,[3] and these include the use of high-pressure TLC and interfacing with detection systems such as Raman spectroscopy and mass spectrometry.

Instrumentation

Figure 13.1 shows a simple thin-layer chromatography apparatus (see Animation 13.1). The most frequently used system is a glass or plastic plate coated with silica gel; for routine applications the silica gel particle size is in the range 2–25 μm. The method of use for this system is as follows:

(i)   A few μl of sample solution are slowly spotted onto the plate at the origin. If more than *ca* 1 μl is applied at once, the spot will spread too far. The spot has to be allowed to dry between each application of 1 μl. Loadings of sample are typically 20 μg.

(ii) The bottom 0.5 cm of the plate is immersed in the mobile phase contained in a tank, and the liquid mobile phase is allowed to travel up the silica gel plate by capillary action.

(iii) The more polar a compound is the more it adsorbs (partitions into) the silica gel stationary phase, the less time it spends in the mobile phase as it

Fig. 13.1
Basic apparatus for thin-layer chromatography.

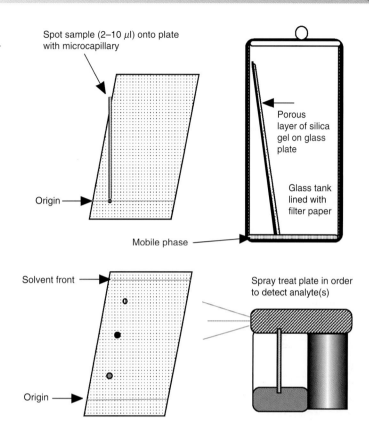

Spot sample (2–10 μl) onto plate with microcapillary

Porous layer of silica gel on glass plate

Glass tank lined with filter paper

Origin

Mobile phase

Solvent front

Spray treat plate in order to detect analyte(s)

Origin

travels up the plate and thus the shorter the distance it travels up the plate in a given time. (see Animation 13.2)

TLC chromatogram

A diagram of a typical thin-layer chromatography plate after development and spraying to locate the analytes is shown in Figure 13.2.

Fig. 13.2
Simple TLC chromatogram with silica gel used as the stationary phase.

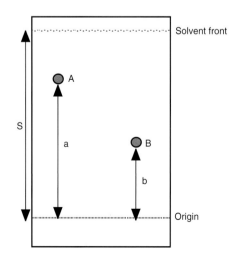

Solvent front

A

S

a

B

b

Origin

In Figure 13.2, compound A is less polar than compound B since it travels further with the mobile phase in the same time. The distance travelled by the compound from the origin (where the compound is put onto the plate) divided by the distance travelled by the solvent from the origin is called the 'Rf value' of the compound. For example, for compound A, Rf = a/S; for compound B, Rf = b/S; the Rf is usually quoted as a Rf × 100 value. The area/intensity of a spot on a TLC plate is logarithmically related to the concentration of the analyte producing it.

Self-test 13.1

Solvent is allowed to move 10 cm from the origin up a TLC plate. The time taken to develop the plate for this distance is 15 min. On the basis of this information, complete the table below.

Distance moved by analyte	Rf × 100 value	Time spent in mobile phase	Time spent in stationary phase
(i) 8 cm			
(ii) 6 cm			
(iii) 4 cm			

Answers: (i) 80, 12, 3; (ii) 60, 9, 6; (iii) 40, 6, 9

Stationary phases

Silica gel (Fig. 13.3) is the most commonly used adsorbant for TLC. The rate at which compounds migrate up a silica gel plate depends on their polarity. In a given length of time, the most polar compounds move the least distance up the plate while the least polar move the farthest (Fig 13.4).

Although silica gel is used widely, some other polar stationary phases are also used in pharmacopoeial tests; silica gel may also be used in modified form. Some examples of stationary phases are given in Table 13.1.

Elutropic series and mobile phases

As described in Chapter 12, the strength of a mobile phase depends on the particular solvent mixture used. Table 13.2 lists common solvents in order of increasing polarity. The more polar a solvent or solvent mixture, the farther it will move a polar compound up a silica gel TLC plate. When non-polar compounds are

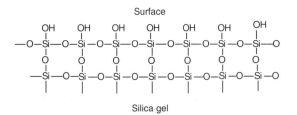

Surface

Silica gel

Fig. 13.3
The surface of silica gel.

Fig. 13.4
Migration steroids on a silica gel
TLC plate.

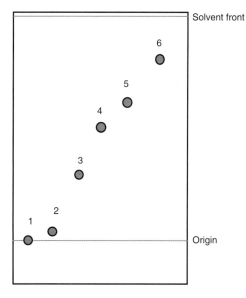

Solvent front

Origin

Table 13.1 Stationary phases which are commonly used in TLC

Stationary phase	Description	Applications
Silica gel G	Silica gel with average particle size 15 μm containing *ca* 13% calcium sulphate binding agent	Use in a wide range of pharmacopoeial tests. In practice commercial plates may be used which contain a different type of binder
Silica gel GF$_{254}$	Silica gel G with fluorescent agent added	The same types of applications as silica G where visualisation is to be carried out under UV light
Cellulose	Cellulose powder of less than 30 μm particle size	Identification of tetracyclines
Keiselguhr G	Diatomaceous earth containing calcium sulphate binder	Used as a solid support for stationary phases such as liquid paraffin used in analysis of fixed oils

---

Table 13.2 Elutropic series

Solvent	Polarity index
Hexane (C_6H_{14})	0
Toluene (C_7H_8)	2.4
Diethylether ($C_4H_{10}O$)	2.8
Dichloromethane (CH_2Cl_2)	3.1
Butanol (C_4H_9OH)	3.9
Chloroform ($CHCl_3$)	4.1
Ethyl acetate ($C_2H_5COOCH_3$)	4.4
Acetone (CH_3COCH_3)	5.1
Methanol (CH_3OH)	5.1
Ethanol (C_2H_5OH)	5.2
Acetonitrile (CH_3CN)	5.8
Acetic acid (CH_3COOH)	6.2
Water (H_2O)	9.0

being analysed, there will not be a marked increase in the distance migrated with increasing polarity of the mobile phase since they migrate toward the solvent front under most conditions. Although water is polar, there are practical difficulties in using pure water as a solvent since many organic compounds are not very soluble in water; thus it is usually used in mobile phases containing a water-miscible organic solvent such as methanol. Quite subtle changes in separation can be achieved by using complex mixtures of solvents. Because of its simplicity, TLC is often used as a preliminary screen for identifying drugs, and thus mobile phases have been developed which ensure that a particular drug will have a quite different Rf value in one system compared with another.

Self-test 13.2

The steroids below are spotted onto a silica gel TLC plate. The plate is developed in methylene chloride/ether/methanol/water (77 : 15 : 8 : 1.2) and under UV light has the appearance shown in Figure 13.4. From your knowledge of the polarity of organic molecules, match the steroids to the spots on the TLC plate shown in Figure 13.4.

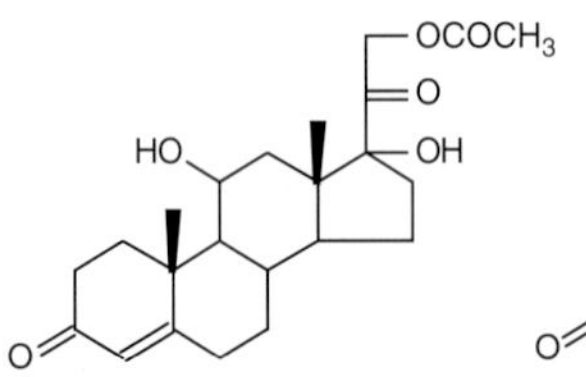

Hydrocortisone acetate

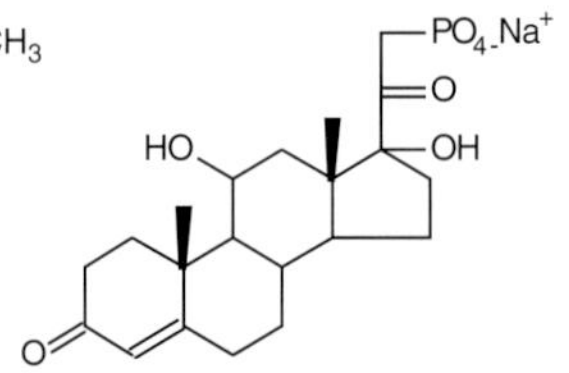

Hydrocortisone sodium phosphate

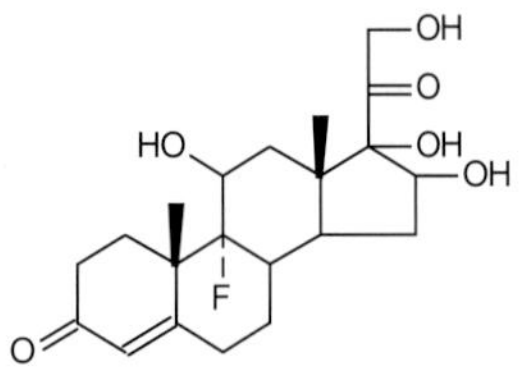

Triamcinolone

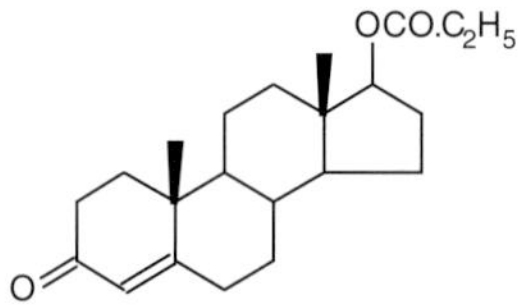

Testosterone propionate

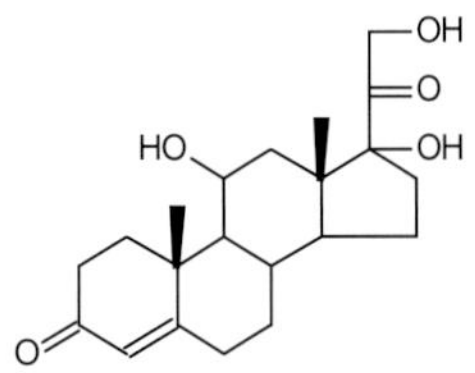

Hydrocortisone

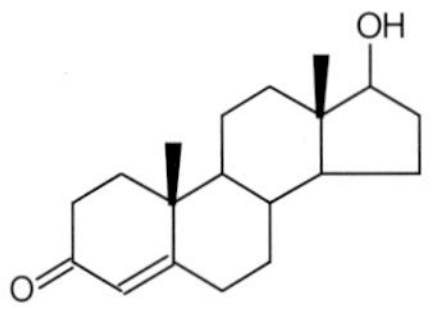

Testosterone

Answer: 1. hydrocortisone sodium phosphate; 2. triamcinolone; 3. hydrocortisone; 4. hydrocortisone acetate; 5. testosterone; 6. testosterone propionate

---

For example, in a general screen for acidic drugs, which includes most of the NSAIDs (Fig. 13.5), three mobile phases may be used.[1] Table 13.3 shows the Rf values obtained for three NSAIDs in three different mobile phases. It can be seen from the data in Table 13.3 that, even for closely related structures, slight differences in polarity and lipophilicity can be exploited to produce separation. For

Fig. 13.5
Some NSAIDs.

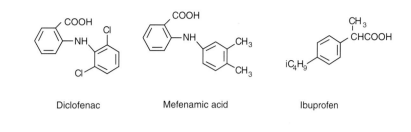

Diclofenac   Mefenamic acid   Ibuprofen

Table 13.3			
Mobile phase	**Diclofenac Rf**	**Mefenamic acid Rf**	**Ibuprofen Rf**
1. Chloroform/acetone (4:1)	25	41	46
2. Ethyl acetate	40	54	54
3. Ethyl acetate/methanol/ strong ammonia solution (80:10:10)	29	32	18

instance, ibuprofen is the least polar drug in system 1 but is the most polar drug in system 3, where the carboxyl groups in the structures will be ionised due to the ammonia in the mobile phase. It can also be seen that the polarity of a mobile phase containing a mixture of chloroform and acetone is similar to that of pure ethyl acetate.

The range of general TLC tests available for different classes of drugs has recently been reviewed.[4]

Self-test 13.3

Considering the three solvent systems (1, 2 and 3) given in Table 13.3, indicate which set of Rf values is most likely to apply to naproxen.

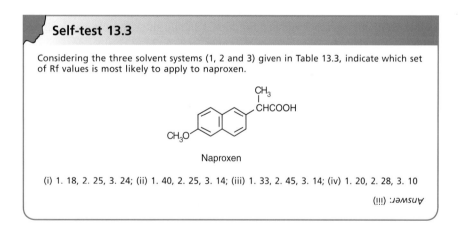

Naproxen

(i) 1. 18, 2. 25, 3. 24; (ii) 1. 40, 2. 25, 3. 14; (iii) 1. 33, 2. 45, 3. 14; (iv) 1. 20, 2. 28, 3. 10

Answer: (iii)

Modification of TLC adsorbant
Treatment of silica gel with KOH

For analysis of basic compounds, silica gel which has been sprayed with a solution of KOH in methanol may be used. Treating the plate with base ensures that basic compounds chromatograph as their free bases rather than as their salts. The salts of the amines have very low mobility in organic-solvent-based mobile phases since basic compounds tend to interact strongly with silanol groups on the surface of the silica; the presence of KOH in the stationary phase suppresses this interaction. The mobile phases used in these type of systems also typically contain a basic component. Examples of the mobile phases used for the analysis of basic drugs on KOH-impregnated silica gel include:

(i)   Methanol/strong ammonia solution (100 : 1.5)
(ii) Cyclohexane/toluene/diethylamine (75 : 15 : 10)
(iii) Chloroform/methanol (90 : 10).

System 2 is quite non-polar and useful for discriminating between highly lipophilic bases, which include many of the antihistamines and narcotics, and sympathomimetic bases, which are often quite polar and move very little in mobile phase 2. The use of selective solvent systems is often combined with use of location agents that are selective for nitrogenous drugs.

Silanised silica gel

The surface of the silica gel can be rendered non-polar by reaction with dichlorodimethylsilane, as shown in Figure 13.6. A wide range of silanising reagents can be used in this type of reaction including octadecylsilanes, which produce ODS silica gel plates analogous to ODS HPLC columns. The BP uses silanised silica gel TLC plates in identity tests for penicillins. For example, a 0.25% w/v solution of ampicillin test material is applied to a silanised silica gel plate along with an ampicillin reference standard (0.25% w/v), Solution 2, and a mixture containing reference standards for ampicillin and amoxycillin trihydrate (0.25% w/v), Solution 3. The plate is developed with a mobile phase consisting of a solution of ammonium acetate adjusted to pH 5.0 with acetic acid and acetone (90 : 10). After development, the plate is stained with iodine vapour; the identity test specifies that the test substance should give a single spot with the same Rf as that seen for Solution 2 and that Solution 3 should show two clearly separated spots.

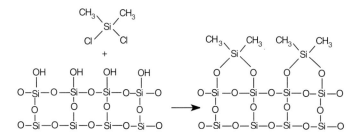

Fig. 13.6
Silanisation of silica gel with dichlorodimethylsilane.

This type of test could be carried out equally well with commercially produced ODS plates. Silica gel plates can be simply modified with reaction with organosilane reagents; the availability of a wide range of reactive organosilanes means that there is potential for producing a wide range of coated TLC plates for specific purposes.

Keiselguhr as an inert support

Keiselguhr in itself does not have strong absorptive properties, but it can be coated with a liquid or waxy stationary phase. The keiselguhr coated with liquid paraffin is used in a pharmacopoeial test for triglycerides and fatty acids in fixed oils. The keiselguhr plate is impregnated with a solution containing liquid paraffin in petroleum ether. This renders the surface hydrophobic. The samples of fixed oil being examined are applied to the plate, and the plate is developed with acetic acid as the mobile phase. Acetic acid is a very polar solvent, and thus the liquid paraffin stationary phase does not dissolve in it appreciably. Furthermore, the triglycerides in the fixed oil are only weakly polar and will partition usefully between the liquid paraffin stationary phase and the acetic acid mobile phase. The longer the chain length of the fatty acids in the triglyceride, the lower the Rf of the triglyceride. The plate is visualised by staining with iodine and then permanently staining the iodine spots with starch solution. The BP shows the typical chromatograms that would be obtained from a number of fixed oils which are composed of mixtures of triglycerides in different proportions. The triglyceride composition of a particular fixed oil does not vary greatly and is very characteristic. A similar test to the one described above is carried out for the fatty acids composing the oil following hydrolysis of the triglycerides.

Other agents used to impregnate keiselguhr include formamide and propan-1,2-diol. In the case of these impregnating agents, the mobile phases used to develop the treated plates have to be of low polarity to avoid washing the agent off the plate.

Detection of compounds on TLC plates following development

A wide range of methods can be used to detect compounds on a TLC plate following its development with a mobile phase.

Ultraviolet light

In order to observe the absorption of UV light by an analyte, silica gel which has been impregnated with a fluorescent material is used to prepare the TLC plate. Light with a wavelength of 254 nm is used to illuminate the plate, and if the analyte absorbs UV light it can be seen as a black spot on a yellow background where it quenches the fluorescence of the background. This method of visualisation is used in many pharmacopoeial tests since most drugs possess chromophores. If a compound is naturally fluorescent, longer wavelength light at 365 nm may be used to visualise the plate. For example, the pharmacopoeial test for anthraquinones in aloes observes the fluorescence of these compounds under UV light at 365 nm.

Location reagents

There is a huge number of location reagents available, and these reagents range from those which are fairly specific for a particular type of analyte to those which will detect many different compounds.

Iodine vapour

The plate is put into a tank containing iodine crystals. This treatment will produce brown spots with many organic compounds; the staining is reversible, so if it is necessary to recover the compound once it has been located, the iodine may be allowed to evaporate by exposing the plate to air, and then the marked spot containing the compound of interest may be scraped off the plate. If a permanent record of the plate is required, it has to be covered to prevent the iodine evaporating, or the iodine spots may be sprayed with starch solution in order to stain them permanently. Iodine is used as a location agent in pharmacopoeial TLC tests of fixed oils and of cetrimide.

Potassium permanganate

Potassium permanganate provides a method for the detection of sugars and sugar-like molecules and drugs with aliphatic double bonds. It is used in TLC identity checks for the antibacterial agents clindamycin and lincomycin and in a check for related substances in spectinomycin.

Ninhydrin solution

This reagent gives pink spots with primary amines and yellow spots with tertiary amines. It is used in pharmacopoeial identity tests for some of the aminoglycoside antibiotics such as gentamycin, in a limit test for aminobutanol in ethambutol and can be used as a general screen for nitrogen-containing drugs in conjunction with Dragendorff reagent. Dragendorff reagent will produce orange spots with tertiary amines and may be used to overspray plates which have been sprayed in the first instance with ninhydrin.

Alkaline tetrazolium blue

This reagent is quite specific for corticosteroids, producing blue spots on a white background. The tetrazolium spray is used in a test for related foreign steroids in fluclorolone acetonide.

Ethanol/sulphuric acid 20%

This reagent is used to produce fluorescent spots from corticosteroids such as dexamethasone or prednisolone by spraying the plate, heating to 120°C and then observing the plate under UV light at 365 nm.

Applications of TLC analysis

Qualitative identity tests

TLC is often used by BP monographs as part of a number of identity tests performed on pure substances. For extra confirmation of identity, more than one solvent system may be used and also different types of spray reagents may be used. Some examples of identity checks based on TLC have been mentioned earlier. Table 13.4 lists a few of the compounds which have their identity checked by TLC, and a variety of location reagents and mobile phases are used to illustrate the fact that there is much less uniformity about TLC methodology than there is in the case of HPLC or GLC methodology.

Limit tests

Where the structure of the impurity is known

TLC is used to perform limit tests for impurities in many pharmacopoeial monographs. A TLC limit test is based on comparison between a concentrated solution of an analyte and a dilute solution of an impurity. The intensities of the spots due to any impurities in the analyte are compared with the intensity of a spot or spots due to standards spotted separately onto the same plate. For the purposes of the examples illustrated as follows, intensity and size are regarded as being interchangeable, which they are to a large extent. For instance, a limit test might be

Table 13.4 Some examples of identity tests based on TLC described in pharmacopoeial monographs

Substance examined	Stationary phase	Mobile phase	Visualisation reagent	Comments
Framycetin sulphate	Silica gel + carbomer binder	10% w/v KH_2PO_4	Naphthalene diol/H_2SO_4	Rf and colour of the sample are compared with a pure standard. The resolution of the analyte from streptomycin is checked
Methyl prednisolone	Silica gel GF_{254}	Ether/toluene/ butan-1-ol saturated with water (85:10:5)	UV light 254 nm then ethanolic sulphuric acid (20%) + heat to 120°C	Rf and colours of the sample and standard are compared. Also Rf of an oxidation product is used as an additional check
Aprotinin	Silica gel	Acetate buffer	Ninhydrin spray	Rf and colour of the analyte spot is compared with standard
Levamisole	Silica gel H with fluorescent indicator	Toluene/ acetone/ 13.5 M ammonia (60:40:1)	UV light 254 nm	Rf and size of the spot obtained is matched to that of a standard.
Pentagastrin	Silica gel G	Analyte is examined by TLC in three different mobile phases	4-dimethyl-aminobenz-aldehyde in methanol/ HCl	The Rf of the analyte in three different mobile phases is determined and the colour of its spot is matched to that of the standard

conducted for hydrocortisone in hydrocortisone acetate as follows: 5 μl of 1% w/v solution of hydrocortisone acetate is spotted onto the origin of a TLC plate; at another position on the plate, 5 μl of a 0.01% w/v of hydrocortisone is spotted on. The TLC plate is developed in the solvent described in Self-test 13.2 and might appear as shown in Figure 13.7 when viewed under UV light. In the example shown, a small amount of hydrocortisone impurity can be seen running below the large spot due to hydrocortisone acetate, which is the main component in the sample. In line with the position where the hydrocortisone standard was spotted onto the plate, there is a very faint spot. In this case the spot for the hydrocortisone impurity in the sample can be seen to be more intense (larger)

Fig. 13.7
TLC limit test for hydrocortisone in hydrocortisone acetate.

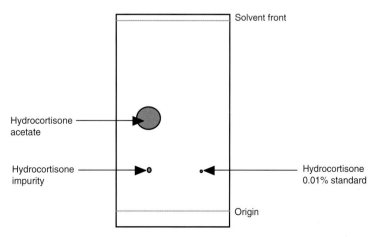

than the spot due to the 0.01% w/v hydrocortisone standard, and thus the sample has failed the limit test. This test is a 1% limit test since $0.01/1 \times 100 = 1\%$.

Self-test 13.4

A limit test is conducted for hydrocortisone in hydrocortisone sodium phosphate. 2 µl of a 1% w/v solution of hydrocortisone sodium phosphate is compared with 2 µl of a solution containing 0.02% w/v hydrocortisone standard using the solvent system given in Self-test 13.2.

(i) What is the percentage limit for hydrocortisone in hydrocortisone sodium phosphate set by this test?
(ii) Would the spot for the impurity appear above or below the substance being examined? (See Self-test 13.2.)

Answers: (i) 2%; (ii) Above

Table 13.5 shows some BP limit tests for known impurities used in pharmacopoeial monographs.

As in the case of hydrocortisone acetate, where hydrocortisone might be expected to occur as a result of hydrolysis of the acetate ester, tests for the presence of known impurities are based on the known manufacturing sequence or on likely degradation pathways. For example, the tests carried out on clotrimazole are based on the last step in its manufacture, as shown in Figure 13.8. Unreacted imidazole is an obvious impurity, and chlorotritanol would be readily formed from unreacted chlorotrityl bromide by hydrolysis, which would occur when the clotrimazole is extracted from the reaction mixture.

Most of the examples given in Table 13.5 have similar obvious origins in the drug manufacturing process.

Table 13.5 BP limit tests for known impurities in pharmaceutical raw materials

Test substance	Impurity	Limit set (%)
Clotrimazole	Chlorotritanol	0.2
Clotrimazole	Imidazole	0.2
Cyclizine	N-methylpiperazine	0.5
Dexpanthenol	3-aminopropanol	0.5
Ethinylestradiol	Estrone	1.0
Loprazolam mesylate	N-methylpiperazine	0.25
Mefenamic acid	2,3-dimethyl aniline	0.01
Mexiletine hydrochloride	2,6-dimethyl phenol	0.2
Phenoxymethylpenicillin	Phenylacetic acid	0.5

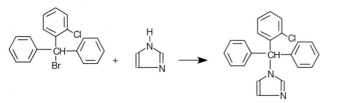

Fig. 13.8 Synthesis of clotrimazole.

Chlorotrityl bromide   Imidazole   Clotrimazole

Where the structure of the impurity is unknown

A related type of TLC limit test is carried out where the identities of impurities are not completely certain. This type of test is used, for instance, on compounds of natural origin or partly natural origin, which may contain a range of compounds related in structure to the test substance which are co-extracted with the raw starting material. For example, the range of synthetic steroids originates from triterpenoids extracted from plants, which are extensively modified by fermentation and chemical synthesis.

The assumption which is made in the type of test described following is that the related unknown substances will produce a similar intensity of spot to the test substance itself at equal concentrations. For example, a limit test is conducted for related (foreign) alkaloids in codeine, which is extracted from the opium poppy, in which a range of alkaloids occurs: thus, the exact identity of the impurities may not be known. To conduct the test, 10 μl amounts of three solutions are applied separately to a TLC plate. The solutions contain 4.0% w/v codeine (Solution 1), 0.06% w/v codeine (Solution 2) and 0.04% w/v codeine (Solution 3). In the test, the dilute solutions of codeine are used as visual comparators for any impurities in the sample. The plate is developed in ethanol/cyclohexane/13.5 M ammonia (72:30:6), is dried and is then sprayed with iodobismuthate reagent, which is specific for nitrogenous drugs. After development and spraying, the plate might look like the diagram shown in Figure 13.9. The conditions set by the limit test are that:

(i)   There should be no secondary spot in the chromatogram of Solution 1 which is more intense than the spot obtained with Solution 2.

(ii) There should be no more than one secondary spot with an Rf value higher than that of codeine which is more intense than the spot obtained with Solution 3.

In this test, two limits are being set: $0.06/4 \times 100 = 1.5\%$ and $0.04/4 \times 100 = 1.0\%$.

This type of test can be a little confusing at first since there are a number of permutations that can lead to the sample passing or failing of the test.

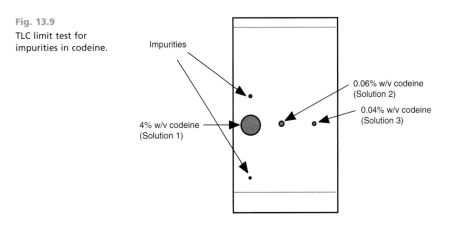

Fig. 13.9
TLC limit test for impurities in codeine.

Impurities

4% w/v codeine (Solution 1)

0.06% w/v codeine (Solution 2)

0.04% w/v codeine (Solution 3)

Self-test 13.5

Three samples of codeine are analysed as described earlier. Indicate whether the TLC limit tests shown below pass or fail the samples. Solutions 1–3 appear in numerical order from left to right.

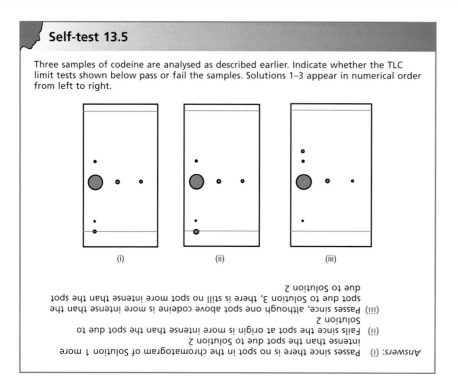

(i)   (ii)   (iii)

Answers: (i) Passes since there is no spot in the chromatogram of Solution 1 more intense than the spot due to Solution 2

(ii) Fails since the spot at origin is more intense than the spot due to Solution 2

(iii) Passes since, although one spot above codeine is more intense than the spot due to Solution 3, there is still no spot more intense than the spot due to Solution 2

Tests in which known and unknown standards are used

Table 13.6 shows some of the other limit tests set in pharmacopoeial monographs, ranging from a simple test for a known impurity to tests in which limits are set for more than one known impurity plus any unknown impurities which might be present.

Perhaps the most detailed pharmacopoeial limit test of this nature is carried out on tetracycline, where a 1% w/v solution is spotted onto the TLC plate with solutions of five structurally related tetracyclines ranging in concentration from 0.02 to 0.005% w/v.

Table 13.6 Some examples of pharmacopoeial limit tests

Analyte solution (Solution 1)	Limit test (Solution 2)	Limit test (Solution 3)	Limit test (Solution 4)
10% w/v procaine.HCl	No secondary spot > 0.005% w/v p-amino benzoic acid	–	–
1% w/v triamcinolone acetonide	No secondary spot > 0.02% w/v triamcinolone acetonide	No other spots > 0.01% w/v triamcinolone acetonide	–
2% w/v promethazine.HCl	No secondary spot > 0.02% w/v isopromethazine.HCl	No other spots > 0.01% w/v promethazine.HCl	–
1% w/v chloramphenicol palmitate	No spot with the same Rf > 0.02% w/v chloramphenicol palmitate isomer	No spot with the same Rf > 0.02% w/v chloramphenicol dipalmitate	No other spots > 0.005% w/v chloramphenicol palmitate

High-performance TLC (HPTLC)

HPTLC is conducted on TLC plates which are coated with purified silica gel with a particle range of 2–10 μm, as opposed to 2–25 μm for standard commercial TLC plates. The narrower particle size range means that a greater number of theoretical plates are available for separation, and thus the spots on the TLC plate remain tighter. These type of plates may be run in a standard type of TLC tank, but optimal performance is obtained from horizontal development of the plates using apparatus of the type shown in Figure 13.10.

The advantages of horizontal development are:

(i)   The mobile phase moves more quickly.
(ii) The proximity of the plate's surface to a saturating solution of mobile phase means that there is little evaporation of solvent from the surface of the plate, which in the case of vertical development can change the composition of the mobile phase as it moves up the plate.
(iii) In the vertical position, if the plate is not in a saturated atmosphere, solvent at the edge of the plate tends to evaporate, drawing solvent from the centre of the plate and causing the solvent at the edge of the plate to migrate more quickly. This does not occur when horizontal development is used.

Fig. 13.10
Apparatus for HPTLC.

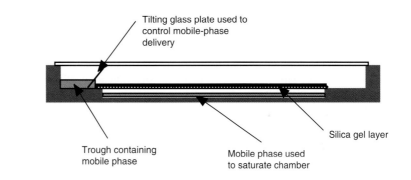

Tilting glass plate used to control mobile-phase delivery

Silica gel layer

Trough containing mobile phase

Mobile phase used to saturate chamber

Applications of HPTLC

It is possible to use TLC as a quantitative method by using a densitometer to read spot intensity. Quantitative TLC is best carried out using high-performance systems. Densitometers can be used to quantify components in a sample on the basis of fluorescence or absorption of UV light. As discussed above, there are a number of advantages in using TLC and a major advantage is the ability to run batches of samples, which gives it an advantage over HPLC. HPTLC with fluorescence densitometry has been applied to the analysis of pharmacologically active thiols including the ACE inhibitor captopril.[5] Compounds such as captopril do not have a strong chromophore and thus require derivatisation to render them detectable, and this would be true whether HPLC or HPTLC were being used. In this example, the thiols were reacted with a thiol-specific reagent which produced fluorescent derivatives (Fig. 13.11) and were then analysed by TLC. Limits of detection for these compounds by this method were in the low picogram range.

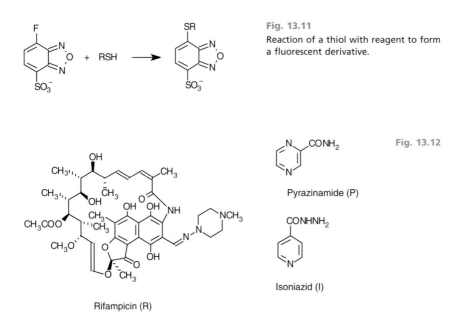

Fig. 13.11
Reaction of a thiol with reagent to form a fluorescent derivative.

Fig. 13.12

Pyrazinamide (P)

Isoniazid (I)

Rifampicin (R)

An HPTLC assay for rifampicin (R), isoniazid (I) and pyrazinamide (P) (Fig. 13.12) in a single dosage form was reported.[6] Pharmacopoeial methods only allow for the determination of each analyte in separate dosage forms. The HPTLC method was also able to resolve rifampicin from two of its named impurities. The analytes were quantified by densitometry by measuring absorbance at two different wavelengths. The precisions reported for quantification of the analytes were $R \pm 1.73$, $I \pm 1.58$ and $P \pm 1.07$, which compared quite favourably with an HPLC method for the same dosage form. Figure 13.13 shows a densitogram for R, its related substances, desacetyl rifampicin (DAR) and rifampicin quinone (RQ), and I and P. Thus HPTLC can be used for the quantitative analysis of mixtures which include large and complex molecules such as rifampicin.

It would be possible to run many current pharmaceutical limit tests with a much higher degree of accuracy and precision if HPTLC methods were used.

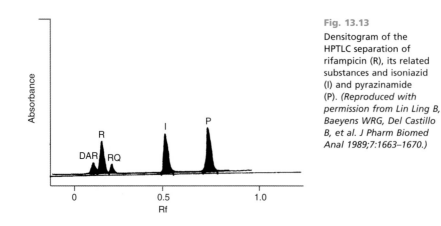

Fig. 13.13
Densitogram of the HPTLC separation of rifampicin (R), its related substances and isoniazid (I) and pyrazinamide (P). *(Reproduced with permission from Lin Ling B, Baeyens WRG, Del Castillo B, et al. J Pharm Biomed Anal 1989;7:1663–1670.)*

References

1. Moffat AC. *Clarke's Isolation and Identification of Drugs*. London: Pharmaceutical Press; 1986.
2. Touchstone JC. *Practice of Thin Layer Chromatography*. 3rd ed. Chichester: Wiley Interscience; 1992.
3. Poole CF. *J Chromatogr A*. 2003;1000:963-984.
4. Poole CF. *Clarke's Analysis of Drugs and Poisons*. Vol 1. Pharmaceutical Press; 2004:392-424.
5. Lin. Ling B, Baeyens WRG, Del Castillo B, et al. *J Pharm Biomed Anal*. 1989;7:1663-1670.
6. Aregkar AP, Kunyir SS, Purandare KS. *J Pharm Biomed Anal*. 1996;14:1645-1650.

Further reading

Bhushan R, Dubey R. Indirect reversed-phase high-performance liquid chromatographic and direct thin-layer chromatographic enantioresolution of (R, S)-Cinacalcet. *Biomed Chromatogr*. 2011;25:674-679.

Casoni D, Tuhutiu IA, Sarbu C. Simultaneous determination of parabens in pharmaceutical preparations using high-performance thin-layer chromatography and image analysis. *J Liq Chromatogr Rel Technol*. 2011;34: 805-816.

Kaale E, Risha P, Layloff T. TLC for pharmaceutical analysis in resource limited countries. *J Chromatogr A*. 2011;1218:2732-2736.

Poole SK, Poole CF. High performance stationary phases for planar chromatography. *J Chromatogr A*. 2011;1218:2648-2660.

Renger B, Vegh Z, Ferenczi-Fodor K. Validation of thin layer and high performance thin layer chromatographic methods. *J Chromatogr A*. 2011;1218:2712-2721.

Vovk I, Simonovska B. Development and validation of a high-performance thin-layer chromatographic method for determination of ofloxacin residues on pharmaceutical equipment surfaces. *J AOAC Int*. 2011;94:735-742.

High-performance capillary electrophoresis

14

KEYPOINTS

Principles

Separation is carried out by applying a high potential (10–30 kV) to a narrow (25–75 μm) fused-silica capillary filled with a mobile phase. The mobile phase generally contains an aqueous component and must contain an electrolyte. Analytes migrate in the applied electric field at a rate dependent on their charge and ionic radius. Even neutral analytes migrate through the column due to electro-osmotic flow, which usually occurs toward the cathode.

Applications

- An accurate and precise technique for quantitation of drugs in all types of formulations.
- Particular strength in quality control of peptide drugs.
- Highly selective and is very effective in producing separation of enantiomers.
- Very effective for impurity profiling due to its high resolving power.
- Very effective for the analysis of drugs and their metabolites in biological fluids.

Strengths

- Potentially many times more efficient than HPLC in its separating power.
- Shorter analysis times than HPLC.
- Cheaper columns than HPLC.
- Negligible solvent consumption.

Limitations

- Currently much less robust than HPLC.
- Sensitivity lower than HPLC.
- More parameters require optimisation than in HPLC methods.

Introduction

Electrophoresis

Capillary electrophoresis (CE) is the most rapidly expanding separation technique in pharmaceutical analysis and is a rival to HPLC in its general applicability. The instrumentation is quite straightforward, apart from the high voltages required, but the parameters involved in optimising the technique to produce separation are more complex than those involved in HPLC. The technique is preferred to HPLC, where highly selective separation is required.

Separation of analytes by electrophoresis is achieved by differences in their velocity in an electric field. The velocity of an ion is given by the formula:

$$v = \mu_e E \qquad \textbf{[Equation 1]}$$

where v is the ion velocity, μ_e is the electrophoretic mobility and E is the applied electric field.

The electric field is in volts/cm and depends on the length of the capillary used and strength of the potential applied across it. The ion mobility is given by the relationship shown below:

$$\mu_e = \frac{\text{Electric force } (F_E)}{\text{Frictional drag } (F_F)}$$

$$F_E = qE$$

where q is the charge on the ion and E is the applied electric field, i.e. the greater the charge on an ion the more rapidly it migrates in a particular electric field.

For a spherical ion:

$$F_F = -6\pi\eta r v$$

where η is the viscosity of the medium used for electrophoresis, r is the ion radius and v is the ion velocity.

When the frictional drag and the electric field experienced by the ion are equal:

$$qE = -6\pi\eta r v$$

substituting this expression into Equation 1:

$$\mu_e = \frac{q}{6\pi\eta r} \qquad \textbf{[Equation 2]}$$

If the applied electric field is increased beyond the point where the drag and electric field are equal, the ion will begin to migrate. From Equation 2 it can be seen that:

(i) The greater the charge on the ion, the higher its mobility.
(ii) The smaller the ion, the greater its mobility. Linked to this, since Equation 2 applies to a spherical ion, the more closely an ion approximates to a sphere, i.e. the smaller its surface area, the greater its mobility. This effect is consistent with other types of chromatography.

Thus the mobility of an ion can be influenced by its pKa value – the more it is ionised the greater its mobility – and its molecular shape in solution. Since its degree of ionisation may have a bearing on its shape in solution, it can be seen that the behaviour of analytes in solution has the potential to be complex. For many drugs the manipulation of the pH of the electrophoresis medium should have a marked effect on their relative mobilities. Thus one would predict that the electrophoretic separation of the two bases (morphine and codeine), which are of a similar shape and size but have different pKa values, would increase with pH. If we assume that morphine and codeine possess the same mobilities at full charge, then Figure 14.1 indicates how their mobilities vary with pH. As can be seen in Figure 14.1, the biggest numerical difference in mobility is when the pH = pKa of the weaker base, although the ratio of the mobilities goes on increasing with pH, e.g. at pH 8.9 the ion mobility of codeine is *ca* two times that of morphine.

Variation of ion mobility with pH is only part of the story with regard to separation by capillary electrophoresis – the other major factor is electro-osmotic flow (EOF).

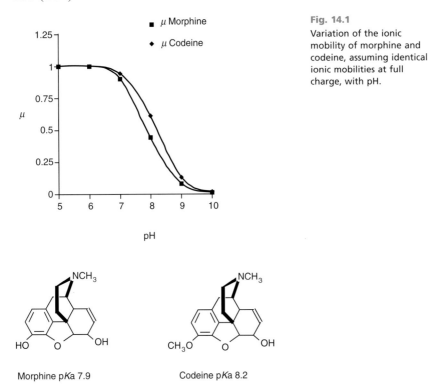

Fig. 14.1
Variation of the ionic mobility of morphine and codeine, assuming identical ionic mobilities at full charge, with pH.

Morphine pKa 7.9

Codeine pKa 8.2

Electro-osmotic flow (EOF) (see Animation 14.1)

The wall of the fused-silica capillary can be viewed as being similar to the surface of silica gel, and at all but very low values the silanol groups on the wall will bear a negative charge. The pKa of the acidic silanol groups ranges from 4.0 to 9.0 and the amount of negative charge on the wall will increase as pH rises. Cations in the running buffer are attracted to the negative charge on the wall, resulting in an increase in positive potential as the wall is approached. The effect of the increased positive potential is that more water molecules are drawn into the region next to the wall (Fig. 14.2). When a potential is applied across the capillary, the cations in solution migrate toward the cathode. The cations in a

Fig. 14.2
Electro-osmotic flow.

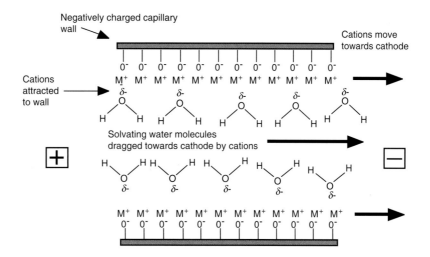

concentrated layer near to the capillary wall exhibit a relatively high mobility (conductivity) compared to the rest of the running buffer and drag their solvating water molecules with them toward the cathode, creating EOF. The rate of EOF is pH dependent since the negative charge on the silanol groups increases with pH, and between a pH of 3 and 8 the EOF increases about 10 times. The EOF decreases with buffer strength since a larger concentration of anions in the running buffer will reduce the positive potential at the capillary wall and thus reduce the interaction of the water in the buffer with the cations at the wall.

The flow profile obtained from EOF is shown in Figure 14.3 in comparison with the type of laminar flow shown in HPLC. The flat flow profile produces narrower peaks than are obtained in HPLC separations and is a component in the high separation efficiencies obtained in capillary electrophoresis (CE).

Fig. 14.3
Flow profiles obtained in CE and HPLC.

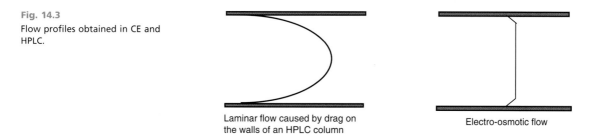

Laminar flow caused by drag on the walls of an HPLC column

Electro-osmotic flow

Migration in Capillary electrophoresis (CE) (see Animation 14.2)

The existence of EOF means that all species, regardless of charge, will move toward the cathode. In free solution, cations move at a rate determined by their ion mobility + the EOF. Neutral compounds move at the same rate as the EOF and anions move at the rate of the EOF – their ion mobility; the rate of EOF toward the cathode exceeds the rate at which anions move toward the anode, by approximately ten times. A typical separation could be viewed as shown in Figure 14.4. The cations in solution migrate most quickly, with the smaller cations reaching the cathode first; the neutral species move at the same rate as the EOF; and

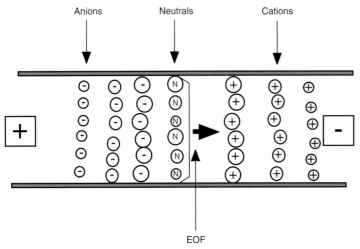

Fig. 14.4
Migration of ionic and neutral species in CE.

the anions migrate most slowly, with the smallest anions reaching the cathode last. The EOF is useful in that it allows the analysis of all species, but it adds complexity to the method in that it needs to be carefully balanced against ion mobility. Table 14.1 shows how EOF can be controlled using different variables and illustrates some of the complexity of CE relative to HPLC.

Instrumentation

A schematic diagram of a capillary electrophoresis instrument is shown in Figure 4.5. The fundamentals of the system are as follows:

(i)   Injection is commonly automated and is usually accomplished by pressuring the vial containing the sample with air.
(ii) Having loaded the sample, the capillary is switched to a vial containing running buffer. The flow rate of the running buffer through the capillary is in the low nanolitres/min range.
(iii) The capillaries are like those used in capillary gas chromatography with a polyamide coating on the outside. The length of the capillaries used is 50–100 cm, with an internal diameter of 0.025–0.05 mm. They are generally wound round a cassette holder so that they can simply be pushed into place in the instrument.
(iv) At the detector end, the capillary has a window burnt into it so that it is transparent to the radiation used for detection of the analyte.
(v)   The most commonly used detector is a diode array or rapid-scanning UV detector, although fluorometric, conductimetric and mass spectrometric detectors are available.

Control of separation
Migration time

As discussed earlier, cations move most quickly toward the point of detection. Time has to be allowed for separations to develop, and the EOF should not exceed the cationic mobility by an amount which is incompatible with achieving separation. The factors which can be used to control EOF have been discussed earlier.

Table 14.1 Variables affecting EOF

Variable	Effects on EOF	Comments
Buffer pH	EOF increases with pH	Most convenient method for controlling EOF but has to be balanced against effects on the charge on the analyte
Buffer strength	EOF decreases with increasing buffer strength	(i) Increased ionic strength means increased electric current flow through the capillary, which can cause heating (ii) At low ionic strength more sample absorption onto the capillary walls occurs (iii) Low buffer concentrations reduce sample stacking following injection
Electric field	Increased electric field increases EOF	Lowering the applied electric field may reduce separation efficiency, and raising the field strength may cause heating
Temperature	Increased temperature decreases viscosity and thus increases flow	Easy to control
Organic modifier	Changes potential at capillary wall – the dielectric constant of the running buffer and the viscosity. Usually decreases EOF	Complex effects – can be useful but best determined experimentally
Surfactant	Absorbs onto the surface of the capillary wall	(i) Cationic surfactants have a high affinity for the silanol groups and thus block access by the smaller cations in solution, reducing EOF. At high concentration they form a double layer, giving the capillary wall an effective positive charge and causing EOF to reverse flow toward the anode (ii) Anionic surfactants reduce the access of the smaller ions in the running buffer to the positive potential at the wall, thus increasing the zeta potential and thus EOF
Covalent wall coating	Can raise or lower EOF depending on the coating	(i) Neutral coatings reduce negative charge of the capillary wall, thus reducing EOF (ii) Ionic coatings will have marked effects on EOF

Fig. 14.5
Schematic diagram of a capillary electrophoresis apparatus (see Animation 14.3).

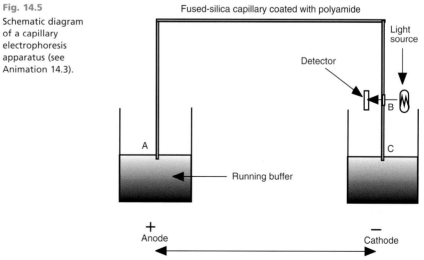

Fused-silica capillary coated with polyamide

Light source

Detector

B

A

C

Running buffer

+
Anode

−
Cathode

Potential difference 15–30 kV

Another factor in allowing separation to develop which is simply controlled is the length of the capillary; however, the longer the capillary in relation to a fixed applied potential, the lower the electric field, which is in volts/cm. Since the detection system is mounted before the column outlet, it is important that the distance between the detector and the outlet is not too great since the effective length of the capillary is reduced.

Dispersion

Longitudinal diffusion

This is generally the most important cause of peak broadening in CE because of the absence of mass transfer and streaming effects seen in other types of chromatography. Thus to some extent CE resembles capillary gas chromatography but with less mass transfer effects and lower longitudinal diffusion since the sample is in the liquid phase. Longitudinal diffusion depends on the length of time an analyte spends in the capillary and also on the diffusion coefficient of the analyte in the mobile phase. Large analytes such as proteins and oligonucleotides have low diffusion coefficients, and thus CE can produce very efficient separations of these types of analytes.

Injection plug length

The capillaries used in CE have narrow internal diameters. For a 100 cm $\times$ 50 μm i.d. capillary, an injection of 0.02 μl would occupy a 1 cm length of capillary space. Automatic injection can overcome difficulties in reproducible injection of such small volumes, but often detection limits require that larger amounts of sample are injected. Typically the injection is accomplished by applying pressure at the sample loading end of the capillary. An important element in accomplishing efficient sample loading, particularly if detection limits are a problem and a larger volume of sample has to be loaded, is stacking. A simple method for achieving stacking is to dissolve the sample in water or low conductivity buffer. The greater resistance of the water plug causes a localised increase in electrical potential across the plug width and the sample ions dissolved in the plug will migrate rapidly until the boundary of the running buffer is reached. By using this method, longer plugs, up to 10% of the capillary length, can be injected, resulting in an increase in detection limit.

Joule heating

The strength of the electric field which can be applied across the capillary is limited by conversion of electrical energy into heat. Localised heating can cause changes in the viscosity of the running buffer and a localised increase in analyte diffusion. Heat generation can be minimised by using narrow capillaries, where heat dissipation is rapid, and by providing a temperature-controlled environment for the capillary.

Solute/wall interactions

Analytes may absorb onto the wall of the capillary either by interaction with the negatively charged silanol groups or by hydrophobic interaction. High ionic strength buffers block the negative charge on the capillary wall and reduce the EOF but also increase heating. If only analysis of cations is required, the pH of the running buffer can be lowered, e.g. to pH 2. The low pH suppresses the charge on the silanol groups, reduces EOF to a low level but ensures full ionic mobility of the cations, which will migrate to the cathode without the aid of the EOF. Full ionisation of the analytes does not allow for differences in pKa to be used in producing separation.

Electrodispersion

The mobility of the running buffer has to be fairly similar to the mobility of the ions in the sample zone. If the mobility of the analyte ions is greater than the mobility of the buffer ions, a fronting peak will result, since the ions at the front of the sample zone tend to diffuse into the running buffer solution, where they experience a greater applied electric field (due to the higher resistance of the buffer compared with the sample) and accelerate away from the sample zone. This effect will be less if the concentration of the running buffer is much greater than that of the sample. Conversely, if the mobility of the sample ions is lower than that of the running buffer ions, a tailing peak will be produced because the ions in the rear of the sample zone will tend to diffuse into the buffer, where they will experience a lower applied electric field (due to the lower resistance of the buffer compared with the sample) and will thus lag further behind the sample zone. This effect will be less if the concentration of the running buffer is much lower than that of the sample zone.

Applications of CE in pharmaceutical analysis

In its simplest form, capillary electrophoresis is termed 'capillary zone electrophoresis'. The conditions used in this type of analysis are relatively simple, and the mobile phase used consists of a buffer with various additives. Many applications focus on critical separations which are difficult to achieve by HPLC. In many cases it is difficult to explain completely the types of effects produced by buffer additives.

Separation of atenolol and related impurities predominantly on the basis of charge

The β-blocker atenolol is shown in Figure 14.6 with its principal known impurities. These impurities are not readily separated from atenolol by HPLC because of their close structural similarity.[1]

The separation was carried out using a 0.05 mm × 50 cm capillary at 15 kV with a phosphate/borate running buffer. Figure 14.6 shows separation at the optimal pH of 9.7 of atenolol (50 μg/ml) from its impurities spiked into solution at concentrations of 5 μg/ml. The elution order is as would be predicted from the ionisable groups in the molecules. Atenolol (AT) elutes first since it bears a positive charge on the basic secondary amine group (pKa 9.6). The dimer (TA) also carries one positive charge but it is a tertiary amine and has a lower pKa than atenolol. It is also a larger ion; thus its mobility will be less than that of atenolol (size was sufficient to cause separation of these two molecules at pH 6.5, where both atenolol and the dimer would be fully charged). The diol (D) is a neutral compound and thus should elute at the same rate as the EOF, which will increase with pH. However, in the paper under discussion the elution time of the diol increased with pH; this may be due to complex formation with the borate in the running buffer, which will tend to form a negatively charged complex with a diol.

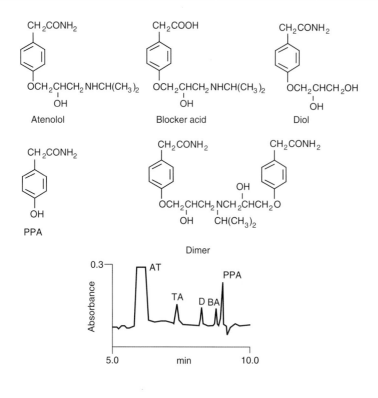

Fig. 14.6

Separation of atenolol and its principal impurities by CE. *(Reproduced with permission from Shafaati A, Clark BJ. J Pharm Biomed Anal 1996;14:1547–54.)*

The blocker acid (BA) bears both a positive and a negative charge, which more or less neutralise each other over a quite wide pH range. As the pH rises toward the pKa of the amine group (*ca* 9.5), the negative charge of the acidic group becomes predominant; although the molecule will still bear some positive charge, the overall negative charge will cause the molecule to lag behind the EOF. Finally, the phenol (PPA) is neutral until its pKa value (*ca* 9.7–10) is approached, and at higher pH values it will develop a negative charge, slowing down its rate of migration; this is consistent with Figure 14.6.

Separation predominantly on the basis of ionic radius

Very small changes in molecular structure can lead to quite marked differences in retention time in CE. An impressive separation of the experimental anti-depressant drug GR50360 from a number of impurities was achieved using isopropanol/0.01 M phosphate buffer pH 7.0 (1:4).[2] In this case the separation is due largely to molecular size or shape since at pH 7.0 the drug and its impurities will be charged to a similar extent.

Figure 14.7 shows the separation of all six components by CE. The *cis* isomer of GR50360A has a completely different molecular shape from the *trans* isomer, resulting in a smaller ionic radius, and thus it runs earlier than the *trans* isomer. Otherwise the compounds elute in order of molecular size, the desfluorocompound being the first of the derivatives of GR50360A to elute. The presence of the isopropanol in the mobile phase slows down the EOF sufficiently for separation to develop.

Fig. 14.7
Separation of GR50360 from its related impurities. *(Reproduced with permission from Smith NW, Evans MB. J Pharm Biomed Anal 1994;12:579–611.)*

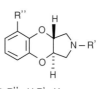

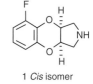

1 *Cis* isomer

2 R'' = H R' = H
3 R'' = F R' = H (GR50360A)
4 R'' = F R' = CH$_3$
5 R'' = F R' = C$_2$H$_5$
6 R'' = F R' = C$_3$H$_7$

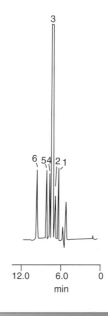

Self-test 14.1

Metipranolol and its possible manufacturing impurities are separated using CE in a buffer at pH 9.5. Suggest the likely order of elution for the components in the mixture.

1 Metipranolol pKa 9.5

2 Tertiary amine pKa 9.1

3 Diamine pKa 9.5

4 Phenol pKa 9.5, 10.0

Answer: Order of elution: 3, 1, 2, 4

Analysis of non-steroidal anti-inflammatory drugs (NSAIDs) by CE and separation of anions on the basis of ionic radius

NSAIDs generally contain a carboxylic acid group, and when ionised they are anions. In CE using an unmodified capillary the EOF is toward the cathode, and the overall mobility of anions is given by the EOF – the mobility of the anions, which is toward the anode. In this example[3] the running buffer used in the analysis was carefully designed with respect to its ionic content to avoid electrodispersion. Glycine was found to have a suitable mobility for the analysis of this class of compound because, although it is a small molecule with a carboxylic acid group which is completely ionised at the pH of the analysis (9.1), it also bears a partial positive charge, reducing its overall mobility toward the anode and giving it a mobility similar to those of the large lipophilic NSAID acids. The cationic component in the buffer was also found to have an important effect on resolution of the components in a mixture containing four NSAIDs. Triethanolamine was found to be the best cationic component since it reduced EOF because of its relatively low ion mobility and also through increasing the viscosity of the running buffer. Figure 14.8 shows the separation of a mixture containing five NSAIDs: sulindac (S), indomethacin (I), piroxicam (P), tiaprofenic acid (T) and aclofenac (A). All the drugs are fully charged at pH 9.1 and the separation was achieved more or less according to molecular weight, with aclofenac, the smallest molecule, migrating most rapidly in the opposite direction to the EOF.

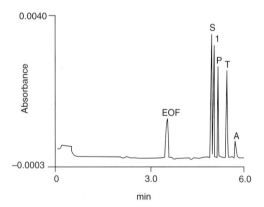

Fig. 14.8

Separation of a mixture of five NSAIDs using a buffer consisting of 0.075 M glycine adjusted to pH 9.1 with triethanolamine. *(Reproduced with permission from Bechet I, Fillet M, Hubert Ph, Crommen J. J Pharm Biomed Anal 1995;13:497–503.)*

Separation of peptides

A particular strength of CE is its ability to separate peptides. The use of therapeutic peptides is increasing rapidly, and their large size and polarity present particular problems in producing separations. Because peptides usually bear two or more charges, the most important factor to optimise in peptide separations is the pH and concentration of the running buffer. The p*I*-value of a peptide is the pH where its positive and negative charges are balanced. An example is provided by the separation of adrenocorticotropic hormone (ACTH) from three of its fragments.[4]

Table 14.2 shows the molecular weights and p*I*-values of ACTH and three of its fragments. The p*I*-value gives some indication of the relative number of acidic

Table 14.2 Characteristics of ACTH and its peptide fragments

Peptide	p*I*-value	Molecular weight	No. of amino acids	Calculated mobility	Migration order
Fragment 1	11.69	1652	14	0.0431	1
Fragment 2	10.05	2934	24	0.0379	2
ACTH	9.24	4567	39	0.0216	3
Fragment 3	7.55	1299	10	0.0151	4

and basic groups in the peptide; a high p*I*-value indicates a peptide with a large number of basic residues such as lysine and arginine, while a low p*I*-value indicates that the balance is in favour of acidic residues such as glutamic and aspartic acids. In this particular example, conditions (pH 3.8) were chosen where the charge on the basic residues was predominant, although, at this pH, acidic residues will still bear an appreciable negative charge, inhibiting migration toward the cathode. In the current example, the separation is consistent with the balance of basic and acidic character in the peptide. The most basic peptide (fragment 1) elutes first whereas the least basic peptide elutes last. Thus in this case the degree of positive charge on the peptides predominates over ionic radius in determining the rate of migration, since ACTH migrates more quickly than fragment 3 despite having a much higher molecular weight. The separation was optimised by increasing buffer strength, as can be seen from Figure 14.9, and increased buffer strength gave increased migration time through its effects in reducing EOF. Another important effect of the increased buffer strength in this case is the reduction of the interaction of these highly basic peptides (particularly fragments 1 and 2 and ACTH) with the silanol groups on the capillary wall, thus resulting in better peak shape.

In this elegant study it was concluded that for all the peptides studied the best separations were achieved in buffers of medium to high strength (0.05–0.1 M), thus allowing manipulation of EOF without moving away from the optimal pH for the running buffer. It was also concluded that acidic pH values in the range of 2.2–3.8 were best for analysis of basic and neutral peptides, whereas acidic peptides were best run at around pH 7.0.

Use of additives in the running buffer

Additives in the running buffer can produce greater selectivity where separation in simple free solution is not possible.

Fig. 14.9
Separation of ACTH and related peptides by CE in buffer at pH 3.8. Buffer strength: (A) 20 mM; (B) 50 mM; (C) 100 mM. *(Reproduced with permission from Langenhuizen MHJM, Janssen PSL. J Chromatogr 1993;638:311–18.)*

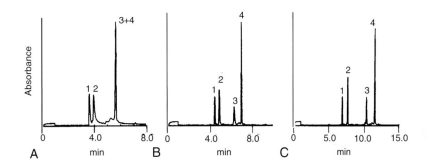

Applications of cyclodextrins in producing improvements in separation

Cyclodextrins are neutral compounds which migrate at the same rate as the EOF. They have large hydrophobic cavities in their structures, into which molecules can fit. The ease with which a molecule fits into the cavity of the cyclodextrin is dependent on its stereochemistry. Cyclodextrins have been used as additives in both chiral, where opposite enantiomers form transient diastereomeric complexes with the optically active cyclodextrins, and non-chiral separations, where the cyclodextrins affect diastereoisomers to a different extent.

Separation of pilocarpine from its epimer

Pilocarpine (P), a drug used in treating glaucoma, can potentially contain its epimer, isopilocarpine (I), as an impurity. In a study it was not possible to completely separate pilocarpine and isopilocarpine by variation of the pH of the running buffer. The optimal pH for separation should be 6.9, where both compounds are *ca* 50% ionised, but even at this pH separation was incomplete.[5]

   Inclusion of 0.01 M β-cyclodextrin in the running buffer resulted in baseline separation of the diastereoisomers. Figure 14.10A shows the separation of the two epimers achieved following addition of the cyclodextrin to the running buffer. In this example capillaries were used where the silanol groups on the capillary wall had been partially blocked by coating, reducing the negative charge on the wall and thus reducing the EOF and allowing more time for separation to develop. In the present example the separation is achieved by the different degree of complexation of the β-cyclodextrin additive with the two diastereoisomers.

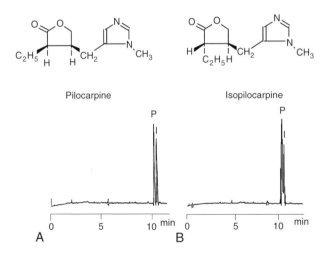

Pilocarpine   Isopilocarpine

A   B

Fig. 14.10
Separation of pilocarpine and isopilocarpine by inclusion of β-cyclodextrin in the running buffer. (A) With addition of cyclodextrin. (B) Without addition of cyclodextrin. *(Reproduced with permission from Baeyens W, Weiss G, van der Weken G, van den Bossche W. J Chromatogr 1993;638:319–326.)*

Separation of chiral local anaesthetics

Cyclodextrins are used in GC and HPLC to effect separation of enantiomers, and they are also very effective in CE applications. The application of CE to chiral separations will undergo rapid growth in the next few years because of the high efficiencies that can be achieved in such separations using this technique and because of the cheapness of the chiral additives compared to the cost of chiral GC and HPLC columns. A series of enantiomers of local anaesthetics was

Fig. 14.11

Separation of the enantiomers of a series of local anaesthetics through their interaction with dimethyl β-cyclodextrin included in the running buffer. *(Redrawn from Sänger-van de Griend CF, Gröningsson K, Westerlund D. Chromatographia 1996;42:263–267.)*

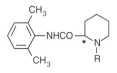

Mepivacaine (M) R = CH_3
EtPPX (E)   R = C_2H_5
Ropivacaine (RP) R = C_3H_7
Bupivacaine (B) R = C_4H_9
Pentycaine (P)   R = C_5H_{11}

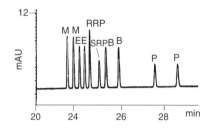

separated by CE using a phosphate buffer at pH 3.0 containing triethanolamine as a cationic additive and 10 mM of a dimethyl β-cyclodextrin.[6] The addition of the cationic additive reversed the EOF (see Table 14.1) toward the anode; however, the analytes still migrated toward the cathode, having an overall mobility in this direction greater than the EOF toward the anode. This allowed increased time for interaction of the analytes with the cyclodextrin, which migrates toward the anode with the EOF. The use of methylated β-cyclodextrin increases the interaction of lipophilic analytes with this chiral selector compared with β-cyclodextrin itself.

Figure 14.11 shows the separation of R and S isomers of a series of structurally related local anaesthetics. Wide separations were achieved for the compounds in this series, where it was proposed that the fit of the hydrophobic portion of the analyte into the cyclodextrin was optimal when one of the substituents at the chiral centre was able to interact with the chiral hydroxyl groups on the rim of the cyclodextrin cavity. Table 14.3 shows the association constants calculated for the interaction of the enantiomeric pairs with the dimethylcyclodextrin.[6] The larger the value of K, the more the enantiomer is retarded by the selector, which in this case is migrating toward the anode. The values in the table also show that the calculated mobilities for each analyte in free solution decrease with the bulk of the N-alkyl substituent.

Table 14.3 Association constants of some enantiomers of some local anaesthetics with dimethyl β-cyclodextrin and their mobilities in free solution

Compound	K_1 (L mol⁻¹)	K_2 (L mol⁻¹)	μ (10^{-8} m²s⁻¹v⁻¹)
Mepivacaine	18	24	1.96
Ropivacaine	18	26	1.82
Bupivacaine	16	26	1.77

Micellar electrokinetic chromatography (MEKC)

This extension of the basic CE technique allows the separation of neutral components to be carried out, but it has also been widely used in achieving separations of ionic species. In MEKC, a surfactant is added to the mobile phase at a concentration above its critical micelle concentration. The surfactants used can be anionic, cationic or neutral. The micelles act in a manner analogous to the stationary phase in HPLC. Anionic micelles migrate in the opposite direction to the usual EOF, which is toward the cathode. Cationic micelles migrate with the EOF, and neutral micelles migrate at the same rate as the EOF. The presence of the surfactant in the running buffer also has an effect on the rate and direction of EOF via interaction with the capillary wall, so the final basis for separation in MEKC may be due to a number of mechanisms. The interaction of the analyte with the micelles may be modified using organic solvent additives in the running buffer, which reduce the partitioning of the analyte into the micelle; at the same time, such organic modifiers tend to reduce EOF. The formation of micelles is illustrated in Figure 14.12.

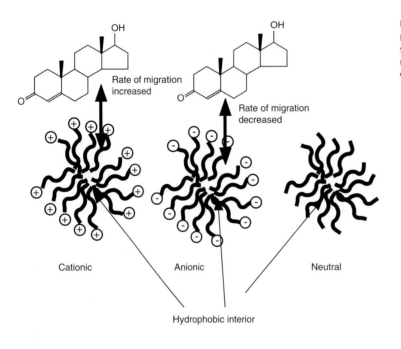

Fig. 14.12
Micelle formation during MEKC and the effect of charged micelles on the rate of migration of a neutral compound relative to the EOF.

Separation of cefotaxime from related impurities

Penicillins and cephalosporins are reactive compounds and may contain a number of degradants; the high selectivity of CE can be advantageous where separation of complex mixtures is required. Some of the impurities may be neutral, and separation of neutral impurities from each other requires partitioning into charged micelles which migrate at a different rate from the EOF. In this particular application, sodium dodecyl sulphate (SDS), an anionic surfactant, was used to conduct MEKC.[7] The pH of the running buffer was 7.2, which was low enough to avoid promoting the degradation of cefotaxime, which is unstable to alkali. Cefotaxime and its related impurities are shown in Figure 14.13.

Fig. 14.13
Cefotaxime and its impurities.

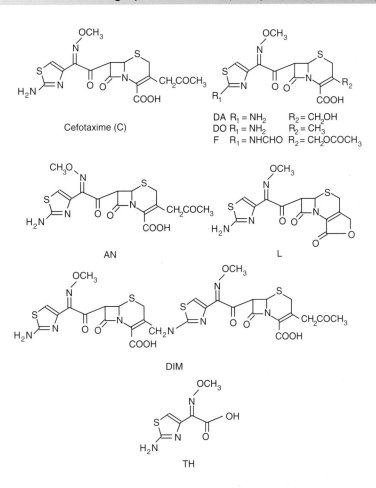

Cefotaxime (C)

DA R₁ = NH₂   R₂= CH₂OH
DO R₁ = NH₂   R₂ = CH₃
F   R₁ = NHCHO R₂= CH₂OCOCH₃

AN

L

DIM

TH

    Figure 14.14A shows the MEKC trace obtained from C, which was spiked
with 0.2% w/w of each impurity, and Figure 14.14B shows an unspiked sample
of C. The slowest migrating compound was the neutral lactone compound L,
which should have the most affinity for the negatively charged and hydrophobic
SDS. The other impurities are carboxylic acids, which will be fully charged at
pH 7.2, thus bearing a negative charge, which will cause some degree of repulsion
between the analytes and the negatively charged micelles. The anti-isomer of C
is late eluting because of its stereochemistry; hence its ionic radius and partition
coefficient are quite different from those of C (this is consistent with a lack of
antibiotic effect for the anti-isomer). The MEKC method was capable of producing separation of all seven impurities from C at the 0.2% level; it gave precision
comparable to a previously developed HPLC method and was more rapid than
the HPLC method.

Analysis of flavonoids by MEKC

Flavonoids are natural products which occur in certain popular herbal medicines
such as *Ginkgo biloba*. They are phenols and are not charged until the pH of the
running buffer is high. Separation by MEKC was carried out using 0.04 M SDS
in a 0.02 M borate running buffer at pH 8.2.[8] At this pH the flavonoids studied

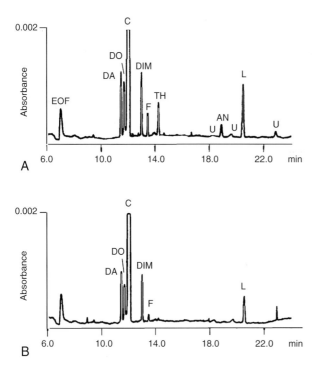

Fig. 14.14
Separation of cefotaxime
and related impurities.
(A) Sample spiked with
impurities. (B) Unspiked
sample. *U,* unknown.
*(Reproduced with
permission from Penalvo
GC, Julien E, Fabre H.
Chromatographia 1996;
42:159–164.)*

are more or less uncharged and in the absence of differential partitioning would migrate at the same rate as the EOF. The presence of SDS in the running buffer slows down the rate of migration of these compounds according to how strongly they partition into the SDS micelles, which are moving toward the anode while the EOF is toward the cathode. Figure 14.15 shows the closely related structures of the flavonoids whilst Figure 14.16 shows the separation achieved for a model mixture of these compounds.

The method gave good precision and rapid separation of the mixture. Chromatography of these types of compounds normally requires the use of gradient HPLC with long elution times.

Capillary electrophoresis with indirect detection

CE provides a useful method for analysing anions or cations which lack a chromophore by using indirect UV detection. This methodology makes use of the fact that if a UV-absorbing anion or cation is included in the running buffer, then the concentration of the UV-absorbing additive will be reduced in zones where analyte ions of the same charge are present. This produces a fall in UV absorbance that is proportional to the concentration of analyte ion; the data system inverts the trace obtained to give positive instead of negative peaks. For example, metabisulphite is used as an antioxidant agent in a number of pharmaceutical formulations. Recently a CE method was developed to simultaneously quantify both metabisulphite and its oxidation product (sulphate) in an injection using indirect UV detection.[10] Ammonium formate was used as an internal standard. The method was found to be capable of resolving the two analyte ions from the large amount of chloride present. Pyromellitic acid (Fig. 14.17) was used as

Fig. 14.15
Some flavonoid structures.

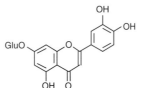

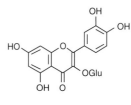

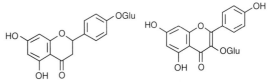

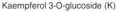

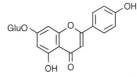

Luteolin 7-O-glucoside (L)
Quercetin 3-O-glucoside (Q)
Narigenin 4'-O-glucoside (N)
Kaempferol 3-O-glucoside (K)
Apigenin 7-O-glucoside (A)

Fig. 14.16
Separation of flavonoids by MEKC. *(Reproduced with permission from Pietta P, Mauri R, Facino RM, Carini M.* J Pharm Biomed Anal *1992;10:1041–1045.)*

0.04
Absorbance
L
I
K
N
A
0
5.0
10.0
min

Fig. 14.17
Pyromellitic acid

HOOC
COOH
HOOC
COOH

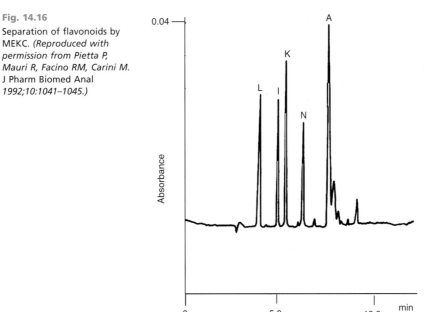

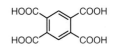

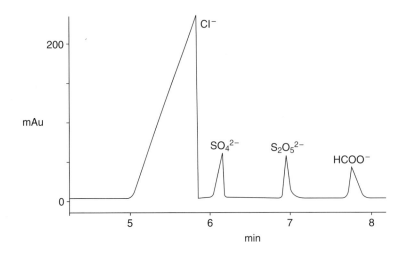

Fig. 14.18
Separation of sodium chloride
(2500 μg/ml), sodium metabisulphite
(150 μg/ml), sodium sulphate
(150 μg/ml) and ammonium formate
(IS, 150 μg/ml) in a pharmaceutical
formulation. Tris buffer pH 8.3
containing 15 mM pyromellitic acid,
indirect UV detection at 225 nm.
*(Reproduced with permission of
J Pharm Biomed Anal.)*

a background electrolyte since it fulfilled the requirement of having a similar electrophoretic mobility to the analytes.

Figure 14.18 shows a trace obtained for the analysis of sulphate and metabisulphite.

Similar type of separations can be carried out on cations using a suitable UV-absorbing cationic additive, e.g. imidazole.

Affinity capillary electrophoresis

Both chiral separations and MEKC involve a type of affinity CE. However, a wide range of interactions that are relevant to both pharmaceutics and medicinal chemistry can be studied by CE.[11] Microemulsion electrokinetic chromatography (MEEKC) provides an alternative to MEKC for achieving separations and has different selectivity in comparison with MEKC. Microemulsions are formed by mixing together a surfactant with polar and non-polar solvents to make a transparent emulsion. A typical mixture consists of sodium dodecylsulphate, butanol and heptane. As well as offering an alternative method of separation, MEEKC also provides a method for investigating solubilisation of drugs by different formulation excipients in a rapid and automated manner. The affinity of a drug for a range of excipients can be investigated using CE, e.g. between oligonucleotides and polycations or water-insoluble drugs and liposomes. Affinity CE can also be used as a tool in drug discovery and has been used to determine the sequence specificity of the binding of experimental drugs to DNA and interaction between proteins and drugs designed to inhibit or modify their activity.

Capillary electro-chromatography (CEC)

In CEC the capillary that is used for achieving separation is packed with a chromatographic stationary phase. Thus separation in this mode combines the high efficiencies achievable with electro-drive flow with partitioning into a stationary phase. The technique can potentially offer very high separation efficiencies. The greatest technical difficulty is in packing the narrow-bore capillary with stationary phase. Perhaps the most promising approach in this area is to form the packing *in situ* by polymerization, e.g. hydrolysis of tetramethoxy silane. Such polymeric packings are known as monoliths, and they are already commercially available as conventional HPLC columns. Monolithic packings have the advantage that they are very porous and can be operated at high flow rates. In CEC mode this means that, by application of a relatively small pressure, mixed-mode separations can be achieved where both electro-drive and pressure-driven flows are used at the same time to achieve rapid separations.

Additional problems

1. Select the most suitable running buffer from those given below to accomplish efficient separation of the following mixtures:
   (i)   Two geometrical isomers of a basic drug pKa 9.7.
   (ii) A mixture of neutral corticosteroids.
   (iii) A mixture of opium alkaloids with pKa values in the range 7.5–8.5.
   (iv) Two enantiomers of a local anaesthetic pKa 8.0.
   (v)   Two proteins both of ca 20 000 MW, one with a pI-value of 5.5 and the other with a pI-value of 7.1.
   (vi) Human and porcine insulin – human insulin differs from porcine insulin by one amino acid, having a more polar threonine residue, in place of an alanine residue, and their pI-values are the same.
   a.   0.05 mM phosphate buffer pH 7.5 containing 0.05 mM SDS.
   b.   0.02 mM borate buffer pH 9.5 containing 0.01 mM β-cyclodextrin.
   c.   0.05 mM phosphate buffer pH 6.5.
   d.   0.05 mM phosphate buffer pH 8.0.
   e.   0.02 mM borate buffer pH 8.0 containing 0.01 mM propylcyclodextrin.

   Answers: (i) b; (ii) a; (iii) a; (iv) e; (v) c; (vi) a

2. Predict the order of elution of the following tricyclic anti-depressants from a CE system with the following running buffer: 0.5 mM buffer pH 9.55/methanol (84.6: 15.4).

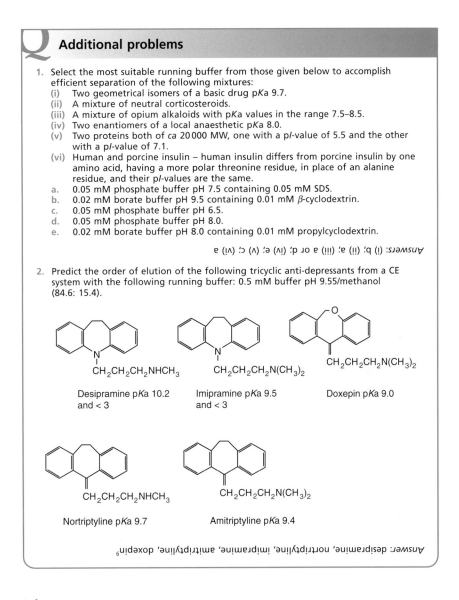

Desipramine pKa 10.2 and < 3

Imipramine pKa 9.5 and < 3

Doxepin pKa 9.0

Nortriptyline pKa 9.7

Amitriptyline pKa 9.4

Answer: desipramine, nortriptyline, imipramine, amitriptyline, doxepin[9]

References
1. Shafaati A, Clark BJ. *J Pharm Biomed Anal*. 1996;14:1547-1554.
2. Smith NW, Evans MB. *J Pharm Biomed Anal*. 1994;12:579-611.
3. Bechet I, Fillet M, Hubert Ph, Crommen J. *J Pharm Biomed Anal*. 1995;13:497-503.
4. Langenhuizen MHJM, Janssen PSL. *J Chromatogr*. 1993;638:311-318.
5. Baeyens W, Weiss G, van der Weken G, van den Bossche W. *J Chromatogr*. 1993;638:319-326.
6. Sänger-van de Griend CF, Gröningsson K, Westerlund D. *Chromatographia*. 1996;42:263-267.

7. Penalvo GC, Julien E, Fabre H. *Chromatographia*. 1996;42:159-164.

8. Pietta P, Mauri R, Facino RM, Carini M. *J Pharm Biomed Anal*. 1992;10:1041-1045.

9. Salomon K, Burgi DS, Helmer JC. *J Chromatogr*. 1991;549:375-385.

10. Geiser L, Varesio E, Veuthey J-L. *J Pharm Biomed Anal*. 2003;31:1059-1064.

11. Neubert RHH, Ruttinger H-H, eds. *Affinity Capillary Electrophoresis in Pharmaceutics and Biopharmaceutics*. Marcel-Dekker; 2003.

Further reading

Baker DR. *Capillary Electrophoresis*. Chichester: Wiley Interscience; 1995.

Cohen AS, Terabe S, Deyl Z. *Capillary Electrophoretic Separations of Drugs*. Amsterdam: Elsevier; 1996.

Jouyban A, Kenndler E. Impurity analysis of pharmaceuticals using capillary electromigration methods. *Electrophoresis*. 2008;29:3531-3551.

Sanchez-Hernandez L, Garcia-Ruiz C, Marina ML, Crego AL. Recent approaches for enhancing sensitivity in enantioseparations by CE. *Electrophoresis*. 2010;31:28-43.

www.separationsnow.com

www.agilent.com

15

Extraction methods in pharmaceutical analysis

KEYPOINTS

Principles of extraction

The analyte is removed from materials in a formulation matrix which would interfere in its analysis using a solvent in which it is highly soluble but in which the matrix interferants have limited solubility. Further solvent partitioning steps may then be used in order to reduce the interferants.

Applications

* Most analyses of pharmaceuticals require an extraction step or extractions steps, and optimisation of these processes has an important bearing on the precision and accuracy of the analysis.
* Widely used in bioanalytical measurements and for concentrating trace amounts of analyte.

Strengths

* A simple and cheap method of removing interferants.

Limitations

* Limited selectivity, limited choice of partitioning solvents, large volumes of solvent required. (See SPE keypoints.)

Introduction

Complex extraction and derivatisation methods are most often applied to bioanalytical procedures and to the concentration of trace impurities in pharmaceuticals rather than to straightforward quality control of active ingredients in pharmaceuticals. Quality control of the active ingredient in a formulation generally utilises a simple extraction procedure, and if there is a problem of interference from excipients following extraction, chromatography is able to resolve the active ingredient from the interferants and permit quantitation. However, there are circumstances where low dosage formulations and advanced drug delivery formulations may require more detailed sample handling.

Commonly used excipients in formulations

The principal reason for conducting extraction prior to analysis is in order to remove materials which might interfere in the analysis. This is a greater requirement if chromatographic separation is not carried out during the analysis. Some non-chromatographic techniques, such as NIRA, aim to avoid all sample preparation through using advanced computing techniques to screen out interference. Even when chromatographic separation is used, extraction of some type has to be carried out prior to analysis in order to remove insoluble tablet matrix materials or oily excipients in creams and ointments. When low levels of drugs are being monitored in biological fluids, extraction procedures may have to be quite detailed in order to remove interference by endogenous compounds. The major types of interferants in formulations are briefly considered in this chapter.

Tablets and capsules

Tablets and capsules usually consist largely of a filler except for high-dose formulations, such as paracetamol tablets and tablets of other non-steroidal anti-inflammatory drugs, where the active ingredient may compose a large part of the formulation. The most commonly used filler in tablets is lactose, and other popular fillers include other sugars or sugar polymers such as cellulose, starch and mannitol. These substances are polar and will dissolve or swell best in water; thus extraction procedures where the drug is water soluble are best carried out in aqueous media so that the drug is efficiently recovered from the sample matrix. The fillers themselves do not absorb UV light so they are not likely to interfere directly in HPLC procedures, where, for instance in commonly used reverse-phase chromatography procedures, they will elute at the void volume with little perturbation of the chromatographic baseline. Similarly, they produce little interference in direct analyses by UV spectrophotometry. If the drug is not completely water soluble, methanol or ethanol may be used for extraction since they will wet the tablet powder quite well and will dissolve many organic molecules.

Lubricants are used in tablet preparation and include magnesium stearate, stearic acid and polyethylene glycol. They only comprise at most 1–2% of the tablet bulk, so their potential to interfere is slight, particularly since their chromophores are weak. The fatty acid lubricants can often be observed if analysis of a tablet extract is carried out by GC–FID. Tablet coatings are often based on modified sugar polymers such as hydroxypropylmethylcellulose. These coatings are used at about 3% of the tablet bulk, are water soluble and do not absorb UV light.

Colourants obviously have the potential to interfere in analysis because they are efficient absorbers of UV/visible radiation. In tablets and capsules, colours tend to be organometallic dyes or metal oxides which are not appreciably soluble in any of the solvents used for extraction and can be filtered off with other insoluble matrix constituents. When capsules are analysed, the coloured outer shell is removed before the contents of the capsule are extracted.

Suspensions and solutions

In suspensions and solutions, the dyes used are water soluble and include natural pigments such as chlorophylls, carotenoids and anthocyanins, and coal-tar-based dyes. More effort may be required to remove interference by these materials. Solid-phase extraction with ion exchange resins may be useful for removing anionic or cationic dyes, although simple extraction of the drug into organic solvent of moderate polarity may leave such dyes in the aqueous phase. Solutions tend to contain anti-microbial preservatives and antioxidants. These are usually either phenols or quaternary amines such as benzalkonium chloride and have strong enough chromophores to interfere in the analysis of a drug. These compounds have to be removed by extraction procedures prior to analysis. Suspensions also contain surfactant materials such as the polyethylene glycol-based detergents, but these compounds do not have appreciable UV absorbance and thus have little potential for interference.

Creams and ointments

Sodium and potassium salts of fatty acids, cationic surfactants and non-ionic surfactants are used in creams and ointments. As discussed above, these compounds do not have strong chromophores but, particularly the fatty acids, may interfere in chromatography, for instance by contaminating reverse-phase HPLC columns, if they are not removed. Contamination of reverse-phase HPLC columns by lipophilic materials can often be observed through a loss of chromatographic peak shape. Creams and ointments contain large amounts of oily triglycerides, which have to be removed to avoid interference with the chromatographic process. Extraction of the cream with methanol can partly remove this type of interference. Partitioning of the extract between hexane and methanol or methanol/water mixtures may also be used; the highly lipophilic material is removed into the hexane layer.

Solvent extraction methods

Solvent extraction procedures provide simple methods for separating the analyte from excipients in formulations. The analytical method applied to the isolated analyte can be, for example, gravimetric, volumetric, spectrophotometric or chromatographic. In most cases in the pharmaceutical industry, chromatographic methods are preferred. The extraction method adopted is governed by the need to remove excipients and by the properties of the analyte.

Extraction of organic bases and acids utilising their ionised and un-ionised forms

Salts of organic bases such as sulphates and hydrochlorides are often highly water soluble, and the free bases are usually quite organosoluble, particularly in

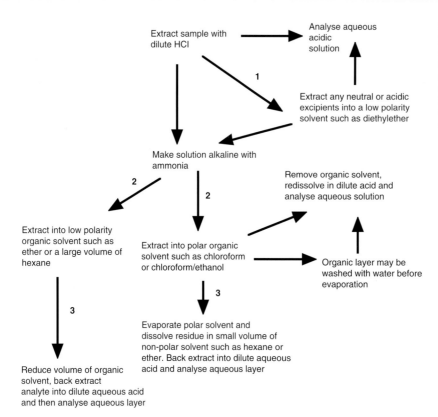

Extract sample with dilute HCl

Analyse aqueous acidic solution

1

Extract any neutral or acidic excipients into a low polarity solvent such as diethylether

Make solution alkaline with ammonia

2

2

Remove organic solvent, redissolve in dilute acid and analyse aqueous solution

Extract into low polarity organic solvent such as ether or a large volume of hexane

Extract into polar organic solvent such as chloroform or chloroform/ethanol

Organic layer may be washed with water before evaporation

3

3

Reduce volume of organic solvent, back extract analyte into dilute aqueous acid and then analyse aqueous layer

Evaporate polar solvent and dissolve residue in small volume of non-polar solvent such as hexane or ether. Back extract into dilute aqueous acid and analyse aqueous layer

Fig. 15.1
Flow diagram for the extraction of an organic base. (1) Direct removal of neutral and acidic excipients. (2) Acidic excipients left behind in aqueous layer. (3) Neutral excipients left behind in organic layer.

relatively polar solvents such as chloroform or mixtures of chloroform and ethanol. Similarly the sodium or potassium salts of organic acids are freely water soluble while the un-ionised acids are usually quite organosoluble. These properties can be used to advantage in designing an extraction procedure. A flow diagram for the extraction steps which can be used for the separation of an organic base from a formulation is shown in Figure 15.1.

This type of extraction is employed in the BP assay of Cyclizine Lactate Injection: the injection is diluted with dilute H_2SO_4, and then neutral and acidic excipients are extracted with ether. The solution is basified and the cyclizine is extracted into ether, leaving the lactate ion, which would not have extracted during the initial ether extraction step, behind in the aqueous layer. For convenience in measurement by UV spectrophotometry and in order to carry out volumetric dilution of the extract, cyclizine is then back extracted into dilute H_2SO_4 and subjected to further dilution.

The same principles apply to the extraction of an organic acid except that in this case high pH values are used to ensure that the acid remains in the aqueous layer and low pH values are used to ensure that it is extracted into the organic layer.

Partitioning between organic solvents

Partitioning between organic solvents is used in the extraction of analytes from oily excipients such as in the extraction of steroid creams prior to HPLC analysis.

The most commonly used systems are methanol/hexane, aqueous ethanol/hexane or acetonitrile/hexane. In the case of analysis of corticosteroids in creams, the cream is usually dispersed by heating in hexane and then extracted with an equal volume of methanol. Methanol and hexane mix only very slightly, and the oily excipients remain in the predominantly hexane layer, while the more polar corticosteroid partitions into the methanol layer. Use of an internal standard with a structure closely related to that of the analyte is essential in order to achieve good precision in this type of analysis through compensating for incomplete recovery of the analyte. Examples of pharmacopoeial methods using this type of partitioning include assays of hydrocortisone acetate cream, fluocinolone cream and beclometasone cream.

Ion pair extraction

Ion pair extraction provides a standard method for estimating ionic surfactants either colorimetrically or titrimetrically. For example, a cationic surfactant such as cetrimide can be estimated by pairing it with a lipophilic anionic dye such as bromocresol purple. The ion pairing creates a coloured lipophilic ion pair, which can be extracted into an organic solvent such as chloroform and a quantitative measurement of the colour extracted can be made spectrophotometrically. This type of assay is described in the BP for Clonidine Injection and Benzhexol Tablets.

Ion pair extraction has also been used to extract polar analytes in bioanalytical procedures. Figure 15.2 exemplifies the determination of the amino acid taurine by gas chromatography–mass spectrometry (GC–MS); this figure also illustrates a useful property of amines (and phenols), which is that they will react more rapidly than water with an acylating reagent in an aqueous environment, thus improving their organosolubility. After acylation and ion pair extraction with tetrabutyl ammonium sulphate, the taurine is converted to an amide prior to analysis by GC–MS.

Fig. 15.2 Extraction and derivatisation of taurine.

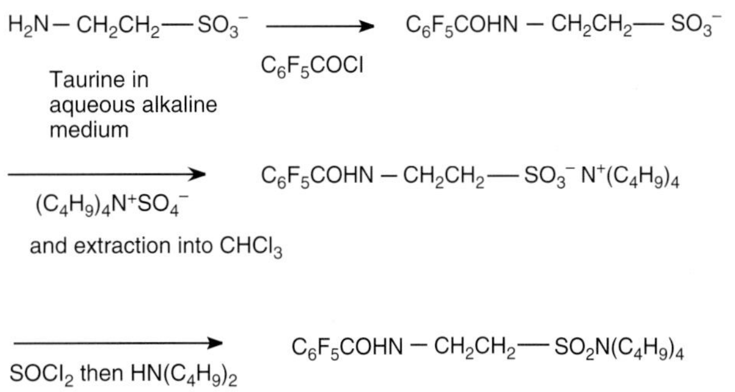

Derivatisation prior to extraction

Figure 15.3 shows aqueous-phase acylation of adrenaline in an injection with acetic anhydride. The reaction is carried out in the presence of aqueous sodium bicarbonate and is used in a gravimetric determination of (-) adrenaline in Adrenaline Injection BP.

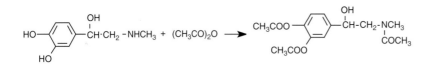

Fig. 15.3
Aqueous-phase acetylation
of adrenaline prior to
gravimetric analysis.

Supercritical fluid extraction

Figure 15.4 shows a schematic diagram of a supercritical fluid extraction apparatus. The advantages of supercritical fluid extraction (SFE) are as follows:

(i)   The solvents are used above their critical temperature and pressure but they function almost as effectively as liquid solvents and have the advantage that mass transfer between sample and solvent, i.e. the rate of extraction, is very fast.

(ii) The solvent strength of supercritical fluids can be increased or decreased by varying the pressure in the extraction vessel, thus providing a simple means of producing selective extraction.

(iii) CO_2, which is frequently used as an extraction medium, is a non-toxic, non-flammable solvent which is readily disposed, of and its low critical temperature ($31.1°C$) means that it can be used as an effective solvent for extracting unstable compounds.

The most efficient method of conducting SFE is via the dynamic process illustrated in Figure 15.4. This process enables the addition of a polar modifier such as methanol, which increases the solvent strength of the non-polar CO_2. The liquid CO_2 with about 5% v/v of modifier is passed though a stainless steel cell containing the sample, which may be mixed with inert material so that the sample occupies the whole cell volume. Two recent examples of the utilisation of SFE in the analysis of pharmaceuticals are discussed as follows.

Vitamin A, vitamin E and their acetate and palmitate esters were determined in tablets.[1] The tablet powder was mixed with sand and loaded into the extraction

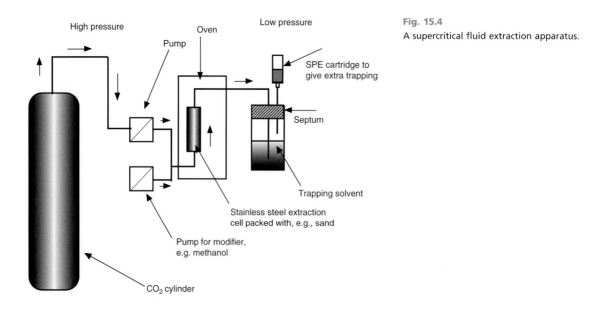

Fig. 15.4
A supercritical fluid extraction apparatus.

vessel; CO_2 alone was used for extraction at 40°C for 15 min. The CO_2 was vented to atmosphere after being passed into a vial containing tetrahydrofuran at 0°C to trap the analytes. The process was found to give good recovery and was more selective for the analytes than an established liquid/liquid extraction process. The sample was analysed by HPLC.

An unstable analogue of prostaglandin, PGE_1 formulated in a polybutadiene polymeric matrix, was placed in an SFE cell and extracted with CO_2/formic acid (95:5) at 75°C.[2] Extraction was continued for 60 min, and then the extract was collected in hexane/ethanol (2:1) at 0°C. The advantages of the SFE method were that the solvent effected simultaneous cleavage of the polymer–prostaglandin bond without instability problems and with improved mass transfer, enabling good recovery from the polymer matrix.

Microdialysis extraction

Microdialysis has become increasingly popular as a method for sampling drugs from biological fluids and tissues.[3] The technique provides protein-free samples that can be analysed directly by techniques such as HPLC. In microdialysis sampling, a probe which is directly inserted into the body is used. The probe has a semi-permeable membrane that will allow small drug molecules to pass through into the buffer within the probe but excludes the proteins in biological fluids. The buffer is pumped through the probe at flow rates of 0.5–5 μl/min, and the fluid collected from the probe may be analysed directly on-line.

Solid-phase extraction (SPE)

KEYPOINTS

Principles

The analyte is dead stopped on the SPE medium by loading it onto the cartridge in a solvent of low eluting power. It may then be washed with other solvents of low eluting power and is then finally eluted with a small volume of a strong solvent.

Applications

- Particularly useful for selective separation of interferants from analytes, which is not readily achievable by liquid/liquid extraction.
- Widely used in bioanalytical measurements and environmental monitoring for concentrating trace amounts of analyte.

Advantages in comparison with liquid/liquid extraction

Solid-phase extraction

- The solid phase is immiscible with solvents, and thus, after loading the sample, a range of washing conditions can be used to remove interferants through having a wide choice of washing solvents.
- Chemical nature of adsorbant can be varied so that it is selective for a particular functional group in the analyte.
- Emulsions are not formed between the two phases.
- A sample in a large volume of solution can be trapped on the column (dead stopped) and thus concentrated.
- Only small volumes of solvent are required for both washing and elution.
- Extraction can be carried out in batches rather than serially.
- The expense of the columns can be offset against savings in solvent purchase and disposal.

(Continued)

KEYPOINTS *(Continued)*

Liquid/liquid extraction
- Solvents must be immiscible; hence there is a limited choice of extraction and washing solvents.
- Emulsions may form.
- Large solvent volumes are required when extraction of large sample volumes is carried out.
- The extract may have to be concentrated prior to analysis and then back extracted into an aqueous phase.
- Extractions have to be conducted serially.

Limitations
- Although recoveries are generally good, it is probably best to use an internal standard in this type of analysis to compensate for any possibility of irreversible absorption onto the extraction medium.
- Silica-gel-based SPE columns are unstable to strongly alkaline conditions.

Introduction

SPE is increasingly being adopted as a useful method of sample preparation where extraction into an organic solvent would have originally been employed. The reasons for this are outlined in the Keypoints box. The technique has been employed more extensively in the 'clean up' of biological samples prior to analysis, but there are increasingly useful examples of its application to the analysis of drugs in formulations.

Methodology

Typically solid-phase extraction is based on the type of system shown in Figure 15.5. The volume of sample which can be loaded onto this small column can be increased using a column with a larger sample reservoir. The sample is usually aspirated through the column under vacuum.

The steps involved in an SPE procedure are shown in Figure 15.6:

(i)   The column is washed with 5–10 bed-volumes of the solvent, which will be used to elute the analyte, and, if an ion exchange adsorbant is to be used, 5–10 volumes of an appropriate buffer.

(ii)   The analyte is loaded onto the column in an appropriate solvent, which is too weak to elute it from the column.

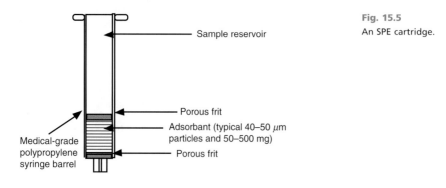

Sample reservoir

Porous frit
Adsorbant (typical 40–50 μm particles and 50–500 mg)
Porous frit

Medical-grade polypropylene syringe barrel

Fig. 15.5
An SPE cartridge.

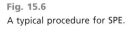

Fig. 15.6
A typical procedure for SPE.

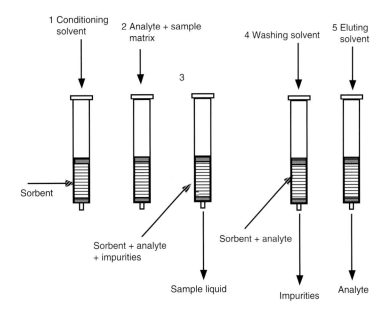

(iii) The sample solvent passes through the column, leaving the analyte + impurities adsorbed on the stationary phase.

(iv) The column is washed with solvent, which will elute impurities while leaving the analyte on the column. This requires a good understanding of the physico-chemical properties of the analyte and the adsorbant.

(v) The analyte is eluted with an appropriate solvent, preferably one which will leave further interferants behind on the column.

A vacuum manifold can be used for conducting multiple extractions simultaneously, as shown in Figure 15.7.

Fig. 15.7
Vacuum manifold for multiple solid-phase extraction.

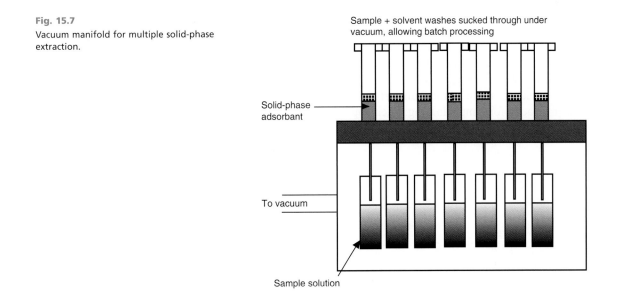

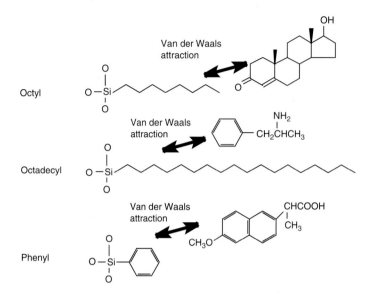

Fig. 15.8
Lipophilic silica gels.

Types of adsorbants used in SPE
Lipophilic silica gels

The lipophilic silica gels shown in Figure 15.8 will retain lipophilic compounds, provided they are in an un-ionised state, through van der Waals interactions and, in the case of amines, through some degree of polar interaction. These phases are generally not completely endcapped so there are free polar silanol groups remaining on the surface.

In the case of amines the type of interaction shown in Figure 15.9 may occur. The shorter the alkyl chain length on the silica gel surface, the more likely it is that adsorption also plays a part in the extraction. It is possible to buy highly endcapped reverse-phase silica gels where most of the residual silanols have been blocked, but it may be better to take advantage of the mixed lipophilic and adsorptive properties of reverse phases which have not been endcapped.

Recently, high-purity styrene divinylbenzene polymeric gels have become available for use in lipophilic SPE extraction; these types of materials formerly contained monomer materials which could interfere in analyses. These types of gels are much more lipophilic than surface-modified silica gels and also have a higher capacity for sample loading. Their applications are similar to those of the lipophilic silica gels.

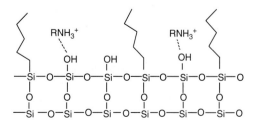

Fig. 15.9
Interaction of amines with residual silanol groups on the surface of lipophilic silica gels.

Typical extraction methodologies using lipophilic silica gels

Typically the columns are conditioned by washing with 5–10 bed-volumes of methanol followed by a 5–10 bed-volume of water or a suitable buffer.

Basic compounds are adsorbed from aqueous solution by adjusting to alkaline pH with buffer, e.g. a buffer of pH 10 would be suitable for most bases. The column can be washed with further aliquots of alkaline buffer, water or, if the compound is highly lipophilic, mixtures of methanol and alkaline buffer can be used. The compound is finally eluted with either an acidic buffer or an organic solvent such as methanol or ethanol. An example of an extraction of an amine using a lipophilic silica gel is shown in Box 15.1.

Box 15.1 Typical example of extraction by reverse-phase SPE

An oral suspension of chlorpromazine has the following composition and must be extracted so that excipients are removed prior to analysis by UV spectrophotometry: Chlorpromazine 0.025% w/v, parahydroxybenzoic acid methyl ester 0.1% w/v, neutral water-soluble dye, lipophilic flavouring agent, sodium lactate buffer.

(i) 5 ml of solution is mixed with 5 ml of 0.5 M ammonia buffer pH 9.5, and the sample is passed through an octadecyl silane (ODS) SPE cartridge. The cartridge is washed with a further 5 ml of ammonia buffer. At this stage the chlorpromazine is in its free base form and has adsorbed onto the lipophilic ODS, and the lactate, the dye and the preservative (which are all water soluble, particularly at high pH) have passed through the column.

(ii) The sample is eluted with 5 ml of 0.5 M phosphate buffer pH 2.0/methanol (95 : 5) and made up to the volume required for analysis by UV spectrophotometry. These conditions elute the basic chlorpromazine and leave behind any neutral lipophilic compounds, e.g. flavouring, on the column.

Acidic compounds are extracted from aqueous solution by adjusting to acidic pH. The column can be washed with dilute acid, water and, if the compound is highly lipophilic, mixtures of methanol and dilute acid. The compound can be eluted with methanol, acetonitrile, tetrahydrofuran (THF) or alkaline buffer.

Neutral compounds can be extracted without controlling pH. Washing can be carried out with dilute acid or alkaline buffer (to remove ionisable impurities) and methanol/water mixtures. The compounds can be eluted from the column with methanol, ethanol or chloroform.

Polar surface-modified silica gels

These silica gels retain analytes through interaction between polar groups; silica gel itself or the surface-modified polar silica gels shown in Figure 15.10 may be used.

Typical methodologies using straight-phase adsorbants

These adsorbants are typically used for polar compounds that are not well retained by reverse-phase adsorbants. The columns are conditioned by washing with 5–10 bed-volumes of the solvent which will be used to elute the analyte. The sample is loaded onto the column in a solvent which is not sufficiently strong to elute it.

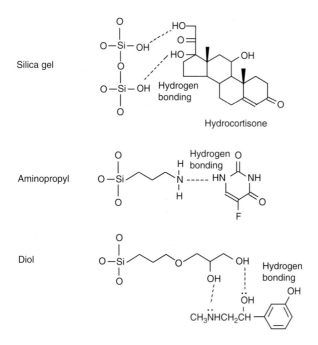

Fig. 15.10
Silica gel and polar surface-modified silica gels.

Washing of the column is often carried out with a moderate-polarity organic solvent, e.g. alcohol-free methylene chloride. Polar compounds are then eluted with methanol or mixtures of methanol and acidic buffer (for basic compounds) or methanol and alkaline buffer (for acidic compounds). Diol columns have been used to good effect in the extraction of polar drugs from pharmaceutical creams.[4,5]

Anion exchangers based on surface-modified silica gels

Ion exchangers based on polymeric resins have been in use for many years. Silica gels coated with ion exchanging groups are a relatively recent innovation. They have the advantage that they have less organosorptive properties than the polymeric resins and thus do not require as high an organic component in the eluting solvent to remove organic compounds after adsorption. Typically the anion exchanger is conditioned by washing with 0.01–0.1 M buffer at the pH of the sample solution. The buffer should contain ions which are relatively easy to displace such as OH, $C_2H_5COO^-$, CH_3COO^-, or F^-. Ions such as Cl^-, Br^-, NO_3^-, HSO_4^- or citrate are not readily displaced. The acidic sample is then applied in a buffer (0.1 M) one or two pH units above its pKa value, e.g. for methicillin shown in Figure 15.11, a buffer pH 3.8–4.8 would be used. Methicillin can be extracted with either a strong or a weak cation exchanger since it is a relatively strong acid. The adsorbant can then be washed with further amounts of the buffer, with deionised water or with organic solvent. The sample can then be eluted with a buffer containing a counter ion at a high concentration, e.g. for methicillin 1 M sodium chloride (NaCl) or 1 M sodium citrate. Many organic compounds are likely to have a high affinity for the lipophilic surface of the SPE medium, and methanol might be included in the elution buffer. Compounds can also be eluted by ionisation suppression; thus methicillin could be eluted at low pH, e.g. with

Fig. 15.11
Silica-gel-based ion exchange SPE media.

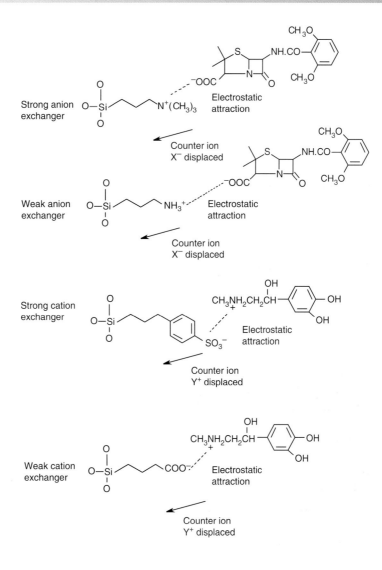

1 M hydrochloric acid/methanol, but this would not be advisable in this example because of the instability of penicillins at low pH.

Cation exchangers based on surface-modified silica gels

The cation exchange column is conditioned by washing with a 0.01–0.1 M buffer at the pH of the sample solution. The buffer should contain K^+, Na^+ or NH_4^+ ions, which are readily displaced from the gel by organic cations; divalent ions such as Ca^{2+} or Mg^{2+} are difficult to displace from the gel. The sample is then applied in a buffer (0.1 M) one or two pH units below its pKa value; e.g. for the extraction of adrenaline (Fig. 15.11) ammonium chloride (NH_4Cl) buffer pH 8.3 might be used. The adsorbant can then be washed with further amounts of the buffer, with deionised water or with an organic solvent such as methanol. Elution is then carried out with a buffer containing a counter ion at a high concentration, e.g.

1 M ammonium chloride buffer. If the sample has limited aqueous solubility a solvent such as methanol or ethanol can be included in the high ionic strength buffer. An alternative to elution at high ionic strength would be suppression of the ionisation of the amine group by elution with methanolic ammonia; however, in this case the time of exposure of the readily oxidised catechol group to high pH conditions should be minimised. This type of elution is useful if GC or GC–MS analysis is to be carried out, because the analyte is eluted in a salt-free solution.

Factors requiring attention in SPE with silica gels

(i)   Too fast a flow rate does not allow sufficient time for equilibration between the extraction medium and the solvent flowing through it; e.g. the solvent may track through the matrix without contacting the whole surface.

(ii) The capacity of sorbent gels is 1–5% of their mass, e.g. for a 100 mg cartridge 1–5 mg.

(iii) Non-selective gels may have reduced sample capacity for dirty sample matrices; e.g. if a small amount of octadecyl gel is used to extract a sample from a matrix containing large amounts of lipophilic materials, the gel capacity may be exceeded.

(iv) Attention must be paid to the control of the pH of the sample and washing solutions.

(v)   A careful choice of washing solvents can produce extensive sample 'clean up'.

(vi) The elution solvent must overcome both the primary interactions of the analyte with the bonded phase and any secondary interactions with silanol groups.

(vii) The number of fines (fine particles of silica gel) generated by different manufacturers' cartridges varies. Ideally very few fines should elute from the column with the sample. Fine particles of silica gel can damage HPLC systems and interfere in derivatisation reactions used prior to analysis by GC.

Borate gels (Fig. 15.12)

These gels are based on immobilised alkyl boronic acids. They have a selective affinity for 1,2- or 1,3-diol groupings such as those found in catechol-containing molecules such as dopamine and in sugars or glycosides.

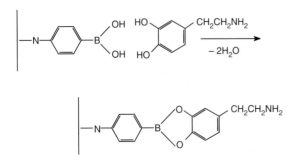

Fig. 15.12
Complex formation with a borate gel.

The analyte is loaded onto the gel in a buffer at *ca* pH 7.0, and the complex formed can then be broken down using a mildly acidic eluent such as 0.1 M acetic acid. This type of extraction has been applied to the determination of dopamine, adrenaline and noradrenaline in plasma and to the determination of the extent of reaction of glucose with serum albumin as a measure of glucose fluctuations with time in diabetics.

Immunoaffinity gels

These adsorbants are based on immobilised ligands, which have a high affinity for a particular analyte (Fig. 15.13). There are examples where antibodies have been raised to an analyte and then bound to the surface of an SPE matrix. Various types of chemistries permit this type of immobilisation, and affinity chromatography is well established in biochemistry. With the proliferation of biotechnological products such as therapeutic peptides, the use of these types of columns for extraction may increase, since they can be designed to be highly selective for such compounds.

An example of a highly specific affinity adsorbant of this type is where a monoclonal antibody to a particular compound is immobilised as shown in Figure 15.13. For instance, a gel with a monoclonal antibody to β-interferon attached has been used in industrial-scale extraction of the compound from fermentation mixtures. In most examples in the literature, polyclonal antibodies are used for preparing such columns, but the increasing availability of monoclonal antibodies (MAbs) should lead to affinity gels based on MAbs becoming available. Such specificity would be particularly valuable where peptide drugs have to be selectively extracted from biological matrices prior to analysis.

Fig. 15.13
Affinity gel with antibodies attached.

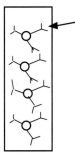

Y-shaped arms bind in a highly specific manner to the analyte

Adaptation of SPE for automated on-line extraction prior to HPLC analysis

Automated extraction can be carried out as illustrated in Figure 15.14. The basics of the system are as follows:

(i) A solvent of low strength loads the sample so that it is trapped at the head of an extraction column. This column could be non-polar if removal of polar impurities is required before chromatography or polar if removal of lipophilic materials is required.

(ii) The sample is back flushed with the same solvent which was used in loading it onto the extraction column and is trapped at the head of the chromatography column.

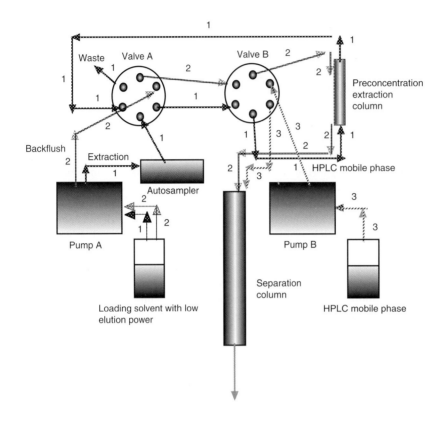

Fig. 15.14
An example of an automated SPE system.

(iii) The sample is eluted with the HPLC mobile phase; e.g. a method was developed for the analysis of macrolide antibiotics.[6] Extraction was carried out by flushing it onto a cyanopropyl cartridge with phosphate buffer pH 10.5/acetonitrile (90:10). The sample was then backflushed with the same solvent onto an ODS analytical column and then eluted with phosphate buffer pH 7/acetonitrile (46:54).

Recent developments in solid-phase and on-line extraction

There has been some development in the range of commercially available SPE media.[7,8] Most usefully a number of polymer-based phases have been produced that can retain polar molecules strongly, e.g. sulphate or glucuronide metabolites of drugs.

Solid-phase micro-extraction has been developed for use in conjunction with HPLC[9] as well as GC. The silica-based extraction fibres are coated with materials such as polydimethylsiloxane or polyacrylate with thicknesses between 7 μm and 100 μm. The fibre is inserted into the sample solution, which is then stirred to promote absorption of the analyte by the fibre. The fibre is then inserted via a septum into a specially designed injection port and is eluted with HPLC mobile phase, which transfers the analyte to the HPLC column.

Restricted access media (RAM) are becoming increasingly popular for on-line SPE.[10] RAM consist of a stationary phase which is hydrophilic on the outside but contains pores which provide a hydrophobic surface. The pores are large enough to allow hydrophobic drug molecules to enter and become trapped, but proteins are too large and are excluded and thus pass straight through the column with minimal interaction. The chemical nature of both the internal and external surface of the RAM can be varied.

References

1. Scalia S, Ruberto G, Bonina F. *J Pharm Sci*. 1995;84:433-436.
2. Royston DA, Sun JJ, Collins PW, Perkins WE, Tremont JJ. *J Pharm Biomed Anal*. 1995;13:1513-1520.
3. Garrison KE, Pasas SA, Cooper JD, Davies MI. *Eur J Pharm Sci*. 2002;17:1-12.
4. Di Pietra AM, Cavrini V, Andrisano V, Gatti R. *J Pharm Biomed Anal*. 1992;10:873.
5. Bonazzi D, Andrisano V, Gatti R, Cavrini V. *J Pharm Biomed Anal*. 1995;13:1321-1329.
6. Hedemo M, Eriksson B-M. *J Chromatogr Biomed Apps*. 1995;692:161-166.
7. Kataoka H. *Trends in Anal Chem*. 2003;22:232-244.
8. Smith RM. *J Chromatogr A*. 2003;1000:3-27.
9. Kumazawa T, Lee X-P, Sato K, Suzuki O. *Anal Chim Acta*. 2003;492:49-67.
10. Souverain S, Rudaz S, Veuthey J-L. *J Chromatogr B*. [In press].

Further reading

Cruz-Vera M, Lucena R, Cardenas S, Valcarcel M. Sorptive microextraction for liquid-chromatographic determination of drugs in urine. *TrAC Trends Anal Chem*. 2009;28:1164-1173.

Kataoka H. Recent developments and applications of microextraction techniques in drug analysis. *Anal Bioanal Chem*. 2010;396:339-364.

Pedersen-Bjergaard S, Rasmussen KE. Liquid-phase microextraction with porous hollow fibers, a miniaturized and highly flexible format for liquid-liquid extraction. *J Chromatogr A*. 2008;1184:132-142.

Thurman EM, Mills MS. *Solid-Phase Extraction Principles and Practice*. Chichester: Wiley Interscience; 1998.

Vuckovic D, Zhang X, Cudjoe E, Pawliszyn J. Solid-phase microextraction in bioanalysis: new devices and directions. *J Chromatogr A*. 2010;1217:4041-4060.

Methods used in the quality control of biotechnologically produced drugs

16

KEYPOINTS

Biologic drugs

The vast majority of drugs produced by using biological systems are peptides or proteins. Insulin was the first protein-based drug to be used and has been used since the early 20th century. The largest number of new drugs currently making it to market are proteins. Monoclonal antibody therapies are the most commonly registered new drugs. The quality control of protein drugs is more complex than the quality control of low molecular weight drugs because of the size and complexity of protein drugs and the complexity of the biological systems which are used to produce them.

Principles and scope of techniques used not covered in previous chapters

- Sodium dodecyl sulphate polyacrylamide gel electrophoresis (SDSPAGE). Proteins are separated according to their molecular weight as they migrate through a gel under the influence of an electric field. Low-resolution technique.
- Isoelectric focusing is used to separate proteins according to their p*I* values using a gel with a pH gradient and with the application of an electric field. The more basic proteins migrate farthest up the gel. Used for determining glycoforms of proteins.

(Continued)

Protein drugs

Proteins have been used successfully as drugs since the early 20th century when insulin was first used to treat diabetes. The isolation of insulin was followed by the development of other protein drugs that were mainly extracted from animal tissues until the 1970s when smaller peptides, which had been discovered by extraction from animal tissues, became available via chemical synthesis. Table 16.1 lists some of these older protein drugs with their therapeutic actions. With the advent of genetic engineering it became possible to insert the genes required to make protein drugs into bacterial and mammalian cells. The cells are then cultured on a large scale to produce the therapeutic peptides. The first peptide drugs to be produced in this way were insulin and human growth hormone which were produced in *Escherichia coli* cultures. This was followed by the production of hepatitis B vaccine in yeast cells and erythropoietin (EPO) in Chinese hamster ovary (CHO) cells. The advantage of using mammalian cells to produce a protein

Table 16.1 Old peptide drugs

Peptide	Physical characteristics	Source	Therapeutic actions
Glucagon	30 amino acids	Bovine or porcine pancreas or synthetic	Reversal of insulin-induced hypoglycaemia
Calcitonin	33 amino acids	Porcine thyroid, salmon or synthesis	Lowers plasma Ca levels in hypercalcaemia
Insulin	51 amino acids, two chains linked by 2 S-S bridges	Bovine or porcine pancreas, *ca* 98% pure	First used in 1922 to treat diabetes
Human growth hormone	191 amino acids	Human pituitary gland	Treatment of short stature resulting from deficiency of the hormone
Blood coagulation factors, e.g. factor VIII	330 kDa	Human blood	Used to treat haemophilia
Vaccines	High molecular weight proteins	Infective organisms. May be live but inactive pathogen, crude extract from dead pathogen or partly purified	Stimulation of the immune system to develop B-lymphocyte memory cells which recognize pathogen
Immunoglobulins	150 kDa or greater	Obtained from pooled human blood	Mixture of antibodies which can confer short-term resistance to a variety of pathogens, e.g. hepatitis A

Table 16.2 Top selling biologics in 2012

Brand name	Production method	Company	Sales (millions of dollars)	Indications
Humira (adalimumab)	CHO	AbbVie	9265	Rheumatoid arthritis, psoriasis, Crohn's disease, ulcerative colitis, ankylosing spondylitis, psoriatic arthritis
Remicade (infliximab)	Murine Myeloma	Johnson & Johnson and Merck & Co.	8215	Rheumatoid arthritis, ankylosing spondylitis, psoriatic arthritis, chronic psoriasis in adults, ulcerative colitis
Enbrel (etanercept)	CHO	Amgen and Pfizer	7963	Psoriasis, psoriatic arthritis, moderate to severe rheumatoid arthritis
Rituxin (rituximab, MabThera)	CHO	Roche and Biogen Idec	7285	Non-Hodgkin's lymphoma, chronic lymphocytic leukaemia, rheumatoid arthritis
Lantus (insulin glargine)	*E. coli*	Sanofi	6648	Once daily treatment for diabetes
Herceptin (trastuzumab)	CHO	Roche	6397	HER2-positive breast cancer and HER2-positive metastatic gastric cancer
Avastin (bevacizumab)	CHO	Roche	6260	Metastatic colorectal cancer (colon cancer), non–small cell lung cancer, glioblastoma, metastatic kidney
Neulasta (pegfilgrastim)	*E. coli*	Amgen	4092	Neutropenia caused by cancer chemotherapy

such as EPO is that they are able to attach sugar chains to the protein after it has been translated from RNA, which may be important for the activity of the protein. Bacterial cells are not able to carry out such post-translational modifications. The field is moving very rapidly, and currently over 50% of new drugs approved are biologics; the most rapidly expanding area is in monoclonal antibody treatments. This is set to increase further. Table 16.2 shows the best-selling biologics, and these can be recognized in Table 16.2 since their generic names always end in 'mab'. Humira is currently the third most valuable drug in terms of revenue, so there are only two low molecular weight synthetic drugs which achieve better sales. Thus a good knowledge of the quality control (QC) for these drugs will be very useful for aspiring pharmaceutical analysts. The major difference between the low molecular weight drugs considered earlier in this book and biologics is the complexity of the molecules, and obviously the more complex the molecule, the greater the challenges in controlling the quality of the molecule.

Protein structure

Amino acids and amino acid sequences

In order to understand the analytical methods used for proteins it is necessary to have some understanding of the structure of proteins. The basic building blocks which make up proteins are the 20 amino acids, and there may be between tens and thousands of amino acids in a particular protein. The simplest amino acid is glycine (Fig. 16.1), which has a carboxylic acid group (pKa 2.5) and a primary

Fig. 16.1
The effect of pH on the charge of amino acids.

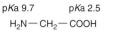

pKa 9.7   pKa 2.5
H_2N-CH_2-COOH $H_3N^+-CH_2-COO^-$

glycine   zwitterion (at pH 5.1 the
                          charges are exactly balanced)

$$\overset{\oplus}{H_3N}-\overset{\underset{|}{R}}{CH}-COOH \qquad H_2N-\overset{\underset{|}{R}}{CH}-COO^-$$

pH 1   pH 13

amine group (pKa 9.7). Like all amino acids in its free state, when not part of a protein chain, it can carry both positive and negative charges depending on the pH of the solution that it is dissolved in, and there is no pH at which it is not charged. A molecule which carries both positive and negative charges in solution is known as a zwitterion, and in the case of a simple amino acid like glycine the charges are equal and opposite at a pH halfway between the two pKa values, i.e. at pH 5.1. This point is known as the isoelectric point, and its value is known as the p*I* of the molecule. As shown in Figure 16.1 an amino acid is completely positively charged only at low pH and completely negatively charged only at high pH. In the case of glycine the side chain of the amino acid is represented by R = H, but the other 19 amino acids occurring in proteins have various R groups.

There are various ways of classifying the amino acids, but perhaps the most useful in terms of protein function is classification into hydrophobic, neutral hydrophilic and charged hydrophilic. Glycine can be classified on its own since it does not fall into any of these categories, although lack of a side chain gives it flexibility. For this reason, it has an important role in protein structure, allowing the protein backbone to bend so that it can form its secondary structure. The hydrophobic, polar and charged categories of amino acids are shown in Figure 16.2 along with their single letter codes which are used as a shorthand method for writing out the primary sequence of a protein.

Polar amino acids

Polar amino acids (Fig. 16.2) have a diverse range of functions. Serine residues are important in enzyme catalysed reactions, cysteine is important in determining the three-dimensional structure of proteins because of its ability to form S-S bridges with another cysteine residue and tyrosine and serine are important because they form phosphate esters which cause an alteration of protein conformation thus triggering other cellular events and even causing the movement of muscle proteins. Asparagine and glutamine are important sites for hydrogen bonding within proteins and with ligands binding to proteins. In addition cysteine is important for its ability to bond to metal ions such as iron or copper which are often present at the active sites of enzymes.

Hydrophobic amino acids

Hydrophobic amino acids (Fig. 16.2) exhibit varying degrees of hydrophobicity depending on how large the hydrophobic side chain is. Alanine is the least hydrophobic and tryptophan is the most hydrophobic, even though it contains a slightly

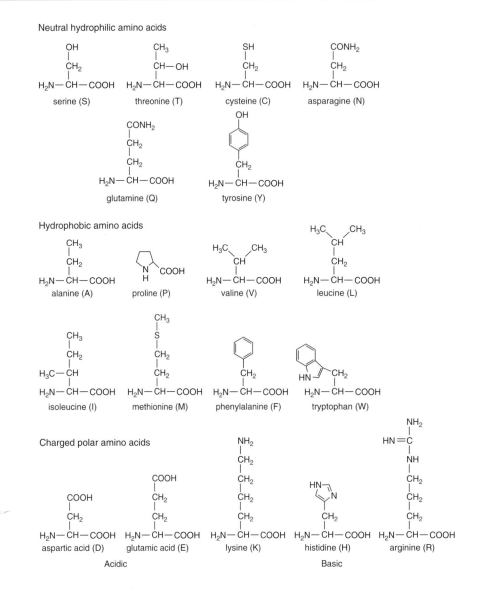

Fig. 16.2
The 19 amino acids in
addition to glycine
occurring in proteins.

polar indole nitrogen. These amino acids are quite water soluble at high or low
pH, but if the pH is adjusted to around their p*I* value, then they are effectively
neutral and their hydrophobicity will cause them to come out of solution. This
class of amino acid is found buried inside proteins avoiding contact with water,
and thus they form the protein core. If the protein has a helical portion which
passes through a lipophilic cell membrane, this portion of the protein will be
found to be rich in hydrophobic/lipophilic amino acids.

Charged amino acids

Charged amino acids (Fig. 16.2) are found predominantly on the surface of proteins in contact with the surrounding solution. Thus they are responsible for the

solution stability of the protein, and if they lose their charge the protein will become unstable and precipitate out of solution. A standard method for removing a protein from a solution is to adjust the pH so that it is strongly acidic so that the negatively charged side chains of the protein become uncharged, thus destabilizing its structure in solution. Often proteins cannot be re-dissolved after such treatment. A more gentle method of removing proteins from solution is to salt them out with concentrated ammonium sulphate, which effectively competes with the protein groups for the solvating water molecules required to keep the protein in solution, thus causing it to precipitate. The charged residues in proteins are important in the action of many drug molecules; many drugs are bases, and they bind to the negatively charged aspartate or glutamate side chains in proteins. Histidine can be classified as a polar neutral amino acid residue since it is only about 4% ionized at physiological pH; however its charge state is important since its pKa value of 6 provides buffering in the pH range 5–7 where many proteins exert their functions. The pI values of the charged amino acids are either higher or lower than those of neutral amino acids such as glycine. The pI value of a protein depends on the balance of acidic and basic residues within its structure. For example a protein such as alpha-1 acid glycoprotein, which is responsible for binding basic drugs circulating in the blood, has a pI value of *ca* 3.0, is referred to as an acidic protein. Lysozyme, which is present in tears and is used to digest bacterial cell walls, is a basic protein containing many arginine residues and has a pKa of 9.0. The pI value of a protein is an important property used in the quality control of protein drugs.

The peptide bond and the primary structure of proteins

The amino acids which make up a protein and the order in which they are joined together is known as the primary structure of the protein. In forming the primary structure the amino group of one amino acid reacts with the carboxylic acid of another amino acid to form an amide: the peptide bond. In the process of the production of the peptide the DNA sequence coding for a particular amino acid is transcribed to produce the RNA sequence corresponding to a particular amino acid. The RNA sequence then binds to a sequence in a tRNA molecule corresponding to a particular amino acid. This process occurs in the cellular ribosomes which contain a binding site which specifies the next amino acid to be added to the growing peptide and recruits the appropriate aminoacyl-tRNA to be added to the growing peptide chain which is held in another binding site within the ribosome. By convention the amino terminal (N-terminal) of a peptide is at the left-hand end of a sequence of amino acids and the carboxyl (C-terminal) of a peptide is at the right-hand end. The structure of the nonapeptide (having nine amino acid residues) vasopressin is shown in Figure 16.3; proteins such as enzymes or antibodies have many more amino acids. However, there are many small peptides which have important biological activities, and vasopressin is important for controlling blood pressure via its anti-diuretic action. Figure 16.3 also shows the short code for vasopressin which has a post-translational modification of its structure at the C-terminus where the carboxyl group in glycine has been converted into an amide. The vasopressin code based on the single letter amino acid codes is shown in Figure 16.3 as well.

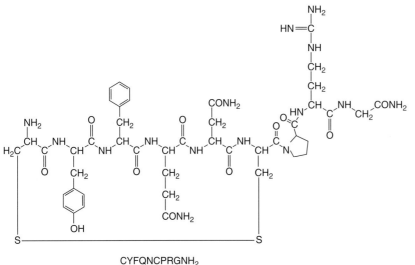

Fig. 16.3
Structure of vasopressin.

CYFQNCPRGNH₂

Self-test 16.1

Draw the structure of the nonapeptide oxytocin based on its single letter code including its S-S bridge.
CYIQNCPLGNH2

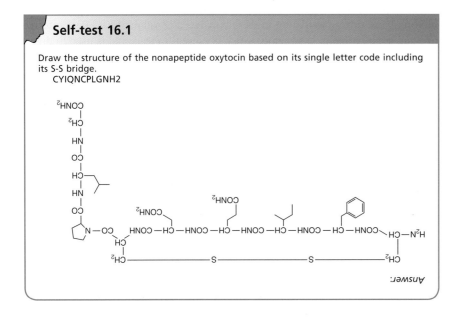

Answer:

As instrumental methods have advanced it has become easier to determine the structure of unknown proteins. Protein molecular weights and sequences can now be rapidly determined by using mass spectrometry (Chapter 9). The protein sequence is most often determined by carrying out a tryptic digest which cleaves proteins at the C-terminus side of either lysine or arginine (Fig. 16.4) except when they are followed by a proline residue. This results in a limited number of peptides which are generally in the range of 500–3000 amu and are thus amenable to analysis by high-performance liquid chromatography (HPLC)-with ultraviolet (UV) or mass spectrometry detection. While proteomics research concerns itself with mass spectrometric elucidation of unknown protein structures, the tests in pharmacopoeial monographs use HPLC-UV to produce a characteristic fingerprint of the protein. Many peptides are likely to contain one of the UV-absorbing amino

Fig. 16.4
Trypsin cleavage points.

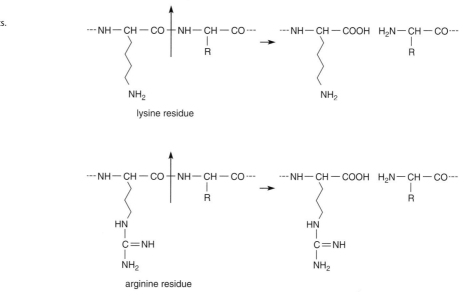

lysine residue

arginine residue

acids phenylalanine, tyrosine, tryptophan or histidine, and the peptide bond itself has weak UV absorption at about 210 nm. Considering the peptide hormone insulin-derived growth factor fragments it is possible to predict that the sequence of peptides shown in Figure 16.5 would be formed following tryptic digest. Cleavage next to the three lysine and two arginine residues should in theory yield the six peptides with the amino acid residues as shown in Figure 16.5. Cleavage does not always proceed according to theory, and sometimes cleavage points are missed by the enzyme, but the fingerprint for a particular protein is reproducible. The short peptide fragments produced by digesting a protein with trypsin or other proteolytic enzyme are quite characteristic of using a basic local alignment search tool (BLAST) to search the peptide against a database which will usually bring up a match against a specific protein. This is illustrated in Self-test 16.2.

Self-test 16.2

Predict the fragments which result from the tryptic digestion of human proinsulin
MALWMRLLPL LALLALWGPDPAAAFVNQHLCGSHLVEALYLVCGERGFFY
TPKTRREAEDLQVGQVELGG GPGAGSLQPLALEGSLQKRGIVEQCCTSICSLYQLENYCN

Answer: MALWMR LLPLLALLALWGPDPAAAFVNQHLCGSHLVEALYLVCGER GFFYTPK TR R
EAEDLQVGQVELGGGPGAGSLQPLALEGSLQK R GIVEQCCTSICSLYQLENYCN

Fig. 16.5
Peptide fragments resulting from tryptic digestion of insulin-derived growth factor-related peptide.

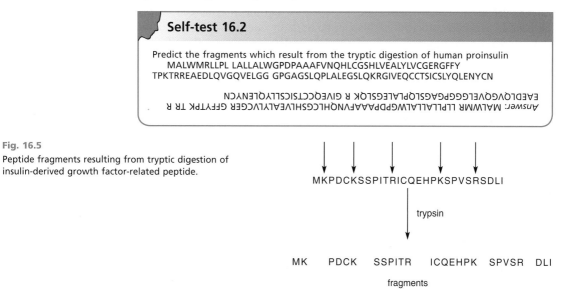

MKPDCKSSPITRICQEHPKSPVSRSDLI

trypsin

MK   PDCK   SSPITR   ICQEHPK   SPVSR   DLI

fragments

Thus the determination of protein primary structure is relatively straightforward, although small alterations in the primary structure due to degradation may be harder to observe.

Protein secondary structure

Determining the primary sequence of a protein is only part of the effort required for structure confirmation. Protein chains fold and this gives proteins a secondary structure. There are two basic formats: the β-sheet format where the protein chains are arranged in a relatively flat sheet, which is the format often found at the active sites of enzymes, and the α-helix format, which is found for instance in membrane spanning receptor proteins or membrane ion channels (Fig. 16.6). The secondary structure is influenced by the protein tertiary structure which includes post-translational chemical modifications such as glycosylation (described in more detail below) and formation of S-S bridges between cysteine residues within the protein. It is also affected by degradation of particular amino acids making up the primary structure of the protein such as hydrolysis of the amino acids glutamine and asparagine which have amide side chains (Fig. 16.7). Small changes in the primary structure can disrupt protein secondary structure and thus may have a large effect on biological activity.

In order for protein digestion to occur efficiently prior to fingerprinting the protein secondary structure has to be disrupted so that the enzyme can access the peptide backbone efficiently. This can be done by addition of a denaturant such as urea, which causes the protein to unfold, and then the protein is unfolded further by reducing the cysteine bridges within its structure using a reagent such

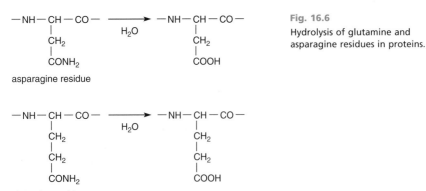

Fig. 16.6
Hydrolysis of glutamine and asparagine residues in proteins.

Fig. 16.7

α-helix and β-sheet forms of protein secondary structure.

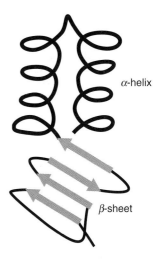

α-helix

β-sheet

as Tris (2-carboxyethyl) phosphine (TCEP), as shown in Figure 16.8. After reducing the S-S bridge reformation of the bridge has to be blocked, and this is typically carried out by reaction with iodoacetamide (Fig. 16.8) which alkylates the SH groups. This process is known as carbamidomethylation. It is possible to predict the fragments which will produced by these processes and the subsequent proteolytic digestion. This is illustrated in Self-test 16.4.

Self-test 16.4

Use Protein Prospector: http://prospector.ucsf.edu/prospector/mshome.htm

From the peptide/protein MS utility programmes select MS digest. Select Uni Prot as the database. Select trypsin as the digest term and carbamidomethyl (C) from the variable mods list. Select Retrieve by: Accession Number, clear the entries box and type in P61278 which is the code for somatostatin. Leave all the other boxes at default, making sure that the variable modifications are deselected by using control-click. Digest your protein. How many fragments do you get? What are the sequences and molecular weights of the fragments from the N- and C-termini of the protein? How many carbamidomethyl groups do these fragments contain?

Change the enzyme to chymotrypsin. How many fragments do you get? Which amino acids does chymotrypsin cleave next to?

Somastatin P61278

1

MLSCRLQCALAALSIVLALGCVTGAPSDPR LRQFLQKSLAAAAGKQELAK YFLAELLSEPNQTENDALEP EDLSQAAEQDEMRLELQRSA NSNPAMAPRE RKAGCKNFFWKTFTSC

116

Answer: 12 fragments, NFFWKTFTSC 1337.5983 (1 carbamidomethyl), MLSCRLQCALAALSIVLALGCVTGAPSDPR 3200.6411 (3 carbamidomethyl). Chymotrypsin produces 52 peptides and cleaves next to leucine, tyrosine and phenylalanine. Trypsin produces the more specific fingerprint in this case

---

Of course the primary structure of the protein tells the analyst nothing about the secondary and tertiary structures, and the control of these complex structures requires methods which differ from those used for low molecular weight drugs. The tests for the quality of protein-based drugs are lengthy and complex in comparison with those used for low molecular weight drugs.

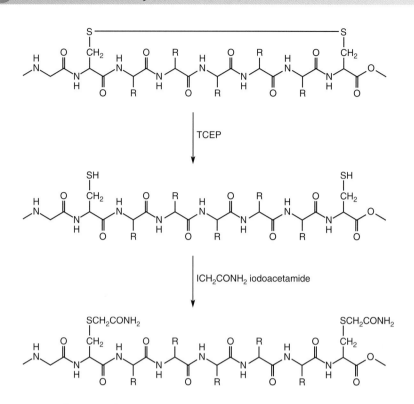

Fig. 16.8
Reduction of an S-S
bridge followed by
carbamidomethylation.

Protein tertiary structure

Protein tertiary structure is formed as a result of post-translational modifications of protein. As mentioned above formation of S-S bridges between cysteine residues in proteins is a common element in tertiary structure. The most common quality control issue in protein tertiary structure is the control of protein glycosylation. Sugar chains in proteins are relatively short, with 5–10 monosaccharide residues being attached to the protein after it has been translated from RNA. For example the sugar chains found on glycoproteins on the surfaces of red blood cells which determine blood group contain just 5–6 sugar residues (Fig. 16.9). There are eight monosaccharides commonly found in glycoside chains in proteins (Fig. 16.9). One of the most important is sialic acid, which affects the p*I* value of a protein.

The common types of post-translational modifications are best illustrated by Figure 16.10, which shows modification sites on a monoclonal antibody. The two halves of the antibody are joined together by S-S bridges, and the antibody contains variable glycoside chains which may affect its half-life within the body. It is the Fab region of the antibody which is responsible for binding to the targeted antigen. Monoclonal antibody therapy is the fastest growing area of drug therapy; MAbs (Fig. 16.10) are very large molecules with molecular weights > 100 000 Daltons. Many of the instrumental methods used to control the quality of these drugs have not found their way into pharmacopoeial monographs since there are no generic versions of these drugs and they are still licensed to only a single manufacturer, but this will change over the next 20 years. Someone wishing to have a career in pharmaceutical quality control would be well advised to get some experience of the methods used in the QC of MAbs.

Fig. 16.9
Monosaccharides commonly found in oligosaccharide chains in glycoproteins and glycoside determinants of blood groups.

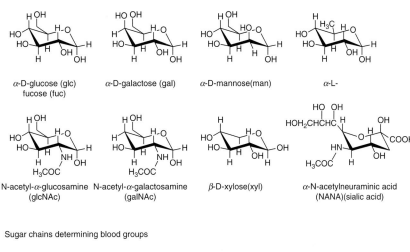

α-D-glucose (glc)
fucose (fuc)

α-D-galactose (gal)

α-D-mannose(man)

α-L-

N-acetyl-α-glucosamine (glcNAc)

N-acetyl-α-galactosamine (galNAc)

β-D-xylose(xyl)

α-N-acetylneuraminic acid (NANA)(sialic acid)

Sugar chains determining blood groups

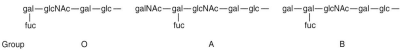

```
gal—glcNAc—gal—glc—     galNAc—gal—glcNAc—gal—glc—     gal—gal—glcNAc—gal—glc—
   |                              |                               |
  fuc                            fuc                             fuc

Group            O                        A                              B
```

Instrumental techniques used in the analysis of biotechnologically produced drugs

Introduction

The production process for biotechnological drugs is complex, and therefore significant levels of impurities may be present in these drugs. Often the 'impurities' arise from variations in the post-translational modifications of the drugs and thus are closely related to the accepted form of the drug but may have different biological properties. Every era of drug development has its disasters, and a notable example in the development of biotechnological drugs was a disastrous clinical trial of an MAb in 2006 which led to six people becoming severely ill due to severe immunological reactions.[1] Thus it is important to ensure that high quality control standards are adhered to in the production of biologics. However, there are a number of other impurities related to the production process, which include host cell protein, host cell DNA, endotoxins (e.g. from *E. coli*

Fig. 16.10
Schematic diagram of a monoclonal antibody. CH1, heavy chain constant region 1; CH2, heavy chain constant region 2; CH3, heavy chain constant region 3; CL, light chain constant region; Fab, antigen binding fragment; VH, heavy chain variable region; VL, light chain variable region.

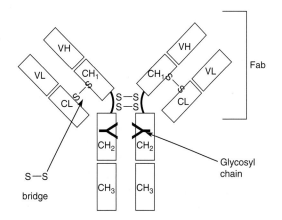

fermentation), process additives such as antifoaming agents, buffer components and enzymes and viruses and prions. In addition, there are impurities related to the drug itself, and these can be classified as equipotent impurities or impurities of higher and lower activity which may include substances such as protein aggregates. For the older drugs there are comprehensive pharmacopoeial monographs, but the registration of new biotech products in recent years has been rapid; thus many of the methods used by companies are not common in pharmacopoeial monographs since the drugs are not yet generic.

Size exclusion chromatography (SEC)

The principle of SEC is briefly described in Chapter 12. As applied to proteins, separation is on the basis that larger proteins are excluded from the SEC matrix to a greater extent than smaller proteins so they elute early. SEC is a low-resolution separation technique in its purest form; this is illustrated in the separation of the proteins shown in Figure 16.11 where there is only 10 ml of elution volume between a protein of MW 12 500 and the smallest amino acid glycine.

The following practical points apply to SEC:

- In order to estimate molecular weight, columns have to be calibrated. Calibration is non-linear.
- Protein conformation affects retention volume.
- Packing is not completely inert and hydrophobic and electrostatic interactions can occur, giving a false molecular weight estimation.
- Mobile phase is an aqueous salt solution, and the salt, and ionic strengths have to be chosen carefully to minimize interactions with the packing.

SEC is a very common basic QC test for non-generic protein drugs. In the pharmacopoeias it is very commonly used to test for protein aggregation in which protein molecules form high molecular weight complexes involving two or three protein molecules which will reduce their efficacy.

The SEC tests used in the pharmacopoeias are based on using HPLC columns packed with hydrophilic silica gels which are coated with a glycol stationary phase. These silica gels work by a combination of adsorption and size exclusion and produce much longer elution times than would be expected from pure SEC. Elution is still in order of molecular size, but the long elution times the retention cannot be due to size exclusion alone, as can be seen in Figure 16.12, which shows the separation of plasma proteins on a diol column. The pore size of these columns can be varied between 6 and 30 nm, with the larger pore size being more suitable for large proteins. The main application of an SEC test in pharmacopoeias is to test for high molecular weight aggregates in proteins. The following tests use a hydrophilic silica gel diol column to carry out the tests:

- The levels of higher molecular weight proteins in erythropoietin. The total of any peaks (higher molecular weight proteins) eluted before the principal peak should not be > 2% of the area of the main peak.
- High molecular weight impurities in aprotinin.
- High molecular weight impurities in human, porcine and bovine insulins.
- Molecular weight size distribution in factor VIII.
- Polyribosylribitol phosphate molecular size distribution and free levels in influenza vaccine.

Fig. 16.11

Separation of mixture of low molecular weight (MW) peptides (column 10x 306 mm dextran based): 1, cytochrome C (MW 12500); 2, aprotinin (MW 6500); 3, gastrin I (MW 2126); 4, substance P (MW 1348); 5, gly$_6$ (MW 360); 6, gly$_3$ (MW 189); 7, gly (MW 75). *(From Irvine G. Size-exclusion high-performance liquid chromatography of peptides: A review. Analytica Chimica Acta. 1997;352:387-397 with permission.)*

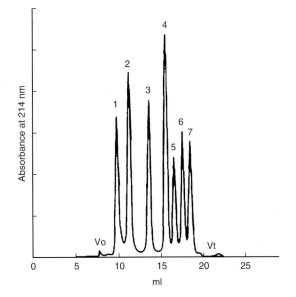

In all cases the high molecular weight impurities will elute before the main peak for the protein drug.

Size exclusion tends to be used less for quality control of monoclonal antibodies, and high performance ion exchange chromatography is more frequently used. Figure 16.13 shows a chromatogram of a monoclonal antibody manufactured by using two different cell lines. The column used is a weak cation exchange column and the forms of the antibody, having a higher content of acidic sugars, elute first because their overall positive charge is lower and hence there is less interaction with the cation exchanger.

Fig. 16.12

Separation of serum proteins on a diol size exclusion column.

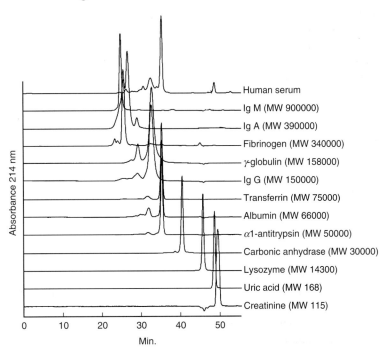

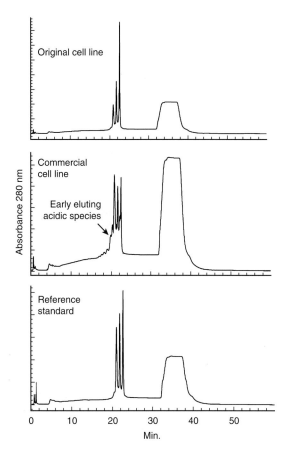

Fig. 16.13
Analysis of monoclonal of a monoclonal antibody produced by two different cell lines by high-performance weak cation exchange chromatography showing earlier eluting impurities with greater acidity in the glycoside chains in the product produced by the commercial cell line. *(From Lubiniecki A, Volkin DB, Federici M, et al. Comparability assessments of process and product changes made during development of two different monoclonal antibodies. Biologicals. 2011;39:9-22 with permission.)*

Self-test 16.5

What would be the order of elution from first to last of the following small peptides from a weak cation exchange column?

1. GYRLIPQD
2. ALWFLLGS
3. KRWFFLSK
4. TWKFYRGG

Answer: Based on the number of basic amino acid residues the order of elution would be 2, 1, 4, 3

Sodium dodecyl sulphate polyacrylamide gel electrophoresis (SDSPAGE)

SDSPAGE was one of the first techniques used for the analysis of proteins. Capillary electrophoresis has been covered in Chapter 14, and the principle of migration under the influence of a high voltage is essentially the same. Figure 16.14 shows the procedure used in SDSPAGE which relies on the fact that all proteins

Fig. 16.14

The process of protein analysis using SDSPAGE.

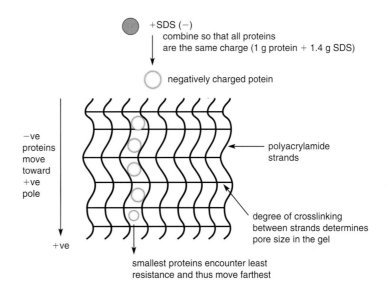

will absorb the anion SDS in exactly the same proportions of w/w basis, giving them an identical negative charge regardless of the type of protein. The proteins are then separated on the basis of their size, with the smaller proteins finding it easier to move through the polyacrylamide gel network under the influence of the applied electric field and thus moving farther up the gel. Using the example of the European Pharmacopoeial monograph for the red blood cell stimulating protein erythropoietin (EPO), EPO is run on a gel which is calibrated by using a series of marker proteins of known molecular weight and is also compared against an EPO reference standard. Having run the gel the next step is to visualize it and various stains can be used. Figure 16.15 shows a stained gel used to analyze several generic batches of EPO in comparison with calibration proteins and Epogen, which is manufactured by the originator of the drug. It is hard to see clear differences between most of the samples with this separation method. The

Fig. 16.15

SDSPAGE gel showing the analysis of different generic batches of EPO in comparison with molecular weight markers and Epogen, the product manufactured the originator of the drug. *(From Federici M, Lubiniecki A, Manikwar P, Volkin DB. Analytical lessons learned from selected therapeutic protein drug comparability studies. Biologicals. 2013;41:131-147 with permission.)*

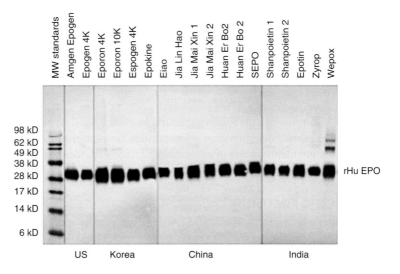

figure also nicely illustrates how rapidly generic products proliferate once a drug is off patent even in the biotech sector. In the pharmacopoeial method for EPO the gel is prepared so that it can be cut in half. Half the gel is stained with Coomassie blue stain, which is a general stain for proteins, and the other half is analyzed by immunoblotting (Fig. 16.16). In order to carry out immunoblotting the gel is laid onto a nitrocellulose membrane, and then a potential is applied between the gel and the membrane so that proteins on the gel are transferred to the membrane (Western blotting). The membrane is then incubated with a blocking protein such as the proteins from dried milk which prevents non-specific binding to the membrane. Then the membrane is developed by incubating with an antibody to EPO which binds specifically to EPO and not to the blocking protein. The detection antibody is conjugated to an enzyme which can be used to locate the place where the antibody has bound. The membrane is incubated with the antibody to EPO, then the membrane is rinsed and the membrane is re-incubated with a secondary antibody which binds to the bound antibody. This antibody is conjugated to an enzyme such as alkaline phosphatase. The membrane is rinsed and then incubated with a substrate for the enzyme-linked antibody; in the case of alkaline phosphatase this is the phosphate of nitrophenol. Nitrophenol is released by the enzyme and stains the EPO spot with a yellow colour. This process is known as enzyme-linked immunosorbant assay (ELISA) and will be described in more detail below.

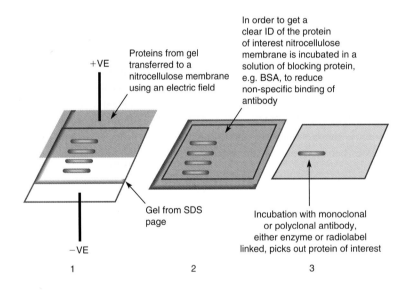

In order to get a clear ID of the protein of interest nitrocellulose membrane is incubated in a solution of blocking protein, e.g. BSA, to reduce non-specific binding of antibody

Proteins from gel transferred to a nitrocellulose membrane using an electric field

+VE

−VE

Gel from SDS page

Incubation with monoclonal or polyclonal antibody, either enzyme or radiolabel linked, picks out protein of interest

1　　2　　3

Fig. 16.16
The process of immunoblotting for the detection of specific proteins (Western blotting).

SDSPAGE is used in the following pharmacopoeial tests: determination of the purity of alteplase, determination of impurities in interferon 2α, impurities in Molgramostim, identification of recombinant factor VIII, identification of recombinant hepatitis B vaccine, identification of adsorbed pertussis vaccine.

Isoelectric focusing

As can be seen in Figure 16.15 SDSPAGE is not exactly a high-resolution test since the spots on the gel for EPO cover quite a wide range of molecular weights. The main cause of variation of the molecular weight of a particular protein is the

Fig. 16.17
Isoelectric focusing.

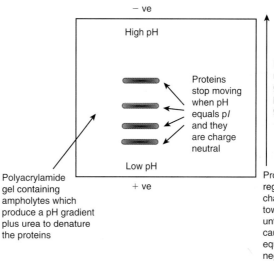

extent to which it is glycosylated. A variation on the SDSPAGE experiment is to use the same gel system but without pretreating the proteins with SDS. Instead the gel is made up so that it contains a pH gradient across the gel. The mechanism of separation in this case is related not to size but rather to pI value (the pH where a protein is equally positively and negatively charged which depends on the relative numbers of basic and acidic side chains in the protein). The protein migrates under the influence of the applied electric field to a point (particular pH) within the gel where it is charge neutral (Fig. 16.17). The usual types of stains are used to visualize the gel. Figure 16.18 shows the separation of the glycoforms of EPO using isoelectric focusing carried out for the same generic batches that were shown in Figure 16.15. The sugar chains attached to any protein carry negative charges in the form of the acidic sugars, sialic acids; the greater number of these sugar acids present in the molecule, the lower the pI of that form of the protein. Thus the lowest spots in Figure 16.18 contain the most sialic acid residues. It can be seen that there is wide variation in the level of glycosylation of the generic forms of EPO, which might have an impact on their biological activity.

The following pharmacopoeial tests use isoelectric focusing.

Fig. 16.18
Analysis of the glycoforms of generic form of EPO using isoelectric focusing. *(From Federici M, Lubiniecki A, Manikwar P, Volkin DB. Analytical lessons learned from selected therapeutic protein drug comparability studies. Biologicals. 2013;41:131-147 with permission.)*

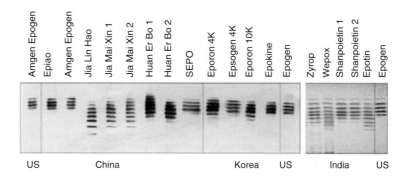

Alteplase glycoforms

- The microheterogeneity of glycosylation of the alteplase can be demonstrated by isoelectric focusing.
- A complex banding pattern with 10 major and several minor bands in the pH range 6.5–8.5 is observed.
- The higher the p*I* value of the variant, the lower its sialic acid content.

Glycosylation is important in alteplase since it affects its half-life in the body.

Molgramostim identification test

- pH gradient over a narrow range 4–6.5.
- The p*I* of the principal band should be 4.9–5.4.
- System suitability: the p*I* markers should be distributed along the length of the gel.
- The position of the test substance should match that of the molgramostim standard.

Other pharmacopoeial tests using isoelectric focusing

- Isoelectric focusing one of a number of tests which may be carried out on monoclonal antibodies for human use.
- Interferon alfa-2 is analysed by isoelectric focusing in the p*I* range 3–10. Bands should match those of standard.
- Characterisation of allergens used in allergy testing, e.g. skin prick tests.

Self-test 16.6

Isoelectric focusing can also be carried out using capillary electrophoresis instrumentation (Chapter 14). The figure shows the electropherogram obtained for an MAb Suba, D.; Urbányi, Z.; Salgó, A., Capillary isoelectric focusing method development and validation for investigation of recombinant therapeutic monoclonal antibody. *Journal of pharmaceutical and biomedical analysis* 2015;114:53-61. with the high pH end of the pH gradient at the detection end of the capillary. A, B and C are p*I* marker compounds with p*I* values of 9, 8.4 and 7, respectively. The other peaks are due to different glycoforms of an MAb. How many glycoforms of the MAb are there? Which component in the MAb has the highest p*I* value? Which component has the highest sialic acid content? What is the approximate p*I* value of the largest peak in the MAb?

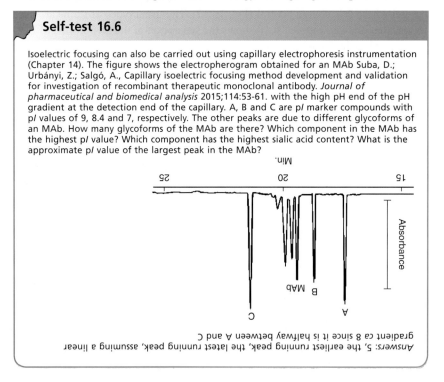

Answers: 5, the earliest running peak, the latest running peak, assuming a linear gradient ca 8 since it is halfway between A and C

Binding assays used in pharmacopoeial tests on protein drugs

Enzyme-linked immunosorbant assay (ELISA)

ELISA has been described above in relation to the location of a specific protein following Western blotting. The assay can be used directly without carrying out the immunoblotting process. ELISA is used in identification tests and also in determination of trace amounts of viral or antigen contamination in various products. The assays are generally carried out in 96-well plates, and the antigen of interest is generally allowed to bind to the plastic of the plate by electrostatic interactions (Fig. 16.19). Sometimes the plate is coated with a capture antibody. The adsorbed antigen is then incubated with an antibody which is specific for it, the antibody solution is then replaced by a solution containing an enzyme-linked antibody which binds specifically to the first antibody. The bound enzyme-linked antibody is then incubated with the appropriate substrate. For example if the linked enzyme is horseradish peroxidase, a solution of tetramethyl diaminobenzene is used which is oxidized by the enzyme to give an intense blue colour which can be measured spectrophotometrically using a plate reader to give an estimate of the amount of antigen present.

Fig. 16.19
The procedure used in ELISA determinations.

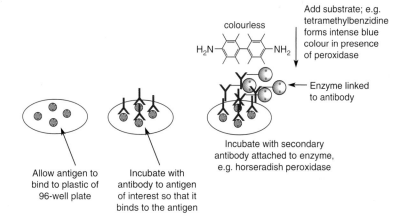

Applications of ELISA in the pharmacopoeias

In pharmacopoeial monographs ELISA is used to check for contaminating proteins in the following products: hepatitis B surface antigen in factor VIII, identification of the inactivated polio virus antigenic components in diphtheria, tetanus, pertussis, polio adsorbed vaccine, identification of hepatitis B surface antigen in recombinant hepatitis B vaccine, identification of antigenic components in adsorbed pertussis vaccine, identification of antigenic components in polio vaccine, determination of the effectiveness of foot and mouth disease vaccine via detection of antibodies raised by the vaccine following inoculation of cattle, determination of pasteurella antibodies in sheep prior to vaccination against the disease.

Radio-immunoassay (RIA)

RIA was the first commonly used binding assay developed. It is based on a simpler concept than ELISA. In the assay a radio-labelled version of the antigen of interest is used; radioactive iodine is generally used since it can be readily reacted with tyrosine residues in proteins. The radiolabelled antibody is mixed with an equivalent amount of antibody specific for the labelled antigen. The sample containing the antigen of interest (which is unlabelled) is then added to the solution containing the antibody bound to the labelled antigen. The unlabelled antigen displaces a proportional amount of radio-labelled antigen. Then following precipitation of the antibody antigen complex the amount of displaced antibody can be measured in the supernatant, giving an estimate of the amount of antigen in the samples (Fig. 16.20).

RIA is used in determination of pro-insulin in human, porcine and bovine insulin and in identification of hepatitis B surface antigen in urokinase and fibrinogen.

Labelled antigen in supernatant can be measured and equals the amount of unlabelled antigen added in the sample

Fig. 16.20
The procedure used for radio-immunoassay.

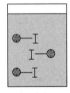 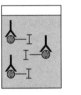

| Antigen is labelled by reaction of its tyrosine residues with radio iodine | Antibody is bound to known amount of labelled antigen | Cold antigen is introduced from the sample of interest displacing the labelled antigen | Antigen bound to antibody is precipitated and removed by centifugation |

Polymerase chain reaction (PCR)

PCR is a method for amplifying traces of mRNA and has been a key technique in the development of biotechnology. It uses a reverse transcriptase to form cDNA from the mRNA which is essentially the DNA from which the mRNA was derived. The cDNA can then be amplified, as shown in Figure 16.21. Heat is used to dissociate the strands of DNA. Then short strands of DNA (primers) which are complementary to a few DNA bases at the ends of the two strands are used to initiate the formation of two DNA duplexes. The formation of the duplexes is carried out using an enzyme from a bacterium such as *Thermus aquaticus* which grows in thermal springs and which catalyses the formation of the duplexes rapidly and can work at the high temperatures required to dissociate the DNA strands. The two primers are bound to a quencher and a reporter dye and at the end of each cycle of duplex formation the reported dye is cleaved from the primer and can be detected spectrophotometrically. The cycle of duplex formation can be repeated many times in order to obtain a measurable reading from trace amounts of mRNA. The technique is not widely applied in pharmacopoeial methods but is crucial for controlling possible viral contamination. PCR is used in determination of hepatitis C virus mRNA in plasma pools, which is a most important test since other blood products are isolated from pooled plasma downstream of this test and in determination of retrovirus contamination in smallpox vaccine.

Fig. 16.21

The use of polymerase chain reaction to detect traces of contaminating mRNA.

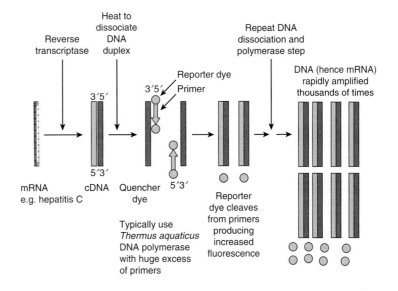

Capillary electrophoresis

Capillary electrophoresis has been covered in Chapter 14. In theory capillary electrophoresis is the ideal technique for the analysis of proteins, but in practice large proteins tend to absorb onto the silanol groups on the capillary wall, and it is not possible to observe any peak for the protein. This explains the buffer used in the method for the assay of EPO by capillary electrophoresis. The buffer contains 7 M urea and 2.5 mM putrescine. The putrescine acts as a dynamic modifier blocking the silanol groups on the wall of the capillary and the high concentration of urea disrupts the secondary structure of the EPO. The combination of these two reagents allows the EPO to pass through the capillary without absorbing onto the walls. Also coating of the capillary wall with polymer may be carried out in order to reduce protein binding. Figure 16.22 shows the electropherogram of the

Fig. 16.22

Separation of glycoforms of EPO comparing a research batch against a European Pharmacopoeia standard using capillary electrophoresis with polymer modified capillaries. *(From Sanz-Nebot V, Benavente F, Vallverdú A, Guzman NA, Barbosa J. Separation of recombinant human erythropoietin glycoforms by capillary electrophoresis using volatile electrolytes. Assessment of mass spectrometry for the characterization of erythropoietin glycoforms. Anal Chem. 2003;75:5220-5229 with permission.)*

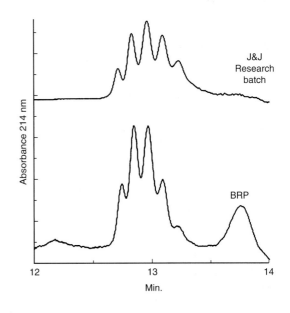

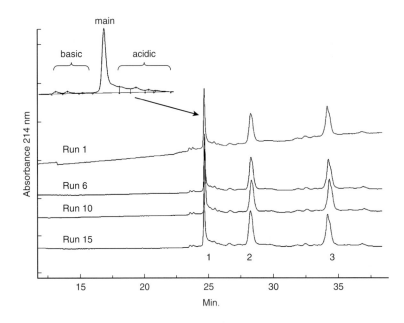

Fig. 16.23
Separation of IgG1 (1) and IgG2 (2 and 3) antibodies by capillary electrophoresis with a zwitterionic buffer. The inset shows the separation of minor glycoforms of IgG1 which are more or less acidic than the main peak. *(From He Y, Lacher NA, Hou W, et al. Analysis of identity, charge variants, and disulfide isomers of monoclonal antibodies with capillary zone electrophoresis in an uncoated capillary column. Anal Chem. 2010;82:3222-3230 with permission.)*

analysis of the glycoforms for EPO using capillary electrophoresis with a polymer-coated capillary; it would be impossible to separate these glycoforms by using HPLC. By careful choice of a buffer it is possible to achieve separations without degradation of the performance of the capillary. Figure 16.23 shows the separation of IgG1 and IgG2 monoclonal antibodies and their minor glycoforms.

Fingerprinting by HPLC and HPLC-MS

A very important piece of information with regard to a protein is its molecular weight, and it is now possible to determine molecular weights of very large proteins by using mass spectrometry. Figure 16.24 shows the deconvoluted mass spectrum for a drug antibody conjugate; such conjugates are used for example for the specific targeting of tumours. The molecular ions for drug-antibody

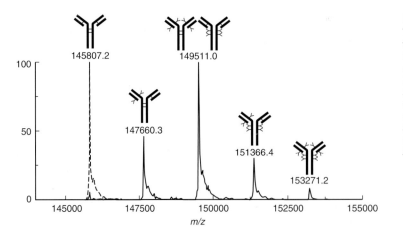

Fig. 16.24
Time of flight mass spectrum showing the molecular weights of an antibody conjugated to different numbers of molecules of a cytotoxic drug. *(From Valliere-Douglass JF, McFee WA, Salas-Solano O. Native intact mass determination of antibodies conjugated with monomethyl auristatin E and F at interchain cysteine residues. Anal Chem. 2012;84:2843-2849 with permission.)*

Fig. 16.25

HPLC chromatograms of tryptic digests from a MAb produced by two different cell lines. Analysis carried out on C18 columns with a gradient between trifluoroacetic acid and trifluoroacetic acid in acetonitrile. *(From Lubiniecki A, Volkin DB, Federici M, et al. Comparability assessments of process and product changes made during development of two different monoclonal antibodies. Biologicals. 2011;39:9-22 with permission.)*

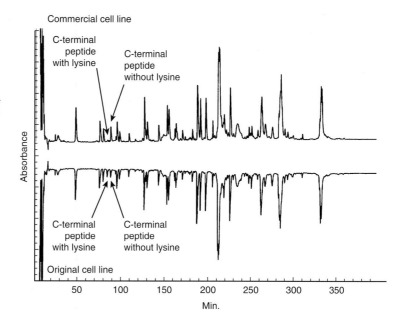

conjugates can be clearly seen, and the molecular weight increases according to how many of the drug molecules have been attached to the antibody. The molecular weight of a protein drug tells us nothing about the sequence of the amino acids making it up. As mentioned earlier the proteolytic enzyme trypsin cleaves proteins at the C-terminus side of the basic residues arginine, lysine or histidine. Cleavage at these points generally reduces proteins to several fragments with MW < 2000. The fingerprints produced are very useful as identification tests. Figure 16.25 shows a tryptic digest of monoclonal antibodies produced by two different cell lines where one of the products is deficient in a lysine residue at the C-terminus of one of the peptides composing the MAb. With such a large molecule long chromatographic elution times are required to get resolution between the huge numbers of peptides generated. However, as can be seen the fingerprint is a very good match between the two products.

The provision of standard digest fingerprints is not currently widespread in pharmacopoeial methods, but there is an example tryptic fingerprint for alteplase included in the European Pharmacopoeia as an identity check. With the advances in chemometric methods it is likely that multivariate statistical comparison of fingerprints will be carried out more widely.

The EP requires tryptic digest tests to be applied to the following drugs: erythropoietin, interferon gamma-1b, molgramostim, and somatropin. Trypsin does not always produce optimal fingerprinting so alternative enzymes are used to digest some drugs. *Staphylococcus aureus* protease (SAP) is used in digest tests for human, porcine and bovine insulin and insulin lispro. The variation of the sequence of amino acids at the C-terminus of insulins is important. SAP cleaves on the C-terminus side of glutamate and aspartate, thus producing more useful mapping fragments for the insulins than trypsin, which cleaves insulins next to the C-terminus. Chemotrypsin is used to map human glucagon.

> ### Self-test 16.7
>
> Refer to the European Pharmacopoeia monograph for alteplase. What are the criteria applied to validate the tryptic digest fingerprint test?
>
> Answer: The monograph includes a chromatogram and states that the resolution between peptides 6 and 7 in the map should be at least 1.5

The Edman reaction

The Edman reaction (Fig. 16.26) cleaves the amino acid at the N-terminus of a protein. The cycle can be repeated by raising and lowering the pH at each cycle. The process can be automated and the instrument programmed to release an amino acid from the N-terminus of a protein at each cycle. The amino acid released at each cycle is identified by automatic injection into a reversed phase HPLC system. As the cycle repeats, more and more amino acids are released into solution, and the HPLC software automatically subtracts the previous runs so that only one amino acid is seen at each cycle (Fig. 16.27).

The Edman degradation is applied in the following in European Pharmacopoeia monographs for EPO, to identify the first 15 amino acids from the N-terminus of the protein, and molgramostim, to identify the first 15 amino acids from the N-terminus of the protein. A test is also indicated for alteplase but without specifying the number of residues to be identified.

Methods used to assess the secondary and tertiary structure of protein drugs

Biotech products are so new that the methods used for their quality control have not yet found their way into the pharmacopoeias. Thus the techniques used to characterize a molecule may be exclusive to the company producing it and general pharmacopoeial methodologies do not apply. A company wishing to obtain a product licence must demonstrate that they understand their product, and to do this a variety of methods will be used. Not all of these methods appear in the pharmacopoeias, but they will eventually as recently established protein drugs become generic. Some of these methods are listed below, and most of them have been covered in previous chapters. However, some of them have not and are discussed below.

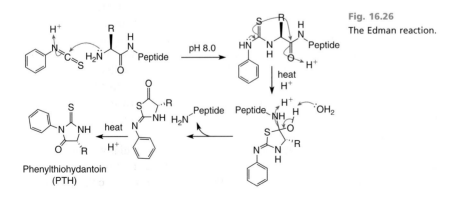

Fig. 16.26
The Edman reaction.

Phenylthiohydantoin (PTH)

Fig. 16.27

Application of the automated Edman degradation to sequencing of a protein from the N-terminus. R = reagent. Analysis is carried out by reverse-phase chromatography with automatic subtraction of the previous run at each cycle.

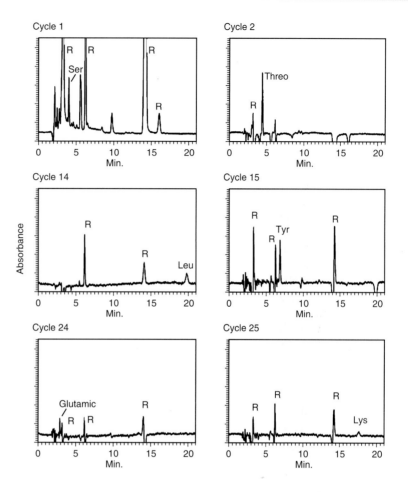

Circular dichroism

Circular dichroism is one of the most sensitive methods for determining protein secondary structure. It is based on an extension of the idea of optical rotation. Plane polarized light can be viewed as being composed of two circularly polarized vectors which rotate to the left and to the right through a 360° sweep during one wavelength. When the light is passed through an optically active sample the left and right polarized components are absorbed to a different extent; in general one of the components is absorbed much more strongly than the other, and the result is instead of being polarized in one plane the light traces an elliptical path. In order to observe the difference the plane polarized light has to be split into its left and right circularly polarized components, and this is achieved by using an electro-optic modulator. This is typically crystalline lithium niobate, which allows left and right polarized light to pass through alternately under the influence of an alternating electric field. Figure 16.28 shows a schematic diagram of a circular dichrometer.

The difference in the absorbance of the left and right circularly polarized light can then be measured as alternately left and right circularly polarized light are passed through the sample and then combined to produce a circular dichroism

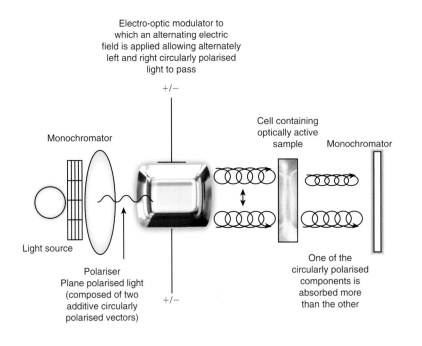

Fig. 16.28
Schematic diagram of a circular dichrometer.

Electro-optic modulator to which an alternating electric field is applied allowing alternately left and right circularly polarised light to pass

+/−

Monochromator

Cell containing optically active sample

Monochromator

Light source

Polariser
Plane polarised light (composed of two additive circularly polarised vectors)

+/−

One of the circularly polarised components is absorbed more than the other

(CD) spectrum which is expressed terms of ellipticity (deg cm^2 dmol^{-1}). The spectra produced are analogous to a differential absorption spectrum. The spectra move between positive and negative values, with a positive value indicating that the left circularly polarized light is absorbed more than the right and negative values indicating that the right circularly polarized light is absorbed more than the left. The spectra obtained are wavelength dependent, and measurements at different wavelengths give different information about the secondary structure of a protein. Figure 16.29A shows the far-UV CD spectra for two batches of EPO produced by different manufacturers. Measurement of the CD spectrum at short wavelengths targets the protein absorption band associated with the peptide bonds in the protein backbone. Figure 16.29A displays two minima at 208 and 222 nm which are typical of an α-helix conformation. The minima for Epogen are slightly lower than those obtained for Eprex, indicating that there is about 5% more of the α-helix form in Epogen. Figure 16.29B shows the near-UV CD spectrum for Epogen, purified Epogen and Eprex. Near-UV CD targets the absorbence of the aromatic residues in proteins, particularly tyrosine and tryptophan. The spectra show that the Epogen is not much affected by the purification process and that there are some differences in the environments of the tryptophan residues between Epogen and Eprex. These differences are confirmed by the fluorescence emission spectra (Chapter 7) for the drugs, which also give an indication of the environment of the tryptophan residues in the molecule.

The far-UV absorbence bands for the α-helix conformation are more intense than those for the β-sheet, as shown in Figure 16.30, and if the α-helix contribution is strong then it may not be possible to see the contribution from the β-sheet component. One solution to observe a stronger contribution from the β-sheet is to work in the vacuum UV region below 200 nm. In the end the CD spectrum is a useful fingerprint, and as the example shown in Figure 16.29 indicates, it can pick up subtle changes in the secondary structure of the protein. This is important

Fig. 16.29
Comparison of two EPO products using far-UV CD, near-UV CD and fluorescence spectrophotometry. *(From Deechongkit S, Aoki KH, Park SS, Kerwin BA. Biophysical comparability of the same protein from different manufacturers: a case study using Epoetin alfa from Epogen® and Eprex®. J Pharm Sci. 2006;95:1931-1943 with permission.)*

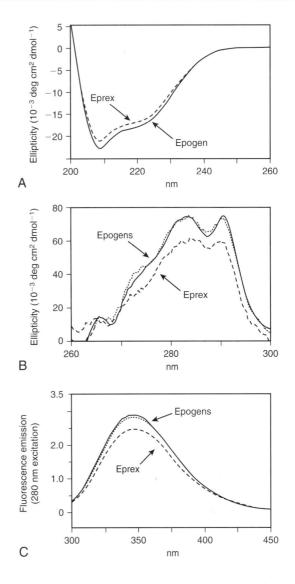

for determining not only that the correct protein is being produced but also that the protein has been formulated in a correct manner that does not cause it to denature.

Other techniques used to assess protein secondary structure

- Differential scanning calorimetry is essentially a very sensitive method for measuring melting point. This technique gives information of thermal stability. The melting point of the protein corresponds with the unfolding of the secondary structure and is thus very characteristic of a particular protein.
- Fourier transform infrared (IR) spectroscopy provides a complex fingerprint giving complementary information to that obtained by CD on the secondary structure of a protein.

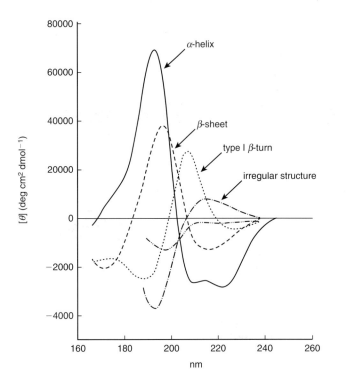

Fig. 16.30
Comparison of the far UV spectra for the different motifs of protein secondary structure. *(From Kelly SM, Jess TJ, Price NC. How to study proteins by circular dichroism. Biochim Biophys Acta. 2005;1751:119-139 with permission.)*

- Raman spectroscopy (Chapter 7) provides a complex fingerprint for protein secondary structure. Unlike IR Raman spectroscopy it is insensitive to water and thus provides complementary information on secondary structure. The use of Raman spectroscopy in the characterization of proteins will expand.
- X-ray crystallography can be used to determine secondary and tertiary structure very precisely. However, it requires good quality crystals.
- Nuclear magnetic resonance (NMR) (Chapter 8) can give information linked to primary, secondary and tertiary structure of proteins. It is a sensitive fingerprint technique, and a range of NMR techniques can be applied in the provision of different fingerprints.

Reference

1. Suntharalingam G, Perry MR, Ward S, et al. Cytokine storm in a phase 1 trial of the anti-CD28 monoclonal antibody TGN1412. *N Engl J Med*. 2006;355:1018-1028.

Further reading

Watson DG. *Pharmaceutical Chemistry*. New York: Churchill Livingstone; 2011 [chapter 27].

17 Electrochemical biosensors

KEYPOINTS

Principles

Biological macromolecules, such as enzymes, act as a transducer to facilitate electron transfer between the analytes of interest and the device at a given potential. The resultant current is measured.

Applications in pharmaceutical analysis

- Biosensors are often utilised in point of care handheld devices for monitoring levels of blood glucose and cholesterol.
- Biosensors have been developed for detection of various pharmaceutical drugs but are not as popular as pharmacopoeial methods for detection.

Strengths

- Provide selective monitoring for a given analyte due to the specificity of the biological macromolecule.
- Offer excellent sensitivity.
- Provide the ability to conduct rapid monitoring of analytes in a remote environment.

Limitations

- Biosensor devices have limited stability and can be prone to biofouling.
- Issues in reproducibility can also be observed due to the influence of environmental factors on the performance of the biological macromolecule.
- Only a select number of analytes can be monitored using this approach.

Introduction

The term 'biosensor' refers strictly to chemical sensors where a biological macromolecule acts as a sensing element that is coupled to a physical-chemical transducer, for the purpose of detecting the concentration or activity of a specific analyte in a sample matrix. The various key elements of a biosensor are shown

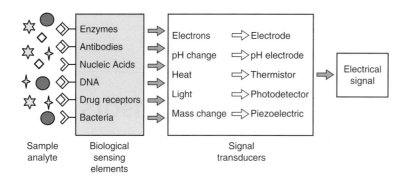

Fig. 17.1
Key components of
a biosensor.

in Figure 17.1. Biosensors can be utilised in portable devices, allowing for real-time measurements in remote environments.

A variety of biological macromolecules have been utilised, such as nucleic acids, antibodies and enzymes, of which the latter is the most commonly used biological sensing element. Due to the various biological sensing elements utilised, a host of compounds from sample organic structures to large biomolecular compounds can be easily monitored using such analytical devices. For the transducer element of the biosensor, a variety of analytical techniques have been utilised. These include electrochemical, optical and piezoelectric. Of the variety of biosensors which can be fabricated for analyte detection, electrochemical biosensors have the most widespread utility in pharmaceutical analysis and the most commercial success to date.

For this reason, this chapter will focus on electrochemical sensors, where the transduction event is the transfer of an electron or ion from the analyte of interest at the interface between the ionic solution (which could be blood, extracellular fluid or cerebrospinal fluid) and an electrified solid, such as a metal, carbon or organic conductor.

Basic principles of electrochemistry

For electrochemical detection, there are two modes of operation: (1) potentiometry, where changes in the voltage can be quantitatively related to the analyte concentration, and (2) amperometry or voltammetry, where a non-equilibrium voltage is imposed on the electrode and the resulting current monitored is related to the concentration of the analyte. Of these approaches, amperometry is the most widely used electrochemical technique for conducting measurements with biosensors.

The fundamental principle governing electrochemical detection is the transfer of electrons to or from an electronic conductor (usually metal or carbon) and to or from a redox analyte species at the electrode surface. Oxidation involves the loss of electrons from the highest occupied molecular orbital, whereas reduction involves electrons being injected into the lowest unoccupied molecular orbital of the analyte. For some arbitrary pair of compounds, where R represents the reduced form and O represents the oxidised form, the electrochemical reaction can be written as:

$$O + ne^- \Leftrightarrow R$$

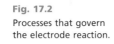

Fig. 17.2
Processes that govern
the electrode reaction.

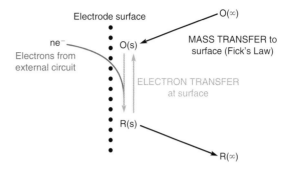

To either oxidise or reduce an analyte of interest, an electrode potential is applied. The electron potential must be sufficiently positive in order to oxidise an analyte and sufficiently negative to reduce an analyte. Each analyte has a specific potential where it can be oxidised or reduced. This potential can be influenced by a variety of factors, such as the nature of the electrode material. The applied electrode potential is measured relative to a reference electrode, with the standard hydrogen electrode (SHE) being given the arbitrary value of 0 volts. Tabulated standard electrode potentials are usually reported relative to this standard.

The relationship between electrode potential (units of volts) and the current is best understood by considering the processes involved in the electrode reaction, which can be seen in Figure 17.2. When a sufficient potential is applied, electron transfer can take place at the electrode surface; this process is governed by two steps. Initially the analyte of interest must reach the electrode surface as electron transfer takes place by electron tunnelling and therefore is restricted to distances of about one bond length. The reactant O must therefore be transported to the electrode surface before electron transfer can take place. This occurs by the process of mass transport, which usually is by diffusion but can be enhanced by either convection or migration. Once the analyte is at the electrode surface, electron transfer can take place. At this point the rate of reaction can be followed either as the rate of change in the concentrations of R or O or by the rate of movement of electrons across the electrified interface. When scaled by the Faraday constant, this rate is equivalent to the electrical current flowing in the electrical circuit. The relationship between flux (J, mol s^{-1} m^{-2}) and current i is given by:

$$i = nFAJ$$

where A is the area of the electrode, F is the Faraday constant and n is the number of electrons transferred.[1] A key feature of electrochemistry is that the rate of the reaction can be directly and continuously measured from the current.

Amperometry is often referred to as a steady-state electroanalytical technique and is the simplest mode of operation of electrochemical detection. In this technique, we impose a fixed potential that is sufficient to drive the electrode reaction, as either an oxidation or reduction, and the resulting current is recorded. In order to accurately utilise amperometry for detection of an analyte, some knowledge of the oxidation or reduction potential of the analyte must be known. Figure 17.3 shows the waveform utilised for amperometry and the resultant data that are

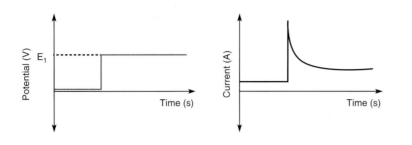

Fig. 17.3
The waveform and result observed when amperometry is utilised to study either an oxidation or a reduction.

generated and presented. The waveform involves applying a fixed potential for a given time. The resultant current over time is monitored. Amperometry has one of the fastest response times of all electrochemical techniques. For electrodes without membranes or biological macromolecules on the surface, the response time is essentially instantaneous since it depends primarily on the diffusion characteristics of the analyte in the test medium. Electron transfer takes place on the femtosecond time scale.

One of the major limitations of amperometry is that the technique can be used to monitor analytes that undergo electron transfer reaction only in a limited potential window (i.e. the analyte must be capable of being reduced at potentials more positive than water reduction to hydrogen or be oxidised at potentials more negative than water oxidation to oxygen). At physiological pH, this potential window is typically -0.9 V to $+1.2$ V depending on the electrode material utilised. Another limitation of this approach is that it has limited selectivity when the analyte of interest is present within a matrix where other compounds can be oxidised or reduced at a potential lower that that applied. However, this limitation can be overcome by using amperometric detection following chromatographic separation as mentioned in Chapter 12 or, as will be discussed within this chapter, by utilising a biological sensing element to provide selectivity.

Types of electrochemical biosensors

There are various types of biosensors that utilise different processes to pass the signal generated from the biological sensing element to the transducer for data acquisition. The majority of all electrochemical biosensors are based on utilising the bioelectrocatalytic activity of a class of enzymes known as oxidoreductases (mainly oxidases and dehydrogenases, see below):

$$\text{Substrate} + O_2 \xrightleftharpoons{\text{oxidase}} \text{Product} + H_2O_2$$

$$\text{Substrate} + \text{NAD}^+ \xrightleftharpoons{\text{dehydrogenase}} \text{Product} + \text{NADH}$$

Early biosensors utilised the product(s) generated from the enzymatic reaction, as they would often be products that could be oxidised or reduced directly on the electrode surface. However, over the years, various types of biosensors have been developed that provide improved performance. Three generations of biosensors that have been utilised for analyte detection are shown in Figure 17.4.

Electrochemical biosensors can be easily developed and maintained and are simple to operate. Biosensors can be made in various geometries, shapes and sizes; therefore these devices have the ability to interface into flow cells or provide specialised high-performance liquid chromatography amperometric

Fig. 17.4
The various types of electrochemical enzymatic biosensors.

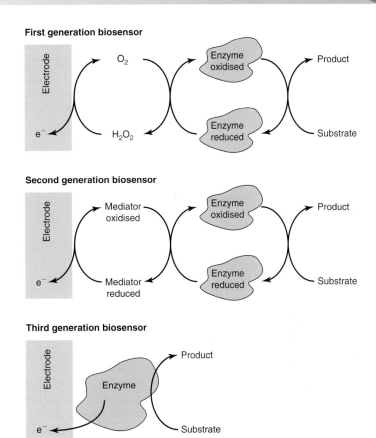

detectors. Due to recent innovations in electrochemical sensor fabrication using screen printing and micromachining, mass production of electrochemical sensors is easily achievable. This therefore provides the ability for biosensors to be produced in large scales for a small cost.

First-generation biosensors

These biosensors are based on either the direct determination of a product generated from the enzymatic reaction or the consumption of a cofactor or substrate utilised within the enzymatic reaction. In Figure 17.4, the first-generation mechanism is shown for a reaction catalysed by an oxidase enzyme. Enzymes are most commonly utilised as they are able to change their redox state as a consequence of the reaction. In the mechanism shown in Figure 17.4, the product generated from the oxidase enzyme is hydrogen peroxide, which is known to be easily oxidised at a metal surface at around + 0.7 V. Applying such a high potential for monitoring is one of the major drawbacks of first-generation biosensors, as they are prone to interference from other electroactive substances in the matrix that can also be oxidised at a lower applied potential. These include substances such as ascorbic acid, paracetamol and uric acid. To overcome these issues, second- and third-generation biosensors have been developed.

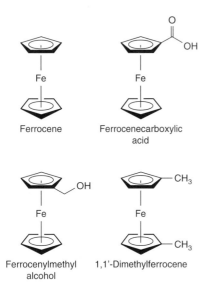

Fig. 17.5
Structure of ferrocene
and commonly used
derivatives as mediators
for second-generation
biosensors.

Second-generation biosensors

In a second-generation biosensor, the electron transfer between the redox centre of the enzyme and the electrode surface is mediated by an electroactive organic compound. These compounds are known as chemical mediators in the biosensor assembly. In these devices electrochemical measurements can be driven at the redox potential of the mediator and therefore a much lower potential can be utilised, which helps to reduce the degree of interference from other electroactive substances in the matrix. The use of the mediator also helps to enhance the sensitivity of the biosensor as the compound utilised for oxidation is more favourable for electron transfer at the electrode surface than some of the products generated from enzymatic reactions of first-generation biosensors.

Various chemical mediators have been utilised, but they all should have the following features: (1) a low redox potential, (2) the ability to allow for rapid reversibility, (3) fast electron transfer rates and (4) good stability over time. Such features are usually found on various chemical mediators, but the most commonly utilised form of mediator has been that which utilises ferrocene derivative compounds. Figure 17.5 shows the structure of some of the most commonly utilised mediators in second-generation biosensors. The majority of ferrocene derivative compounds has oxidation potentials ~ 0.2 V.

Third-generation biosensors

Third-generation biosensors offer more advantages than the other two formats but are often the most difficult type of biosensor to develop. Within this form of biosensor there is direct electron transfer from the enzyme to the electrode surface (Fig. 17.4). This is a major advantage as these biosensors offer more enhanced selectivity than first- and second-generation biosensors. In third-generation biosensors, the detection potential is closer to the redox potential of the enzyme itself and thus can be much lower than 0.2 V. Despite the clear advantages, direct electric connection between the enzyme and the electrode is difficult due to the location of the redox centre within the protein and its vicinity to the electrode surface. This limits the ability in developing this type of sensor, as the appropriate enzyme is needed; if this is not feasible, the sensitivity is impaired.

Instrumentation

Steady-state amperometry requires a stable voltage source which can respond rapidly to a current load that may vary by many orders of magnitude. To achieve this, a three electrode setup is utilised. This composes of the working electrode (in this case acting as the biosensor), the reference electrode and the counter (also known as the auxiliary) electrode. The electrode potential applied to the working electrode is with respect to the reference electrode, and the counter or auxiliary electrode serves to provide a current path between itself and the working electrode. This can be visualised in Figure 17.6. As shown, the working electrode and reference electrode are connected by a voltmeter, and the working electrode and counter electrode are connected by an ampmeter. This is the most common setup

---

Self-test 17.1

You have developed a first-generation oxidase biosensor. Which of the following compounds below that are present in the background matrix could cause an increase in the current at the electrode surface if a potential of +650 mV is applied?

1. Paracetamol (acetaminophen)
2. Short chain fatty acids
3. Proteins
4. Oxygen

Answer: 1

Fig. 17.6
Instrumental components that are utilised to conduct electrochemical measurements.

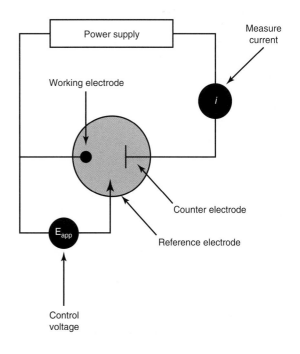

for amperometry; however, in the case where low currents are observed (nA or less), it may be possible to use a simple two electrode setup where the counter electrode also serves as a reference electrode.

A suitable reference electrode is of a known potential and acts to measure and control the working electrode's potential. The potential must be stable over time, must not change experimental variables at the reference electrode and at no point should it pass any current. The agreed international reference electrode is the standard hydrogen electrode (SHE), which has arbitrarily been assigned a potential of 0 V. Hydrogen electrodes are temperamental and difficult to set up and, these days, are rarely seen outside of the undergraduate chemistry laboratory. Fortunately, several suitable alternatives exist, of which the most common are the calomel electrode (SCE) and silver–silver chloride electrode. The calomel electrode (Hg_2Cl_2, 'calomel') is based on the reaction between elemental mercury and mercury (I) chloride. The reaction takes place in a saturated solution of potassium chloride in water. The electrode is 0.268 V more positive than the SHE. The silver–silver chloride electrode consists of a silver wire that has a thin film of silver chloride deposited on the surface by either anodisation or sputtering. This is also placed in a saturated solution of potassium chloride in water. The electrode is 0.222 V more positive than the SHE.

Counter electrodes are most commonly made from inert noble metal wire or gauze, usually platinum or carbon-based materials such as graphite. The counter electrode is there simply to provide a current path to balance the current observed at the working electrode. The counter electrode is used to assure that current does not pass through the reference electrode. The counter electrode also always has a larger surface area than the working electrode (approximately five times greater). When the working electrode is held at a positive potential, the counter electrode reaction is likely to be hydrogen generation. Similarly, when the working electrode is held at a negative potential and passing a reduction current, the counter electrode reaction will cause a decrease in the local pH.

Examples of biosensors utilised for pharmaceutical analysis

Biosensors are not well known in pharmaceutical analysis, particularly industrial pharmacy; however, they have been widely used in clinical and community pharmacy as sensors that are utilised in point of care diagnostic kits. Given that the pharmacopeial methods are often time consuming and expensive, biosensors have become an interesting alterative that also provides the scope for high throughput. The majority of biosensors utilised for pharmaceutical analysis are based on using enzymes as the biological sensing element. However, antibodies, drug receptors and DNA have also been utilised in biosensor development for drug analysis.

Detection of blood glucose levels

Blood glucose monitoring is a means of testing the concentration of glucose in blood (glycemia). It is used to aid the management of patients suffering from type 1 and 2 diabetes. The aim of the measurement is to understand how fluctuations of blood glucose relate to environmental behaviours and medication and thus help to guide and direct management of these conditions.

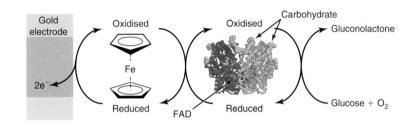

A glucose biosensor utilises the enzyme glucose oxidase and over the years from conception to current use has been refined from a first-generation biosensor to a second-generation biosensor. The concept of a second-generation biosensor was shown by Cass et al. using dimethyl ferrocene.[2] The ethanolamine derivative of ferrocene is the mediator utilised in the original glucose biosensor by Medisense, the ExacTech system. It is the use of a ferrocene derivative mediator on the glucose strip that explains why it is orange in colour. Figure 17.7 shows the mechanism by which the blood glucose biosensor works.

However, like all analytical devices, there are particular limitations also to the blood glucose biosensor, which are mainly associated with the key elements of the biosensor. Due to the use of an enzyme for facilitation of the detection of glucose, there will be a point at which the concentration of glucose is at saturation. As the level of the substrate increases, then the enzymes on the device become saturated and the rate reaches the V_{max} (the enzyme's maximum rate). Therefore when concentrations of glucose are present above the saturation point, there will be no perceived change in the response observed. This can be influenced by the amount of enzyme/mediator that is loaded on the device; however, in all instances there will always be a saturation point. Although the response for enzyme kinetics shows a saturation point, the relationship between the observed current response and the area of the enzyme/mediator is linear. Therefore changes in the area of mediator/enzyme load can influence the current observed.[3] The relationship of the enzyme/mediator to the concentration of blood glucose is shown in Figure 17.8.

Like all devices, there are errors that can decrease the accuracy of the result observed. This could be from a variety of issues, such as error in the preparation of the device and interferences. Tables 17.1 and 17.2 show some common

Fig. 17.8
The relationship between
amount and area of
mediator/enzyme to the
concentration of blood
glucose monitored.

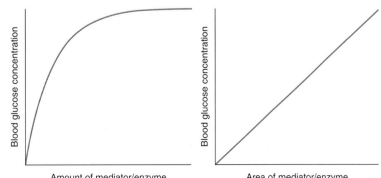

Table 17.1 Sources of instrumental error that can decrease the accuracy of a blood glucose measurement

Biosensor device error	Consequence
Expired reagents	A reduction may be observed.
Inaccurate calibration	A reduction may be observed.
Low/high amount of mediator	A reduction may be observed in the case of low mediator, but no change may be observed if high amounts of mediator are used.
Low/high amount of enzyme	A reduction may be observed in the case of low enzyme, but no change may be observed if high amounts of enzyme are used.
Varying size of the electrode	If the electrode is made smaller, then a lower response will be observed; if the electrode is larger, an increased signal will be observed.
Blockage of the electrode	A reduction in the observed response
Malfunction	A reduction in the observed response due to reductions in mass transfer

Table 17.2 Physiologic and drug interactions that can decrease the accuracy of blood glucose measurements

Physiologic/drug interactions	Consequence
Decreased hemotacrit	Seem in anaemia, which would decrease the concentration of glucose due to increased fluid volume
Increased hematocrit	Observed in neonates, which would increase the concentration of glucose due to decreased fluid volume
Oxygenation	Oxygen can interfere with the response, as it is required as part of the enzymatic reaction.
pH	The voltage required for the oxidation of the mediator is influenced by pH shift, where based on the Nernst equation the oxidation potential changes by 59 mV per pH unit. This could over- or underestimate the amount of glucose depending on the mediator.
Water content	Changes in water content can change the concentration of blood glucose in cases such as dehydration.
Maltose	Found usually as an additive in medicines but can compete for the enzyme and increase the response
Mannitol	Found usually as an additive in medicines but can compete for the enzyme and increase the response
Paracetamol	Known to be easily oxidised; however, with a mediator which requires low potential for oxidation, this interaction can be negated.
Ascorbic acid	Known to be easily oxidised and present in high concentrations; however, with a mediator which requires low potential for oxidation, this interaction can be negated.
Uric acid	Known to be easily oxidised and is elevated with severe gout; however, with a mediator which requires low potential for oxidation, this interaction can be negated.

Self-test 17.2

The glucose biosensor is commonly used by patients suffering from diabetes to regularly check their blood sugar levels. Which of the biosensor construction errors below would explain an overestimation of blood sugar levels?

1. Too much enzyme loaded
2. Too much of the mediator present
3. An increase in the size of the electrode on the device

Answer: 3

interferences to blood glucose biosensors and the potential consequences these could have on the actual result.

Detection of cholesterol

Cholesterol is a lipid that is vital for normal functioning of the body. It is mainly formed in the liver but can also be found in certain foods. Having excessive amounts of lipids in your blood (hyperlipidaemia) can have a detrimental effect on your health. There is evidence to suggest that elevated levels of cholesterol can increase the risk of atherosclerosis (narrowing of the arteries), ischaemic heart diseases, heart attack, stroke, transient ischaemic attack and peripheral arterial disease.

Cholesterol testing is now readily available as a point of care detection device for homecare testing and is also widely used in community and clinical pharmacy. Biosensors are one of the methods being utilised for detection of cholesterol. Cholesterol esters in the presence of water can be catalysed to cholesterol and fatty acid by cholesterol esterase. The resultant cholesterol in the presence of water and oxygen is converted to cholesterol-4-en-3-one and hydrogen peroxide in the presence of cholesterol oxidase. The hydrogen peroxide can be oxidised at an electrode surface or the electrons generated can be transferred to a mediator for detection. The reaction process can be seen in Figure 17.9. Although it can be detected electrochemically, the peroxide can also be detected using a chromogen. The cholesterol enzymatic biosensor offers a degree of complexity when compared with the glucose biosensor, as two enzymatic steps are needed to generate a product that can be detected at the electrode surface.

Fig. 17.9
Biosensor mechanism by which cholesterol is monitored in blood.

$$\text{Cholesterol ester} + H_2O \xrightarrow{\text{Cholesterol esterase}} \text{Cholesterol} + \text{fatty acid}$$

$$\text{Cholesterol} + H_2O + O_2 \xrightarrow{\text{Cholesterol oxidase}} \text{Cholesterol-4-en-3-one} + H_2O_2$$

Detection of pharmaceutical drugs

At present there are no methods that utilise biosensors as the technique of choice for analysis of drug concentrations in pharmaceutical analysis. Pharmacopoeial methods of choice are mainly chromatographic or spectroscopic. However, these approaches are often time consuming and expensive; therefore biosensors are becoming an interesting alternative for sensitive and selective detection of pharmaceutical drugs. The major attraction of using biosensors for analysis is that current approaches utilised for the analysis of drugs, such as high-performance liquid chromatography and UV-visible spectroscopy, require one or more sample preparation steps. Biosensors on the other hand require limited sample preparation and can often be utilised in complex matrixes.

However, there are various published methods that showcase the ability to detect various drugs. Various biosensors have been developed for the detection of salicylate using salicylate hydroxylase. The mechanism is shown in Figure 17.10. In this reaction process, catechol is generated as the product which is known to undergo an oxidation at the electrode surface.[4] Various researchers have

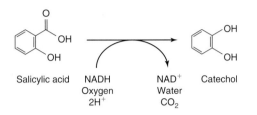

Fig. 17.10
Mechanism by which salicylates can be detected using biosensors.

focused on developing biosensors for detection of drugs, in particular, devices that could be of benefit for drug therapeutic monitoring. Biosensors have also been developed for the detection of paracetamol, methylxanthines, benzodiazepines, antidepressants, and beta-lactam antibiotics.[5] Most of these developed biosensors are based on enzymatic biosensors, as it is very difficult to obtain drug-target receptors in quantities sufficient to create a biosensor.

Limitations of biosensors in pharmaceutical analysis

Although there are many benefits to using biosensors for pharmaceutical and clinical analysis, there are also major limitations. These are stability, reproducibility and usability limitations.

The stability of biosensors can be influenced by the nature of the device itself and also by other components present within the sample matrix. As mentioned within this chapter for pharmaceutical analysis, the majority of biosensors utilise enzymes for the biological sensing element. Enzymes, like any other biological macromolecule, can behave differently in varying conditions, and if the conditions for its viability are not preserved then the stability of the enzyme will be lost eventually. Therefore most biosensors have a limited shelf life and are prone to drift in response over time. This can be overcome by two measures, initially by assuring a calibration is always conducted prior to an analytical measurement so that changes in the behaviour of the biosensor are accounted for. Secondly, the stability of the enzyme can be improved by utilising additives such as polyethylene glycols and synthetic polymers. These additives provide a microenvironment around the enzyme that promotes stability.

The reproducibility of enzymatic electrochemical biosensors can vary from sensor to sensor. This is mainly due to the issues in development of biosensors and the *in*ability to create devices that have identical performance. The error in the reproducibility of biosensors is mainly due to performance variations in strains of the same enzyme and also in varying loading of the enzyme on the electrode surface. This is something that is common for all analytical assays that utilise biological elements such as immunoassays. Therefore compared with chromatography or spectroscopy, the precision of biosensors is limited.

Biosensors are specific for analytes, which is one of their core advantages for measurement, especially in complex matrixes. However, as biosensors are based on the activity of specific enzymes, receptors or other biological recognition elements, the ability to monitor all analytes through this approach is limited by the specificity and availability of biological recognition elements.

Q Additional problems

1. Based on the biological matrixes listed below, which generation of biosensor would be the single best option for selective and sensitive chemical monitoring of the given analyte? In each case you can assume the generated product is electroactive:

(i) Detection of glucose in blood samples
(ii) Detection of digoxin in an glucose infusion
(iii) Monitoring of caffeine in a medicine for colds
(iv) Detection of vitamin E in a multi-vitamin supplement
(a) First-generation biosensor
(b) Second-generation biosensor
(c) Third-generation biosensor
(d) Either first- or second-generation biosensor

Answers: (i) b; (ii) d; (iii) b; (iv) c

References

1. Bard A, Faulkner LR. *Electrochemical Methods: Fundamentals and Applications.* New York: John Wiley & Sons; 2001.
2. Cass AEG, et al. Ferrocene-mediated enzyme electrode for amperometric determination of glucose. *Anal Chem.* 1984;56(4):667-671.
3. Ginsberg BH. Factors affecting blood glucose monitoring: sources of errors in measurement. *J Diabetes Sci Technol (online).* 2009;3(4):903-913.
4. Frew JE, et al. Amperometric biosensor for the rapid determination of salicylate in whole blood. *Anal Chim Acta.* 1989;224:39-46.
5. Gil EdS, Melo GRd. Electrochemical biosensors in pharmaceutical analysis. *Brazilian J Pharma Sci.* 2010;46:375-391.

Further reading

Bard A, Faulkner LR. *Electrochemical Methods: Fundamentals and Applications.* New York: John Wiley & Sons; 2001.

Cooper J, Cass A. *Biosensors.* Oxford University Press; 2004.

Eggins BR. *Chemical Sensors and Biosensors.* Wiley; 2002.

Index

Page numbers followed by '*f*' indicate figures, '*t*' indicate tables, '*b*' indicate boxes, and '*e*' indicate online content.